IEA WIND RECOMMENDED PRACTICE FOR THE IMPLEMENTATION OF RENEWABLE ENERGY FORECASTING SOLUTIONS☆

CORINNA MÖHRLEN
WEPROG
Assens, Denmark

JOHN W. ZACK
MESO Inc.
Troy, NY, United States

GREGOR GIEBEL
Technical University of Denmark
Department of Wind and Energy Systems
Roskilde, Denmark

ELSEVIER

ACADEMIC PRESS
An imprint of Elsevier

☆ Coordinated by Task 36 Wind Energy Forecasting and Task 51 Forecasting for the Weather-driven Energy System

Academic Press is an imprint of Elsevier
125 London Wall, London EC2Y 5AS, United Kingdom
525 B Street, Suite 1650, San Diego, CA 92101, United States
50 Hampshire Street, 5th Floor, Cambridge, MA 02139, United States
The Boulevard, Langford Lane, Kidlington, Oxford OX5 1GB, United Kingdom

ISBN: 978-0-443-18681-3

For information on all Academic Press publications
visit our website at https://www.elsevier.com/books-and-journals

Publisher: Charlotte Cockle
Acquisitions Editor: Peter Adamson
Editorial Project Manager: Naomi Robertson
Production Project Manager:
Paul Prasad Chandramohan
Cover Designer: Greg Harris

Typeset by VTeX

IEA WIND RECOMMENDED PRACTICE FOR THE IMPLEMENTATION OF RENEWABLE ENERGY FORECASTING SOLUTIONS

This IEA Wind Recommended Practice guideline is dedicated to the renewable energy industry, especially those who are seeking ways to obtain the most value from wind and solar forecasting information for their applications. These include the pioneers who have courageously found innovative ways to extract value from forecasting information as well as those that are still in doubt about the value of forecasting, or those who are still trying to understand how to best and most efficiently integrate wind and solar forecasting into their business processes.

In short, it is dedicated to all those that have to use forecasting of wind and solar energy and can see the benefit of standardizing business processes for the integration of wind and solar energy connected to the electric grid and, to a large extent, participating in power exchange markets.

This guideline is also dedicated to all those that took part in the process of assembling and refining the recommended practices presented in this document. Many valuable contributions have been made by those who have brought up relevant issues in the discussion forums that we organized at various workshops and conferences and thereby helped us to formulate common and internationally acceptable procedures.

In addition, the authors want to acknowledge those that guided us to publicly available information, provided relevant pictures and graphs and also made us aware of proprietary information that otherwise is only available to those in contractual relationships. By anonymizing the latter type of information, we are now able to provide a compendium with comprehensive and practical information of how to optimally integrate wind and solar generation forecasting in a wide range of business processes.

Contents

List of figures

List of tables

Biography

Dr. Corinna Möhrlen

Dr. Corinna Möhrlen is co-founder, managing director and research coordinator of WEPROG, a firm which has been providing world-wide operational weather & energy ensemble forecasting services with their 75 member multi-scheme ensemble prediction system (MSEPS) since 2003. It is highly specialized in forecasting services for the integration of renewable energy into the electric grid.

She is also a member of the German engineering society (VDI, 1994), the int. IEEE Power & Energy Society (2008), a member of the management board and task leader in the IEA Wind Task 36 "Wind Energy Forecasting" (2016–2021) and IEA Wind Task 51 "Forecasting for the Weather driven Energy System" (2022–2026).

She has been participating and coordinating forecasting projects on the national and international level for over 20 years and actively writes and reviews journal articles related to forecasting of renewables and their integration into the electric grid. She earned a MS degree in Civil Engineering from Ruhr-University Bochum, Germany, and a MEngSc and PhD degree in Civil & Environmental Engineering from University College Cork, Ireland. In her PhD studies she focused on the atmospheric science and meteorology part of the forecasting process by advancing the multi-scheme ensemble approach into an operational forecasting system. In 2020, she received an ESIG excellence award for contributions to advances in the use of probabilistic forecasting.

Dr. John W. Zack

Dr. John W. Zack is the President, Chief Scientist and co-founder of MESO, Inc., a small business established in 1985 that specializes in the development and application of physics-based and statistical geophysical models in a wide range of industries. In 1993 he was a co-founder of Meteosim, SL, a meteorological services company based in Barcelona, Spain, and currently serves on its Board of Directors.

He was one of the founding partners of AWS Truepower, a global leader in renewable energy consulting services, and served on its Board of Directors until its acquisition by UL, Inc in 2016. He is a co-chair of the

Renewable Energy Committee of the American Meteorological Society and is also a task leader in the IEA Wind TCP Tasks 36 "Wind energy Forecasting" (2019–2021) and 51 "Forecasting for the Weather Driven Energy System" (2022–2026).

He is the author of numerous articles on atmospheric modeling, forecasting and renewable energy applications of meteorological information that have appeared in scientific journals and trade publications. He earned a BS degree in meteorology and oceanography from New York University and a Ph.D. in atmospheric sciences from Cornell University, USA.

Dr. Gregor Giebel

Dr. Gregor Giebel has worked for over 25 years with short-term forecasting of wind power, large-scale integration of wind power into electricity grids, wind farm flow control and standardization within the IEC in various positions in the Wind Department of the Danish Technical University (formerly known as Risø National Laboratory).

He was the Operating Agent for IEA Wind Task 36 "Forecasting for Wind Energy" and is the Operating Agent of the IEA Wind Task 51 "Forecasting for the Weather Driven Energy System". He heads the EU Marie Curie Initial Training Network Train2Wind (train2wind.eu) and the Forecasting for Renewable Energy in Egypt research project.

His main claim to fame is a report on the state of the art in short-term forecasting, with 1000 citations. He is an accomplished writer of research proposals, with a funding quota of over 50% for a total amount of about 25 million euro. He earned his MS in Physics at the Technical University of Munich and his PhD from the Carl von Ossietzky University Oldenburg, Germany.

Preface

This IEA Wind Recommended Practice is the result of a collaborative work that has been edited and authored in alignment with many discussions at project meetings, workshops and personal communication with colleagues, stakeholders and other interested persons throughout the phase 1 (2016–2018) and phase 2 of the IEA Wind Task 36 "Wind Energy Forecasting" (2018–2021) and as part of work packages 2.1 and 3.3 and IEA Wind Task 51 "Forecasting for the Weather Driven Energy System" (2022–2026).

Part 4 of this recommended practice has been established in close collaboration with the IEA Photovoltaic Power Systems (PVPS) Task 16 and the IEA Wind Task 32 Lidar Systems.

The recommended practice document in all four parts has undergone a public review as well as a review by the IEA Wind Executive committee, that approved the recommendations for publication in January 2022.

The authors and editors want to thank everybody that contributed in our meetings, workshops and sessions to the discussions, provided feedback, reviewed the guideline or parts of it or provided other input throughout the past 6 years.

The authors specifically want to acknowledge and thank the contributing authors and those that have provided example code and input to our reference material at the companion website[1] of this book for their dedication, time spent writing, and discussing the best way to incorporate their specific experience and contributing information: namely Aidan Tuohy, Anton Kaifel, Caroline Draxl, Craig Collier, Ines Würth, Jakob W. Messner, Jan Remund, Jeffrey Lerner, Jethro Browell, Jie Yan, Joseph Lee, Justin Sharp, Martin Felder, Mathias Blicher Bjerregård, Mikkel Westenholz, Ricardo J. Bessa, Rui Pestana, Stephan Vogt and Stefan Wilbert.

Last but not least, the authors want to thank Yves Gagnon for encouraging us to publish our work with Elsevier, the Elsevier Team supporting us throughout the publishing process and our funding source, the Danish Energy Technology Development and Demonstration Programme (EUDP) (Grant Number 64018-0515 and 134-22015).

Corinna Möhrlen, John W. Zack, and Gregor Giebel

[1] https://www.elsevier.com/books-and-journals/book-companion/9780443186813.

About the IEA Wind TCP and Task 36 and 51

The International Energy Agency (IEA) was formed in 1974 as an autonomous body within the Organization for Economic Co-operation and Development (OECD). The IEA works to ensure reliable, affordable and clean energy for both its member countries and nations around the world. The agency has established a legal framework for international collaboration, which takes place under 39 Implementing Agreements, or Technology Collaboration Programmes (TCPs).

The IEA Wind TCP is an international co-operation of 23 countries to advance the technological development and global deployment of wind energy technology. The IEA Wind TCP is a vehicle for member countries to exchange information on the planning and execution of national large-scale wind system projects, and to undertake co-operative research and development (R&D) projects called Tasks.

IEA Wind Task 36 "Forecasting for Wind Energy" (2016–2021) and its successor Task 51 "Forecasting for the Weather-Driven Energy System" (2022–2025) have been established to facilitate communication and collaborations among international research groups, forecast vendors and forecast users. The Task members are engaged in the improvement of forecast accuracy and optimization of the value of forecast information for a range of decision-making applications encountered by stakeholders in the electric power industry.

PART ONE

Forecast solution selection process

Editors (1) and Authors (2):
Dr. Corinna Möhrlen, WEPROG, DK, DE[1,2]
Dr. John W. Zack, MESO Inc., USA[1,2]
Dr. Gregor Giebel, Technical University of Denmark, DK[1]

Contributing Authors (Version 1, 2019):
Dr. Jethro Browell, University of Glasgow, UK
Dr. Jakob W. Messner, MeteoServe Wetterdienst, AT
Dr. Aidan Tuohy, EPRI, USA
Dr. Craig Collier, Energy Forecasting Solutions, USA

Contributing Authors (Version 2, 2022):
Dr. Jeffrey Lerner, ENFOR, DK
Mikkel Westenholz, ENFOR, DK
Dr. Ricardo J. Bessa, INESCTEC, PT
Dr. Jie Yan, North China Electric Power University, CN

CHAPTER ONE

Forecast solution selection process

1.1. Before you start reading

This is the **first part** of this IEA Wind recommended practice for the implementation of renewable energy forecasting solutions.

In this **first part**, *Forecast solution selection process*, the design of a customized process to select an optimal forecast solution for a user's specific situation and application is addressed. In the **second part**, *Design and execution of benchmarks and trials*, the design, execution and analysis of customised forecasting benchmarks and trials is addressed. In the **third part**, *Forecast solution evaluation* methods and guidelines for the meaningful evaluation of alternative forecasts, operational and non-operational forecasts and entire forecast solutions are presented. In the **fourth part**, *Meteorological and power data requirements for real-time forecasting applications* guidance for the selection, deployment and maintenance of meteorological sensors, power measurements and associated data quality control relevant to real-time forecasting is provided.

If your main interest is in (2) testing or evaluating different forecasting solutions against each other, (3) verifying the quality of your forecast solution, or (4) setting up meteorological sensors or power measurements for real-time wind or solar power forecasting, please move on to part 2, part 3 or part 4 of this recommended practice guideline to obtain recommendations on any of these specific issues, respectively.

It is recommended to use the table of contents actively to find the topics that are most relevant for you.

1.2. Background and introduction

The effectiveness of forecasts in reducing the variability management costs of the variable power generation from wind and solar plants is dependent upon both the accuracy of the forecasts and the ability to effectively use the forecast information in the grid management decision-making process. Therefore, there is considerable motivation for stakeholders to try to

https://doi.org/10.1016/B978-0-44-318681-3.00011-8

obtain high-quality forecasts and effectively use this information as input to operational business processes.

This document is intended to provide guidance to stakeholders who are seeking a forecasting solution that fits their purpose and enables them to work efficient and economically responsible. It provides important input into business processes, for those starting from scratch to build a forecasting solution, consider renewal of your IT infrastructure, require new forecasting products, or need to extend or reduce the amount of vendors engaged. An overview of the decision support tool to help develop structured processes in the design and planning of a new or updated forecasting solution including its associated data communication, can be found in chapter 3 and 4, while chapters 1 and 2 provide background information and initial considerations.

In recent years, carrying out trials or benchmarks seemed to be an industry practice with an easy and straightforward decision process for many. In reality, trials are often expensive for both the end-user and the vendor, and are often neither straightforward, nor entirely conclusive. Benchmarks have little value for commercial vendors, except in their start-up phase, and end-users can often not count on results to indicate the state of the art for their application. Furthermore, if trials and benchmark studies lead to a dissatisfying result, forecasting solutions become increasingly criticized for their value. Providers that may have had the most technically qualified solution at hand, but did not score best at a specific (maybe oversimplified) test, may be deselected. This recommended practice document will therefore focus on the key elements to consider when establishing or updating a forecasting solution to obtain maximum value for a user-specific application. The objective is to provide a decision support tool (chapter 3) and data communication recommendations (chapter 4) to enable the user to establish procedures for an effective selection process.

1.3. Objectives

This document is intended to serve as guidance and a reference standard for industry, academia and government for the process of obtaining an optimal wind or solar power forecast solution for their applications and, in particular, for the specification of requirements and the design of effective renewable energy forecasting solutions.

These guidelines and best practices are based on years of industry experience and intended to achieve maximum benefit and efficiency for all parties involved.

1.4. Definitions

In the discussion of the process of obtaining the best possible forecasting solution, there are a number of terms and concepts that are used. Several of the key terms and concepts are defined in the following.

Note, these definitions are as general as possible with a focus on forecasting processes in the power industry and may not have such a completely general character to be applied to other areas of business.

- **Request for Information (RFI)**: a RFI is a formal document through which a forecast user or potential user requests information about the state-of-the-art business practices and available commercial products in the preparation or design of a forecast application or solution for a specific target process. By providing information about the target application, a client can ask vendors for their recommendations and experience to solve specific tasks. Such information is useful in the preparation and design of a new system, but also for systems that need to be rebuilt due to changing requirements.
- **Request for Proposal (RFP)**: a RFP is a tender process, where the client prepares a document laying out the system design of a forecasting solution and asking vendors to propose a solution and price quote. Usually, a set of minimum requirements are provided that become part of a contractual agreement for the awarded vendor.
- **Renewable Energy Forecast Benchmark**: an exercise conducted to determine the features and quality of a renewable energy forecast, such as wind or solar power. The exercise is normally conducted by an institution or their agent and usually includes multiple participants from industry forecast providers or applied research academics.
- **Renewable Energy Forecast Trial**: an exercise conducted to test the features and quality of a renewable energy forecast solution, such as wind or solar power. This may include one or more participants and is normally conducted by a private company for commercial purposes. A trial is a subset of a Renewable Energy Forecast Benchmark.

CHAPTER TWO

Initial considerations

Key points

This part provides guidelines for the task of formulating a plan and the justification for a forecasting solution selection process. It intends to assist in finding the necessary information when navigating through the vast jungle of information, opinions and possibilities and ensures that crucial details are being considered.

2.1. Tackling the task of engaging a forecaster for the first time

The most important consideration, at the start of a search for an optimal forecast solution, is a clear definition of the desired outcome. A lot of time and resources can be wasted for all parties involved in trials and benchmarks that are (1) not aligned with the requirements of the intended application, and/or planned and conducted by personnel with little or no experience in the forecast solution evaluation and selection process. To avoid this, the recommended practice is to carry out a market analysis in the form of a "request for information" (RFI) and to establish a requirement list (see also Appendix B). In some cases, it can be beneficial to test vendors or solutions prior to implementation. The difficulty with this method lies in the evaluation of tests, especially, when limited time is available for the test and the evaluation of its results. In many cases the test of the vendors do not answer the questions an end-user needs answered, because such tests mostly are simplified in comparison to the real-time application but still require significant resources. For such cases, this guideline provides other methods for an evaluation of different forecast solutions and vendors. The pitfalls and challenges with trials and/or benchmarks are the topic of part 2 of this series of recommended practices. The following table summarizes some aspects and provides guidance on where and when such pilot projects, trials or benchmarks may not be the best approach for the selection of a forecast solution. The column "recommendation" in Table 2.1 provides other methodologies that may be used to evaluate a forecast solution. Additionally, a typical set of questions to be asked to service providers is provided in Appendix A.

https://doi.org/10.1016/B978-0-44-318681-3.00012-X

Table 2.1 Recommendations for initial considerations prior to forecast solution selection for typical end-user scenarios.

Scenario	Limitation	Recommendation
Finding best service provider for a large portfolio (> 1000MW) distributed over a large area	Test of entire portfolio is expensive for client and service provider in terms of time and resources. Simplifying test limits reliability of result for entire portfolio.	RFI and RFP, where service provider's methods are evaluated and include an incentive scheme in the contract terms to provide more security for performance (see information about incentive schemes in section 3.9.3.3 and Part 3).
Medium sized Portfolio (500MW< X <1000MW) over limited area	Test of entire portfolio is expensive for client and service provider in terms of time and resources. Simplifying tests limits reliability of result for entire portfolio.	RFP, where service provider's methods are evaluated. Building a system that facilities an efficient change of service provider and include an incentive scheme (see information about incentive schemes in section 3.9.3.3 and Part 3) in the contract terms may be more efficient than conducting a trial.
Finding best service provider for small-sized portfolio (< 500MW)	Test of portfolio requires significant staff resources, a budget and a minimum of 6 months.	Difficult to achieve significance on target variable in comparison to required costs and expenses – trial costs makes solution more expensive. Test is possible, but expensive. Cheaper to setup an incentive scheme (see information about incentive schemes in section 3.9.3.3 and Part 3) and a system, where the suppliers may be exchanged relatively easily.
Micro portfolio (< 100MW) or single plants	Cost of a trial with many parties can easily be higher than the cost of a year of a forecasting service. Time for a trial can delay real-time experience by up to a year.	Evaluation of methodologies and setting up the internal system with an incentive scheme (see information about incentive schemes in section 3.9.3.3 and Part 3) and ease of service provider exchange is more beneficial.

continued on next page

Table 2.1 (*continued*)

Scenario	Limitation	Recommendation
Sale of generation at power market	Best score difficult to define, as sale is dependent on market conditions and a statistical score like RMSE or MAE cannot reflect the best marketing strategy, considering the uncertainty of a forecast and the associated costs.	Strategic choice of forecast provider and incentive scheme better than real-time test. Strategic choice may be: choice of vendor in comparison to others that use different, uncorrelated weather forecasts, uncorrelated weather-to-power model, unique forecast methodology, flexibility, expandable, etc. Incentive scheme ensures resources and incentive for continuous performance improvements (see section 3.9.3.3).
Market share of service provider is high	Monopolies in the power market can develop easily in new markets, when "do-what-all-others-do" mentalities start prevailing and result in correlated forecast errors among generators.	This situation often leads to increased balancing costs, even though the forecast error might be low in general, the costs for errors may be disproportionately high due to the correlations. Ask about the market share of a provider and do not choose one with a share > 30% as the only provider!
System operation in extreme events	Today, extreme (or rare) events are better forecasted, when considering weather uncertainty.	Statistical approaches relying solely on historic information may not be sufficient. A *PoE*50 (probability of exceedance of 50%) needs to have equally high probability in every time step above and below. The IEA Task 36 WP 3 has been dealing with uncertainty forecasting and provides recommendations for such situations (see workpackage 2.2 Uncertainty,[a] [1–6] and section 15.1). Forecasting solution needs to be weather and time dependent, i.e. only physical methodologies (ensemble forecast systems) fulfill such tasks

continued on next page

Table 2.1 *(continued)*

Scenario	Limitation	Recommendation
Critical Ramp forecasts	Critical ramp forecasts are part of an extreme event analysis and require probabilistic methods with time dependency.	Consider difference between a ramp forecast and a critical ramp as extreme event analysis that requires time + space dependent prob. methods such as ensemble forecasts. See references for uncertainty forecasts ([3–6]).
Blind forecasting, i.e. no measurement data available for the park or portfolio	Only useful for portfolios, where small errors are canceled out and indicative regarding performance. Without measurements, forecast accuracy will be non-representative of what accuracy can be achieved by training forecasts with historical data.	Evaluation can only be carried out for day-ahead or long-term forecasts, if measurements are collected throughout the trial. If you have a portfolio > 500MW, a blind test against a running contract can provide an inexpensive way to test the potential of a new provider. For single sites, the benefits of training are so large (>50% of error reduction at times) that blind forecasting is not recommended. It wastes resources for everybody without providing useful results.
Dynamic reserve	Deterministic forecasts cannot solve reserve requirements.	It is necessary to apply probabilistic methods for reserve calculation for variable resources such as wind and solar (see sec. 3.10.4 and C.1).

[a] https://iea-wind.org/task36/task36-work-packages/wp2-power-and-uncertainty-forecasting/wp2-2-uncertainty/.

2.2. Purpose and requirements of a forecasting solution

Once the limitations are defined, the next step is to define the objectives of the forecasting solution. As outlined in Table 2.1, very different forecasting strategies are needed for different application objectives such as maintaining system reliability by balancing supply and demand for a system with a large amount of renewable generation or maximizing revenue by seeling generated electricity into the power market. In the system balance task, extremes must be considered and risks estimated; mean error scores are not that important. Large errors are most significant, as they could potentially lead to lack of available balancing power. In the case of selling electricity into the power market, it is important to know the uncertainty of the forecast and use a forecast that is uncorrelated to others. The mean error of a forecast is important, but not a priority target, if the target e.g. is to use a forecast that generates low balancing costs. This is not always the same, because errors that lie within the forecast uncertainty are random. Such errors can only be reduced by strategic evaluations and decisions, not by methodology. If the objective is to calculate dynamic reserve requirements, probabilistic forecasts are required and should be part of the requirement list. When choosing a forecast solution, understanding the underlying requirements is key. It is not enough to ask for a specific forecast type without specifying the target objective. For this reason, defining the objective is most important. If there is no knowledge in the organization regarding the techniques required to achieve the objective, it is recommended to start with a RFI (see Appendix B) from different forecast providers and thereby gain an understanding and overview of the various existing solutions and their capabilities.

2.3. Adding uncertainty forecasts to forecasting solutions

In any power system that is in the transition to carbon neutrality, wind and solar generating resources are part of the solution. In order to integrate larger amounts of these variable energy resources, forecast uncertainty needs to be considered in grid related operational decision-making processes. Future renewable energy systems cannot be economically operated without the consideration of uncertainty in grid management decisions.

In the World Meteorological Organization's (WMO) guidelines on ensemble prediction [7], the WMO warns about ignoring uncertainty in forecasts in situations in which an end-user receives a deterministic forecast. The WMO argues that if a forecaster issues a deterministic forecast the underlying uncertainty is still there, and the forecaster has to make a best guess at the likely outcome. Unless the forecaster fully understands the decision that the user is going to make based on the forecast, and the impact of different outcomes, the forecaster's best guess may not be well tuned to the real needs of the user.

Therefore, weather-related decision-making requires a deeper understanding of weather uncertainty, the way any weather service provider produces uncertainty of weather forecasts, and how such forecasts are to be translated into end-user applications. In [1], [2], [3] and [4] reviews of uncertainty forecasting techniques, methods and applications have been made. These reviews will be the basis for the following definitions and recommendations for the selection of forecast solutions in which uncertainty forecasts are incorporated. Other work on decision-making under uncertainty [5,6] has indirectly also gone into these recommendations. It will describe how to best apply uncertainty forecasts in power system applications and identify potential gaps and pitfalls.

2.4. Information table for specific topic targets

Table 2.2 lists a number of topic targets and provides references to specific chapters of this document or other parts of this guideline series where the topic is addressed in detail.

Table 2.2 Information table for specific targets.

Target	Information
How to find the best forecast solution	Section 3
Creating a requirements list	Sections 3.3, 2.2, 3.2.1, and 3.2.2
Deterministic versus Probabilistic Forecasts	Sections 3.2.2 and 3.9.1.2
Decision support tool and practical guide to forecasting	Fig. 3.1
Evaluation of vendors: interviewing or conducting a trial?	Section 3.9 and reference material[a]
Is there need to test reliability and consistency?	Sections 3.2.1 and 3.9.2.1
How do I know which forecast solution fits my purpose best?	Sections 2.2 and 3.1, Appendix A
How do I build up sufficient IT infrastructure for a trial?	Chapter 4 and RP Part 2: Trial execution
Which metrics for what purpose?	RP Part 3: Evaluation of forecasts
Step-by-step guide for trials and benchmarks	RP Part 2: Trial execution
Are there differences of carrying out a trial or benchmark with deterministic versus probabilistic forecasts?	RP Part 2: Trial execution, Chapter 9

[a] Reference material is available at the companion website accompanying this book (https://www.elsevier.com/books-and-journals/book-companion/9780443186813).

continued on next page

Table 2.2 (*continued*)

Target	Information
Which requirements are needed for meteorological measurements in real-time forecasting applications?	RP Part 4: Meteorological and power data requirements for real-time forecasting applications
Which met and power measurements and data quality are required for real-time forecasting applications	RP Part 4: Meteorological (Chapters 18 and 21) and power data (Chapter 19) requirements for real-time forecasting applications

CHAPTER THREE

Decision support tool

Key points

Practical usage of the Decision Support Tool: The decision support tool in Fig. 3.1 provides a high-level overview of the process for finding the most suitable forecast solution and vendor, respectively. The sections provide guidance in how to use the decision support tool with detailed descriptions and explanations of the low-level information for the detailed planning and design of the decision process.

Note for the efficient usage of the Decision Support Tool: the numbers in the boxes of Fig. 3.1 correspond to the headings in the following sections that provide detailed information about each item.

From an end-user perspective, it is a non-trivial task to decide which path to follow, when implementing a forecasting solution for a specific application. Whether this is at a system operator, energy management company, a power producer or power trader, there are always multiple stakeholders involved in the decision-making process. A relatively straight forward way to formulate a specific approach for this process is to use a decision support tool.

Visualization of the decision support tool

Fig. 3.1 shows a decision support tool designed for the high-level decisions of managers and non technical staff when establishing a business case for a forecasting solution. The high-level thought construct shown in Fig. 3.1 is targeted to assist in planning the required resources and involvement of departments and staff for the decision process. The decision tool is constructed to begin with initial considerations to establish a "Forecast System Plan". The tool is designed to assist in making a decision on the major dependencies to the planned item. There are cross-references in the decision tool and referrals to different decision streams depending on the answer at each step of the decision flow.

IEA Wind Recommended Practice for the Implementation of Renewable Energy Forecasting Solutions
https://doi.org/10.1016/B978-0-44-318681-3.00013-1

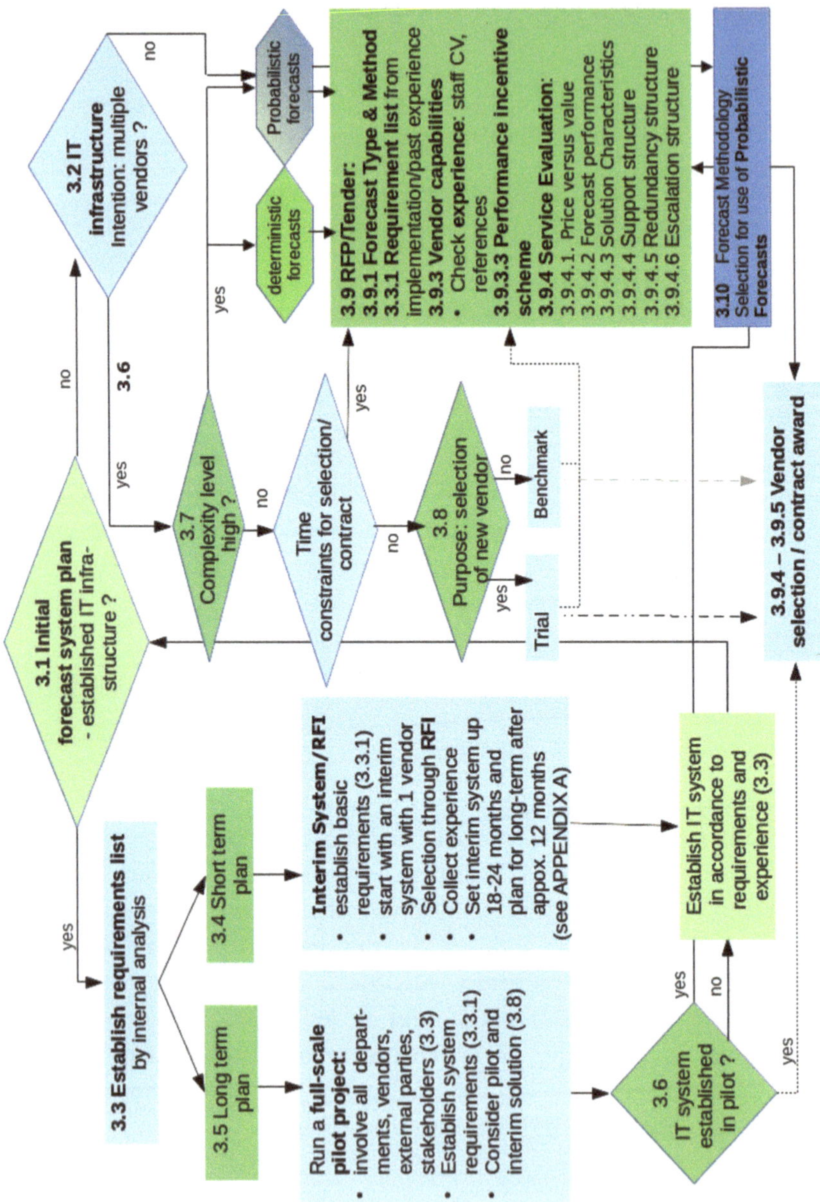

Figure 3.1 Decision Support Tool.

Starting at the very top, the first major dependency when planning a new or updated forecasting system is the IT infrastructure. The recommended procedure follows different paths depending on the status of the IT infrastructure. This is not to be understood that the IT infrastructure has higher priority over the forecasting solution itself. It is rather to sharpen the awareness that if the IT infrastructure is not in place yet or needs to be updated with new technology, the IT needs to be part of the decision process from the very beginning. The decision support tool in Fig. 3.1 provides a high-level overview of the process for finding the most suitable forecast solution and vendor, respectively. The following sections provide guidance in how to use the decision support tool with detailed descriptions and explanation to provide the low-level information for the detailed planning and design of the decision process.

3.1. Initial forecast system planning

The planning of a forecasting system for renewable generation is a complex task and highly specific to applications and organizations. This guideline therefore focuses solely on the aspects of general planning and management tasks specific to the implementation of wind power or solar power forecasts into an operational environment. Note that the limited information and considerations about forecast technologies or methodologies has the objective to provide guidelines on the impacts of commonly implemented technologies in the implementation and decision process. On the other hand, there is a strong focus on the IT infrastructure as one of the most crucial tasks in the implementation and integration of forecast solutions that are prone to become limiting factors for changes at later stages. For that reason, it is recommended that the IT infrastructure be established or, if already available, evaluated together with the planning of the forecast solution and methodology, in accordance to its ability to develop along with changes in forecast practices, possible statutory changes, etc. Databases are prone to have limitations that often make it difficult and costly to incorporate additional types of information or change the structure of how information is stored. Such consideration need to be part of the decision process and the requirements list (see section 3.3).

3.2. IT infrastructure considerations

The starting point of the tool is the IT infrastructure. If a company has already built an appropriate infrastructure, finding a solution or vendor is more straightforward. The reason for this is that in this case, for example, the forecast provider will need to conform to existing file formats, communication protocols or security constraints. If an IT infrastructure for the forecasting solution is to be established or updated, it needs to closely follow the technical requirements of the solution.

In the other case (no IT infrastructure has been built yet) an internal analysis of the needs is required. In this analysis, it is important to know whether there is a short-term goal with an objective to be reached with time constraints, or whether it is a long-term plan that needs to be satisfied. Usually, such differentiation is dependent on the policies for the development of renewable generation in the target country.

The important aspects in the IT infrastructure to be considered are:

- database structure
- communication layer
- monitoring and error handling
- data storage and historic data accessibility

In general a forecast system interface, whether in-house or outsourced requires multiple data streams, starting with measured power and weather variables. Usually, there is a connection to the power unit's SCADA (Supervisory Control and Data Acquisition) system. However, the measurement data needs storage and a data flow to the forecaster needs to be added as an additional internal data flow process.

It needs to be decided, whether there is a need to access other external data sources, such as numerical weather prediction (NWP) data, or the forecast data itself.

Dependent on the setup of the forecasting solution, it is necessary to evaluate how fast the access to historical data has to be, for example to carry out internal analysis, external data delivery to vendors, etc.

3.2.1 IT requirements for single versus multiple forecast vendors

IT infrastructure impacts for multiple vendor solution:

- infrastructure more complex
- database requirements are higher due to higher data volumes
- requires a forecast strategy: mixing versus primary/secondary forecaster

IT infrastructure impacts for single vendor solution:

- reliability requirement of solution high
- monitoring requirement higher for up-time
- higher requirements for quality control of forecasts
- less data volume than for multiple-vendor solutions
- database structure less complex than for multiple-vendor solutions

3.2.2 IT requirements for deterministic versus probabilistic forecasts

From an IT infrastructure and architectural perspective, deterministic and probabilistic forecasting solutions are quite different. The database requirements are typically higher by a factor of 10 to 100 for the latter. Therefore, depending on what components of a probabilistic forecasts are used and archived, the storage requirements can increase significantly.

Nevertheless, the available storage and computational resources are changing with changing requirements in industry and hence should not immediately be considered a barrier or limitation for the integration or implementation of new forecasting technologies. However, careful consideration and planning is needed.

The advantages and disadvantages of the deterministic versus the probabilistic solution from a IT perspective are similar to single versus multiple providers in section 3.2.1.

3.3. Establishment of a requirement list

Establishing a requirement list for a forecasting solution is highly specific to the characteristics of the application and the user's institution, and depends on many factors. Each end-user will have very specific needs. There are however common areas that require consideration, and the following recommendation list should be interpreted from that perspective.

The three most fundamental aspects when establishing a requirements list are:

1. Description of the current situation
   In this process, it is imperative to describe exactly all processes in which forecasting is required and how these processes are interlinked. Here, it is essential to get all departments involved, also the IT department, that will use forecasts. The more accurate you can describe the situation at hand, (e.g. integration plans, use of forecasts, market situation, statu-

tory aspects, IT restrictions, existing limitations and methods for data exchange, current and/or future challenges, etc.), the more straightforward it will be to (1) ask questions to the vendors regarding forecasting methodology and also (2) get information about the processes that are required and the time until the forecasting for the client can commence.

2. Engagement with vendors, stakeholders and independent consultants

   Questions to vendors should be of technical character regarding forecast methodology, but also on available data exchange methodologies, required input data for the models and system support.

   If you already have a forecast vendor, it is recommended to engage with the forecaster to discuss the current situation and where the forecaster sees limitations and potential for improvements. Often, forecast providers need to adopt their forecasts to a specific need and even though a new technology may be available, it is not used due to current limitations. Other vendors, stakeholders and independent consultants may at any stage be engaged, not only when it comes to establishing a new or renewal of a forecasting system. For new systems, it is recommended to engage different forecast vendors and stakeholders to provide insight from a variety of experiences.

   In all cases, it is essential to describe the planned objective and specify limitations if they are already known. The more information that can be shared the better a vendor, stakeholder or consultant can evaluate what is considered the most appropriate solution.

   Appendix A contains an additional listing of recommended considerations that are also applicable for RFIs.

3. Description of the envisioned situation

   The description of the envisioned situation is most important for the implementation of a solution. Analysis of the current situation, the forecast vendor(s) input and other organizational and statutory requirements should lay the basis for the vision of a new system. It is recommended to put as much detail into this part as possible. The following requirements list assists in defining all aspects for the planning phase of a forecasting system.

   Recommendation in short: Describe (1) the current situation, (2) engage vendors and stakeholders and (3) describe the envisaged situation in great detail. Ask specific questions that are required to get the highest possible level of detail for the decision process.

Recommendation: Describe (1) the current situation, (2) engage vendors and stakeholders and (3) describe the envisioned situation in great detail. Ask specific questions that are required to get the highest possible level of detail for the decision process.
The following Requirement List and Appendix A contain listings of recommended considerations.

3.3.1 Requirement list

It is recommended that the following items be considered:

IT infrastructure:

- communication/data exchange with the forecast vendor(s)
- communication/data exchange with assets (wind/solar parks)
- database and storage implications
- accessibility of data information of internal users
- application interfaces to internal tools (e.g. graphics, models, verification, metering)
- information security policies

Forecast Methodology and Attributes:

- weather input
- methodology of weather to power model
- application/model background for each forecast product
- forecast time horizons
- forecast frequency
- forecast uncertainty

Support and Service:

- service level for each product (e.g. 24/7, business hours etc.)
- system recovery
- failure notifications and reporting
- escalation procedures
- service documentation
- contact list for different services
- staff training

Contracting:

- contract length
- amendment possibilities

- additional work outside contract
- licenses (hardware, software, services, etc.)
- confidentiality (NDA)
- insurances
- subcontracting
- price table for each product category

Performance and Incentivization:

- verification methods
- verification parameters
- definition of payment structure (boolean or sliding areas)
- expected accuracy for each forecast horizon

3.4. Short-term solution

In this case, current requirements should be listed and analyzed in accordance with possible time limitations. It is recommended that a short-term solution be sought, if the political situation does not seem to be stable to make long-term investments, or a here-and-now issue needs to be solved and experience gained. In such cases, a relatively simple methodology that can be implemented fast and easy is the best way forward. Today, this can be found by carrying out a RFI, where vendors can suggest the best approach to fulfill very specific needs with the lowest level of cost and effort. Due to IT constraints in many organizations, such solutions are sometimes set up with delivery by email. This is not a recommended practice for security and reliability reasons, but can help to fill a gap between a long-term solution and an urgent need.

Despite the shortcomings, interim solutions are recommended as they are valuable in respect to experience with the handling of forecasting data inside an organization. If such solutions are employed while a long-term plan is being developed, it can be of great benefit for the long-term solution. Such solutions should last approximately 18–24 months. Planning for a long-term solution should ideally start after 12 months.

The danger lies in staying with an interim solution, if it has real limitations on security (e.g. email delivery) and reliability. Such limitations may not be problematic for a long time, but reliance on non-redundant systems can cause sudden uncontrollable situations. For this reason, the question about the IT system is raised at the end of the short-term solution, as this is a crucial part in the next step. It is recommended that this should be a priority topic, once practical experience with forecasting has been gained.

3.5. Long-term solution

Developing a long-term solution can be cumbersome and difficult, as many aspects have to be considered, from policies to governmental plans or corporate strategies.

A practical way forward is to conduct a full-scale pilot project in which different solutions are tested and verified over a period of at least one year. The advantage of such a pilot project is that there is the possibility to verify and evaluate different solutions and their fit for purpose over a longer time span.

A pilot project is characterized by:

1. Involvement of all relevant internal and external stakeholders
2. Establishment of system requirements
3. Possible use as interim solution

The disadvantage of a pilot project is that it takes a long time and hence is costly, and it is not certain that it will produce a very clear winning solution for a specific area or task. On the other hand, to find the most appropriate long-term solution needs many considerations, not only technically, but also economically and whether a solution is future compatible.

The experience of the vendor in adjusting, maintaining and developing a solution with changing needs may be a challenge for some and not part of the business philosophy for others. Such vendor policies can be identified and clarified when carrying out long-term tests. The box therefore feeds into the question about an appropriate IT system. If this has not been established, it is recommended to prioritize the IT before going further.

Optional paths at the end of a pilot project:

1. Vendor selection
2. Redefining requirements to start a solution bottom up
3. Carrying out a RFP with the identified requirements.

3.6. Going forward with an established IT system

In the case that an IT system has been established and new vendors or an update of an existing system is the objective for the project, there are various possibilities to move forward. Crucial in this phase is again to set a target and objectives.

If the objective is to determine if there are forecast vendors in the market that may provide high quality forecasts with other methods or for a lower price, a benchmark/trial or an RFP are possible approaches. The best choice in a specific situation will depend on the structure and/or complexity of the system and time constraints, a benchmark/trial or a RFP are alternative approaches. One crucial factor when deciding between an RFP or a trial/benchmark is whether the existing IT structure can handle multiple suppliers.

If this is not the case, any evaluation against an existing supplier can be cumbersome and at times impossible. Part 2 provides details on this topic, which is mostly related to the design of tests that are:

- **representative** (including consistency)
- **significant** (including repeatable)
- **relevant** (including fair and transparent)

These are the key points when carrying out a forecast performance comparison.

3.7. Complexity level of the existing IT solution

In addition to the accuracy or statistical skills of forecasts, there are other important aspects to be considered when choosing a forecast supplier. It has been observed that evaluations based on non-technical skills or skills leading to forecast performance for a specific purpose have been underestimated in their importance. One important factor is the ability to improve. This is typically excluded when a trial/benchmark is employed because the short duration of such an exercise effectively eliminates an assessment of the ability to improve over time and pushes the solution selection criteria to be predominantly current performance and price.

It is often forgotten that long-term experience in a specific area can provide significant advantages. On the other hand, verifying only a small part of a complex system for practical reasons may result in a misleading result (see section 12.1 "representativeness", section 12.2 "significance" and section 12.3 "relevance").

The complexity of a system that a forecast solution must adapt to, but also the data flow that complex systems inherit, is seldom easy to simulate in trials and will almost always disqualify some participants, when it comes to the real system. To conclude, the complexity of a system and the purpose of a forecast within a complex corporate structure are significant aspects to consider in a forecast solution selection.

Recommendation: In case of complex structures and requirements it is best to employ a RFP process in which the core capabilities of potential forecast solutions are evaluated.

3.8. Selection of a new vendor versus benchmarking existing vendor

If there are no time constraints and the complexity level of the operational system is not too high, or a new system is in the process of being built, a trial or a benchmark exercise can be very useful in order to acquire experience in the building process.

Recommendation: A trial should be conducted in cases in which a new vendor will be selected and a trial can be executed in a manner that yields results that are fair, transparent, representative and significant.
A benchmark should be conducted, if the initial objective is not to engage a new vendor, but to compare the capabilities of an existing vendor to other vendors or to newer forecasting technology. In both cases the invited vendors should be notified of the purpose of the exercise.

3.9. RFP evaluation criteria for a forecast solution

If complexity levels are high and if time constraints do not allow for a lengthy trial or benchmark, the RFP should be compiled with care in order to address all requirements and yet not ask for more than is needed.

The most important evaluation criteria to be defined in an RFP are:

- required type of forecast (e.g., hours-, day-, or week-ahead)
- the methodology that is applied to generate these forecasts
- compliance to requirements

It is recommended that this first step should be vendor independent. And, if this cannot be defined, it is recommended to first conduct an RFI to survey the industry on their capabilities and their recommendations on the forecast type and methodology that should be employed for the specific needs of a user's application. Appendix B contains typical questions for an RFI. Input from specific vendors should only be used after the forecast type and methodology have been defined via a vendor-independent process. At this point, the important vendor-related factors to consider are:

- capabilities (experience)
- support and maintenance services

The following sections describe these considerations in detail.

3.9.1 Forecast solution type

Most users will agree that they want to obtain forecasts with the best possible forecast accuracy for their application. A benchmark or a trial has in the past often been viewed as a way to determine which provider is most likely to deliver the best possible forecast performance. In theory, this is a reasonable perspective. In practice, it is strongly recommended that a solution selection decision should not be based solely on results from a trial or benchmark.

The following subsections will address a number of key issues associated with the dilemma of finding the best forecasting solution with a simple and low-cost exercise for both the end-user and the forecast provider. Appendix F.6 provides some hints on the definition of a "good" forecast (see also Table F.1).

3.9.1.1 Single versus multiple forecast providers

It has been widely documented (e.g. [8,9]) that a composite of two or more state-of-the-art forecasts will often achieve better performance (accuracy) than any of the individual members of the composite over a statistically meaningful period of time. Indeed, many of the forecast service providers (FSP) internally base their approach and services on that concept. There are certainly significant reasons for an end-user to consider the use of multiple FSPs to achieve better forecast accuracy.

However, in a practical sense, there are several advantages and disadvantages that should be considered. When building a solution, it is recommended to consider the following aspects:

Benefits of using multiple vendors:

1. There are a number of FSPs in today's forecast market that exhibit performance that is close to the state-of-the-art. It may be advantageous for reliability to assemble a set of state-of-the-art forecasts.
2. Higher forecast accuracy can often be achieved by blending forecasts from multiple state-of-the-art FSPs whose forecast errors have a relatively low correlation.

Challenges of employing multiple forecast vendors:

1. Increased internal costs, even if two "cheap" vendors may be less costly than one high-end forecast vendor, employing multiple vendors increases internal costs significantly due to increased amounts of data and IT processes.
2. Blending algorithms need to be intelligent in order to consistently obtain performance benefits from combining multiple forecasts. The algorithm must be able to appropriately adjust to variations in forecast availability (e.g. one forecast is missing, more than one forecast is missing etc.) and also automatically (or be easy to manually) update when forecast statistics indicate the relative performance of forecast providers changes. Another issue is that blending is only easily applied to deterministic forecasts (or probabilistic forecasts have been reduced to deterministic forecasts, for example, by taking the mean or median of the probability distribution). Benefits of blended probabilistic forecasts have been reported for time-lagged ensembles [10]. Other methods to blend e.g. ensemble prediction systems (EPS) with other EPS or other probabilistic forecast systems are maybe possible, but its use and benefits are unknown, because it is a much more expensive and complex task to implement an algorithm that produces a valid blend of multiple probability distributions.
3. Forecast improvements are more complex and difficult to achieve with a multi-provider solution. When improvements are achieved on the vendor side, the blending algorithm becomes inconsistent with those changes, and this can result in worse performance for the composite forecast unless long-term historic data can be delivered to retrain the blending algorithm.
4. It is more difficult to incentivize multi-vendor solutions to achieve continuous performance improvement over time. Although incentive schemes can be a good way to provide resources to the FSP for continuous improvements, this can be counter-productive in a multi-vendor environment, because changes to the statistical characteristics of forecasts can have a negative influence on the resulting blended forecast. An end-user needs to be aware of this pitfall, when choosing a multi-vendor solution, and take mitigating measures.
5. Multiple points of failure – with multiple forecast providers, the IT infrastructure needs to contain more logic to deal with one or more data streams when there are, for example, delivery disruptions, timeliness, or quality issues.

3.9.1.2 Deterministic versus probabilistic

Many forecasting applications need a discrete answer. For that reason, most users have historically employed deterministic forecasts for their applications. Although weather forecasts and hence also power forecasts of variable resources such as wind and solar power, contain inherent uncertainties, probabilistic forecast products have been associated with forecasts not being discrete. The probability of a generic power generation at time x cannot be used in a trading application with the purpose of bidding into the market. As the penetration of variable generation resources increase and digitalization increases, the uncertainty information for decision-making can and is being processed by algorithms, including those who yield a discrete answer for the ultimate decision-making process. Deterministic forecasts by default ignore the underlying uncertainty in the forecasts. By using probabilistic forecasts, this uncertainty can be taken into consideration in the decision processes.

The most common products of uncertainty or probabilistic forecasts are the probability of exceedance (PoE) values, typically given as PoE05, PoE50 and Poe95, quantiles or confidence bands (see Glossary for definitions).

The advantage of probabilistic/uncertainty forecasts in comparison to the deterministic "best guesses" is the possibility to act upon the probability of an event, rather than being surprised, when the deterministic forecast is wrong. In power markets, for example, a probability of exceedance of 50% (PoE50) is an important parameter for a system operator, because such forecasts prevent the market from skillfully speculating on system imbalance. Extreme ramping, high-speed shut-down risk, unit commitment and dynamic reserve allocation are other examples, where probabilistic forecasts are beneficial or required (see Table 15.3). In other words, in situations in which there is sufficient forecast uncertainty to have a significant impact on a decision or the costs of a process, probabilistic forecasts provide the necessary information to an end-user to make a decision with a consideration of objective uncertainty information.

Recommendation: When establishing or updating a forecasting system, the question should not be posed on advantages and disadvantages of a deterministic or probabilistic forecast solution, but rather whether a deterministic solution can achieve the objective of the application. Section 3.10 describes uncertainty forecasts and how to select the appropriate probabilistic methodology for specific applications.

Two thorough academic reviews about probabilistic methodologies and the uncertainty through the entire forecasting chain can be found on IEA Wind Task 51's publication webpage (https://iea-wind.org/task51/task51-publications/task51-articles-and-reports/).

3.9.1.3 Forecast horizons

The forecast horizons play a major role in the ability to plan using forecasts. Today, there are 5 general classes of forecast horizons widely used and defined by a new IEC standard (IEC 62934:2021 [11]) in the power industry:

1. Minute-ahead forecasts or now-casts (0–120 min)
2. Hours-ahead forecasts (0–12 hours)
3. Day-ahead forecasts (0–48 hours)
4. Week-ahead forecasts (48–180 hours)
5. Seasonal forecasts (monthly or yearly)

The **Minute-ahead forecasts** are also sometimes referred to as "ultra-short term forecast" or "now-cast" in the technical literature. These are mainly used in areas with high penetration and high complexity in system operation or significant risk for high-speed shut down and extreme events. These forecasts are either based on a statistical extrapolation of power generation measurements or a combination of weather input and high frequency (e.g. 1 minute) measurements of generation. The recommended practice depends on the severity and costs of the target value. For situational awareness, a simple extrapolation of measurements may be sufficient. For extreme events (e.g. ramps, high-speed shut down) the involvement of weather related forecasts in high time resolution is recommended.

Hours-ahead forecasts are sometimes referred to as short-term or intra-day forecasts. These are typically used to correct a day-ahead forecast by using real-time measurements. These forecasts extrapolate from recent real-time power generation data and local area real-time weather observations to obtain a more accurate representation of the current state and the anticipated changes over the next few hours.

There are different methods available, from simple extrapolation of measurements to advanced weather and distance-dependent algorithms. It's recommended to get details of a short-term forecast methodology described by the vendors, as quality and usability can differ strongly with availability of data, quality of measurement data etc.

If the target is e.g. ramp forecasting, system control, a very large fleet or quality issues with measurement data not dealt with by the end-user, simple algorithms are often not capable of providing a good enough picture of the next few hours.

The **Day-ahead forecasts** are widely-used forecasts for general system operation, trading and short-term planning. Traditionally, they are based on a combination of weather models and statistical models.

Week-ahead forecasts are sometimes referred to as long-term forecasts and are usually applied in cases where the focus is not on forecast accuracy, but on forecast skill, e.g. in situations, where trends are more important than granularity. These forecasts are most valuable as a blending of a number of different forecasts or from an ensemble predication system, where the small-scale variability is reduced. If this is done, such forecasts can serve to reduce reserve costs and generate more dynamic reserve allocation as well as auctions.

Seasonal forecasts are sometimes referred to as ultra-long-term forecasts and predict longer-time-scale variations due to seasonal and or climate variability. They may be derived based on climatology, correlation to various climate indices and oscillatory phenomena, climate models, or a combination of these methods. Ensemble methodologies are the most preferable method due to the inherent uncertainty on such time frames. The simplest method is to identify trends or typical variations by analyzing past measurements.

Recommendation: A key component of choosing a methodology is a careful analysis of the accuracy requirements of the target application. For trading of futures in a trading environment a simple methodology may be sufficient. Tasks such as grid balancing, grid infrastructure planning or long-term capacity planning however require more advanced methodologies. It is recommended to choose the method according to the need to capture quantities only (simple method) or also capture climatic extremes (advanced method).

3.9.2 Vendor capabilities

3.9.2.1 Experience and reliability

Experience is a crucial element of a successful vendor implementation of the forecasting solution. It can usually be evaluated by the selected references that are provided and measured by conducting interviews with similar types of customers or by asking for information about the vendor's background and experience with similar customers. If a vendor is new to the market that may not be possible. In this case, staff resources and the experience of the key staff are a useful indicator of whether the experience level for the minimum requirements is present.

Reliability is often associated with experience, as it implies the reliable implementation and real-time operation of a forecasting service. It is an important aspect and may be assessed by requiring examples of similar projects and interviewing references. It can also save a lot of work and resources in comparison to carrying out a trial, if reliability and experience with respect to e.g. complex IT infrastructure, security aspects, reliable delivery and provision of support etc. are a more crucial aspect than specific statistical performance scores.

Recommendation: Ask vendors to describe their experience, provide user references and also the CV of key staff members.

3.9.2.2 Ability to maintain state-of-the-art performance

The previous section provided an overview of all the considerations for the technical aspects of forecast type and methodology. In order to assure that the forecast vendor can maintain state-of-the-art performance, it is recommended to determine the extent of a provider's ongoing method refinement/development and forecast improvement activities. Recommendation: Evaluate by asking the vendor to provide information about

- research areas and engagement
- references to staff publications such as methodology documentation or project reports
- references of participation in conferences/workshops
- percent of revenue reinvested into research and development

3.9.2.3 Performance incentive schemes

A performance incentive scheme is the most effective way to ensure that a forecaster has an incentive to improve forecasts over time and also allocates resources to it. By setting up a performance incentive scheme, the client acknowledges that development requires resources and vendors have not only an economic incentive to allocate resources for further developments, but can also influence their reputation. Incentive schemes do not have to be enormously high, but usually range between 10–30% of the yearly forecast service fee.

A key attribute of an effective performance incentive scheme is that it reflects the importance of the forecast performance parameters that are most critical for a client's application. The evaluation of such forecast parameters should be selected according to:

1. the objective of the forecasting solution
2. the use/application of the forecasts
3. the available input at forecast generation time

The **first objective** in this context is defined as the purpose of the forecast. For example, if a forecast is used for system balance, an evaluation should contain a number of statistical metrics and ensure that there is an understanding of the error sources that the forecaster can improve on. A typical pitfall is to measure performance only with one standard metric, rather than a framework of metrics reflecting the cost or loss of a forecast solution in the context of a user's application. For example, if the mean absolute error (MAE) is chosen to evaluate the performance in system balance, an asymmetry in cost for forecast errors will not be taken into account. Also, if, for example, large errors pose exponentially increasing costs, an average metric, such as the mean absolute error (MAE), is unsuitable.

The **second objective** (use or application of forecasts) is defined in the context of where forecasts are used in the organization and where these have impact and influence on internal performance metrics or economic measures. For example, a wind power forecast that a trader uses for trading the generation of a wind farm on a power market has two components: revenue and imbalance costs. The revenue is defined by the market price for each time interval, whereas the cost is defined by the error of the forecast, the individual decision that may have been added to the forecast and the system balance price. When evaluating a forecast in its application context, it is important to choose an evaluation that incentivies the vendor to tune the forecast to the application. A forecast that is optimized to avoid large errors may create lower revenue. However, if income is evaluated rather than revenue, such a forecast may be superior due to lower imbalance costs. On the other hand, if the end-user makes changes to the forecast along the process chain, the forecast evaluation must not include forecast modifications that are outside the forecast vendor's influence.

The **third objective** (available input at forecast generation time) is most important when evaluating short-term forecasts that use real-time measurements. For example, if the forecast is evaluated against a persistence forecast with corrected measurements rather than with the measurements that were available at the time of forecast generation, the evaluation is to the disadvantage of the forecaster. The same applies, if aspects that affect the forecast such as curtailments, dispatch instructions or turbine availability, are not taken out of the evaluation either by excluding periods when these occur or by correcting the measured data to eliminate their impact.

Additionally, the use of single standard statistical metrics (e.g. MAE or RMSE) alone is not recommended. More details on the purpose and interconnection of statistical metrics for evaluation of incentive schemes can be found in part 3, especially section 15.1 and in Appendix F.

The structure of performance incentive scheme is an individual process and contractual matter between parties. When establishing the structure of a performance incentive it is recommended to consider that by choosing a maximum and minimum, the maximum value provides budget security to the end-user, also when e.g. changing from a very simple solution to an advanced one with much higher performance. The latter provides security to the forecaster to ensure that the basic costs for generation of forecasts are covered. Adding a sliding structure between these limits ensures the forecaster always has an incentive to improve even when it is foreseeable that the maximum may not be achievable.

Recommendation: When a performance incentive is formulated and implemented, the evaluation needs to consider the non-technical constraints in the forecast and the parts that are beyond the control of the forecaster. A fair performance incentive scheme needs to measure the performance of a forecast by blacklisting any measurement data that is incorrect or corrupt, that contains curtailments, dispatch instructions, reduced availability or other reductions outside of the forecasters influence. Evaluation against persistence forecasts also need to be done with the available data at the time of forecast generation in order to not give advantage to persistence.

It is recommended to apply a maximum incentive payment and a maximum penalty or minimum incentive. A sliding incentive payment between these limits is preferable over a boolean (yes | no) scheme, as it always encourages forecast improvement efforts.

3.9.3 Evaluation of services

The recommended practice in any evaluation is to consider a number of factors that contribute to the value that a user will obtain from a forecast service. It is not possible to provide a complete list of factors to consider. However, the most important factors that should be addressed are:

- Price versus value and quality
- Forecast performance
- Solution characteristics
- Speed of delivery
- Support structure
- Redundancy structure

The issues associated with each of these aspects will be addressed in the following subsections in more detail.

3.9.3.1 Price versus value and quality

The value of a forecast may or may not be directly measurable. In most cases however, the value can be defined in terms of cost savings or obligations and in that way provide an indication of the expected value from a certain solution.

Prices are difficult to evaluate. A low price often indicates that not all requirements may be adequately fulfilled in operation or not all contractual items are accepted and left to the negotiations. For these reasons, care has to be taken in the evaluation process.

Some services and methods are more expensive than others, because of computational efforts, required licenses, database requirements, redundancy to insure reliability and other factors. Unless prices are driven by competition in a overheated market, a service price is normally coupled to the requirements and acceptance of contractual items. Some items such as reliability, customer support or system recovery can have high prices, but can always be negotiated to a different level. In an RFP end-users need to be aware of the relationship between cost, value and associated service level to prevent vendors from speculating on negotiable items in the requirement list.

Recommendation: Following a decade of experience in the forecasting industry, the recommended practice on price evaluation is to connect technical and contractual aspects to the price and let vendors provide proposed contractual terms that may be associated with high service costs separately, especially, if a fixed cost price is requested. An example could be the requirement of full system recovery within 2 hours in a 24/7/365 environment. If there is no penalty associated, a vendor may ignore this requirement, which may result in a much lower price. Requesting transparent pricing makes the evaluation process easier and makes sure that negotiable aspects of a service can be clearly compared.

3.9.3.2 Forecast performance

Forecast performance evaluation should contain a number of metrics that are representative of the needs of the forecast user. It is recommended that an evaluation framework for the performance evaluation be established. The process of establishing such a framework is addressed in Part 3, section 15.1 of this recommended practice.

3.9.3.3 Solution characteristics

The solution characteristics of a forecast service also contain much value for an end-user and should get attention in the evaluation. It can be defined in terms of the available graphical tools, ease of IT services for retrieving data or exchanging data in real-time as well as historical data, customer support setup and staff resources connected to the forecasting solution. This can be a key factor for the operational staff of the forecast user to accept and be comfortable with a forecast service, as well as having confidence in the service. Additional work that may be connected, but outside the scope of the operational service, can also be key elements for a well-functioning service.

Recommendation: Ask the vendor to describe how the forecast system will be constructed, their vision for communication and support, and to provide examples of forecast graphics (if applicable).

3.9.3.4 Support structure

Customer service is often under-estimated and in most cases second to an accuracy metric when selecting a vendor. Support can be a costly oversight if, for example, costs are related to a continuously running system or extreme events, where the user needs an effective warning system and related customer service. Support can have a relatively large cost in a service contract and may provide a false impression of service prices, if, for example support is only offered during business hours.

Key elements for the customer support are:

- the responsiveness of the provider, when issues arise
- live support in critical situations

A support structure and it's management for operational processes additionally need to bind the following strategic areas together:

1. Customer Support
2. Operations Software and Service
3. IT Infrastructure

Customer support (1) should be handled by a support platform, ideally with different forms for contact, e.g. a telephone hotline and an email ticket system.

End-users should ensure that third-party software used in the operational environment (2) is licensed, renewed in a timely manner and maintained according to the licensing party's recommendations.

The IT infrastructure (3) should ideally be ISO 9001 and ISO 27001 certified in cases, where real-time operation and security is of paramount importance.

> **Recommendation:** Definition of the required support structure should be part of the requirement list for any forecasting solution. For real-time forecasting solutions the end-user needs to ensure that there is an appropriate support structure in place. Considerations of the real-time environment, the user's resources and which of the forecasting business practices are of significance to the user should be carried out. Especially, where processes are expected to run every day in the year.

3.9.3.5 Redundancy structure

Redundancy depends very much on the end-users needs to maintain a frictionless and continuous operation. Forecasting is mostly carried out in real-time, which has an inherit requirement of being functional all the time. While there are many processes and targets for forecasting that may not require large redundancy and permanent up-time, the following recommendation is targeted to those end-users where forecasting is to some extend mission critical. There are a number of different redundancy levels that need consideration and that can be achieved in various ways:

1. Physical delivery of the service – IT infrastructure
2. Content of the delivery – Forecasting methods

The delivery of the service (1) is connected to the IT infrastructure. Redundancy measures may be a combination of any of these:

- Delivery from multiple locations to mitigate connectivity failures
- Delivery from multiple hardware/servers to mitigate individual server failure
- Delivery with redundant firewalls to mitigate hardware failure
- Delivery through an ISP using Email, etc.

The redundancy of the forecast content is equally important as the physical delivery of the data, but often neglected. It is recommended to consider any combination of the following redundancy measures for correct forecast content:

- redundant providers of weather input
- redundant/multiple providers of forecast service
- redundant input and mitigation strategy for weather models
- redundant input and mitigation strategy for power conversion models

Recommendation: Define the required redundancy level according to the importance of a permanent functioning service and the impact of delivery failure on other internal critical processes.

3.9.3.6 Escalation structure

It is recommended for high-level contracts, where forecasting is critical to the end-users processes to get information about escalation structures in case of failure. This is especially important when employing only one forecast provider.

An end-user needs to have a description about structure and corresponding responsibilities for their operations staff in order to incorporate such information into own escalation structures in case of emergencies. Table 3.1 provides recommendations of a three tier escalation structure.

Each level of escalation ideally contains the following structured process:

- Formulation of the problem/failure
- Root cause analysis
- Coordination of action plan for troubleshooting responsibilities
- Coordinated action plan progression
- Escalation to the next level or closure of escalation procedure.

Table 3.1 Recommendation of a three tier escalation structure.

Escalation level	Forecast service provider coordination	End-user coordination
Level 1: failure to deliver service	Technical Staff	Operations Staff Project manager
Level 2: failure to recover or implement service	Project manager	Project/Department manager
Level 3: failure to solve failure/recovery	General management	General management

3.10. Forecast methodology selection for use of probabilistic forecasts

Methodologies used to generate probabilistic uncertainty forecasts for the power industry are proven concepts and integrated in current business practices. Looking into these applications, it becomes apparent that uncertainty forecasts have found their place in the power industry, but are on the other hand far from being optimally exploited in most applications. As the level of penetration of variable generation resources increases, the value of uncertainty information in operational processes will increase and provide greater incentive to optimize their use in these processes.

The following definitions and recommendations are intended to assist in the implementation of uncertainty information in the form of probabilistic forecasts into operational processes. While this guide aims to be comprehensive, it is not possible to provide all the details that may be necessary for a first time implementation or for the planning of a fully integrated probabilistic forecast solution. Nevertheless, the information provided is taken from existing documentation, partially coordinated by the IEA Wind Task 36, but also from general publications. This information can be found in the References Material,[1] and in the reviews on probabilistic methods for the power industry [1], on uncovering wind power forecasting uncertainty origins and development through the whole modeling chain [4] and on decision making under wind power uncertainty [5,6].

[1] Reference material is available at the companion website accompanying this book (https://www.elsevier.com/books-and-journals/book-companion/9780443186813).

3.10.1 Definitions of uncertainty

In order to establish a common language of uncertainty forecasts, some of the most frequently used terms (see e.g. [1]) are defined below:

1. **Forecast error spread:**
   The historically observed deviation of a forecast from its corresponding observation at a specific time. It can also refer to a reference error magnitude provided by an error metric, e.g. variance or standard deviation.
2. **Confidence interval:**
   The probability that an observed value will fall between a pair of forecast values around the mean. Confidence intervals measure the degree of uncertainty in a *sampling method*, not the forecast.[2] They are often constructed using confidence levels of 5%, 95% etc.
3. **Forecast uncertainty:**
   The possible range of forecast values in the future. In meteorology this range is defined by the uncertainty of the atmospheric development in the future and represented in ensemble forecasts by applying perturbations to initial and boundary conditions and expressing model physics differences.
4. **Forecast interval:**
   Determined uncertainty band representing **forecast uncertainty** and containing the respective probability of the real value being contained in the range of forecasted values, which will only be observed in the future.

Forecast intervals are the most commonly used visualization for forecast uncertainty. They can be derived from:

(a) parametric (e.g. Gaussian distribution)
(b) non-parametric (e.g. empirical distribution functions, kernel density estimation) representations of uncertainty
(c) a larger number of NWP forecasts in an ensemble forecasting system that represent the forecast uncertainty of the target variable

From these probability density functions (PDFs), quantiles or percentiles[3] can be extracted and higher-order statistics such as skewness and

[2] One of the common misunderstandings is that a **confidence interval** is showing the uncertainty of a forecast. This is not the case. By adding and subtracting for example one standard deviation to the deterministic forecast of wind speed and converting it to wind power, such intervals represent a measure of the deviation to climatology and do not represent current or geographically distributed uncertainty.

[3] In statistics and the theory of probability, quantiles are cut points dividing the range of a probability distribution into contiguous intervals with equal probabilities. The 100-quantiles are called percentiles.

kurtosis can be calculated. This is where the distinction is most pronounced: from a statistical error measure like standard deviation, it is not possible to derive quantiles or percentiles. For applications like reserve predictions, ramp constraints or optimization tasks for storage applications, this distinction is imperative. Such applications also require that the geographical distribution of the variables are captured by scenarios of ensembles of possible outcomes of a pre-defined value.

3.10.2 Uncertainty forecasting methods

The estimation of forecast uncertainty for application in the power industry is currently based on three primary methods (Fig. 3.2):

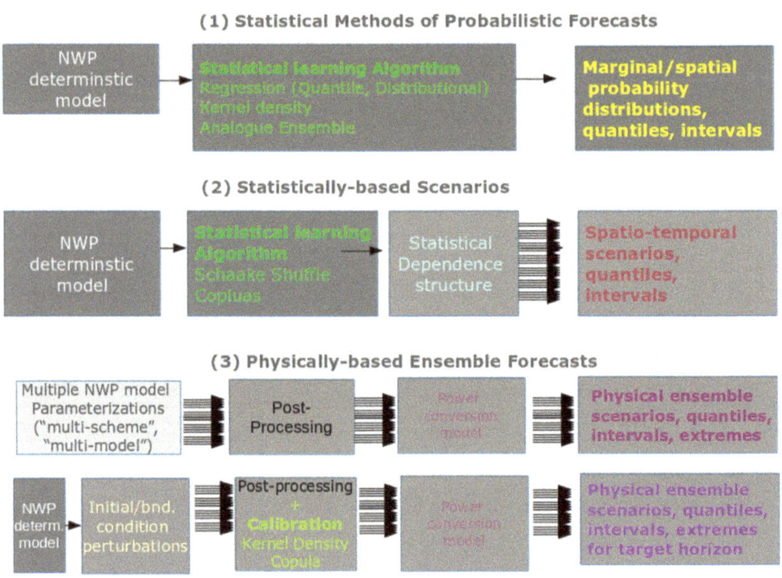

Figure 3.2 Standard methods of uncertainty forecast generation to be used in wind power and PV forecasting. The black arrows indicate whether the so-called "ensemble members" stem from a statistical procedure or are individual scenarios. Image is a reprint with permission from [3].

1. **Statistical methods:**
   This approach is based on statistical processing of past (historic) data in order to derive a probability density function of the possible forecasting spread. The advantage of such methods is that they are computationally extremely cheap and simple to apply. The disadvantage is that none of these methods produce a realistic representation of the forecast uncertainty in a spatial and temporal manner. There is also no physical

dependency on the forward results, as the spread is based on past climatology. Typically, statistical learning algorithms (e.g., neural networks, machine learning) are used to fit historical time series of weather parameters from a NWP model to their corresponding power generation data. From the fitting process, a PDF can be derived and used forward in time. A newer, more intelligent method is the analogue ensemble method (AnEn) that searches through historical forecasts for those past events that are most similar or "analogous" to the current forecast (e.g. [12]). The observations with the best fit form the probability distribution of the forecast uncertainty. So far the method is one-dimensional and hence does not take geographical or temporal aspects of uncertainty into account. To be able to benefit from integration of information from geographically distributed time series or from a grid of NWP the method needs to add a second dimension. Another approach is to use copula theory, which offers a flexible approach to the probabilistic power forecast taking the spatial correlation of the forecast errors into account [13,14].

2. **Spatial-temporal statistical Method:**
In this approach scenarios are produced by a statistical scenario generation method from the probability distributions produced by statistical models based on the copula theory [13,14]. We define them as scenarios, as the further processing of the approach contains x independent results in contrast to the statistical method, producing a PDF function. Such scenarios are quite similar to the third type of methods, the physically-based ensembles. However, the uncertainty representation of the statistical scenarios today only capture the spacial variability of the forecast, like ramps. We therefore distinguish them here as scenarios rather than ensembles. Outliers that indicate extreme events, for example above cut-out wind speeds of wind turbines, can only be detected with probability characterization and require an extreme event analysis. This is due to the conversion to power taking place in the first step of the statistical training in the same way as for deterministic forecasts. Extremes in wind power are in that way difficult to detect, because the flat part of the power curve prevents extremes that would be visible in the wind speeds to show up in the power scenarios. Additionally, events that are not present in the historic data cannot be forecasted.
The clear advantage of the statistically based scenarios is that they are computationally much cheaper than physical ensembles, as they are built from a deterministic weather forecast. They also generate a much

more realistic uncertainty representation than the pure statistical approach, while only being slightly more computationally costly.

3. **Physically based ensemble forecast Method:**
   The third type of methodologies, the "physically based ensembles" can be sub-divided into 2 types:
   a. The **first type of ensemble** is generated by perturbing a deterministic NWP forecast model's initial conditions. Often ensemble prediction systems (EPS) are found to be "under-dispersive", i.e. the uncertainty spread under-estimates the true uncertainty of the target variables (i.e. the ensemble spread is too narrow meaning it is "too confident" relative to the observed outcomes, see also 14.5). This can be attributable to many factors. Some of the more common causes are:
      - the ensemble is not targeted to the variable of interest of the end-user
      - the time or spatial resolution is too coarse to capture the small scale phenomena of the target variable
      - insufficient information is extracted or used in the conversion to wind power to represent a realistic uncertainty. Mostly such deficiencies can be mitigated by calibration methods (see e.g. [1], [15]).
   b. The **second type of ensemble** can be considered a post-processing of a set of NWP ensemble members. The ensemble members are a set of deterministic NWP forecasts produced by perturbing the initial or boundary conditions (i.e. input data for a specific forecast) and/or the formulation of model physics. The perturbations of the model physics can be in the form of alternative sub-models (e.g. for radiative processes or water phase changes associated with clouds and precipitation) within a single NWP model (referred to as a "multi-scheme" approach) or a set of different NWP models (referred to as a "multi-model" approach). The meteorological variable output from each ensemble member is converted in a subsequent phase into power with a curve fitting method (see e.g. [1]).
      The NWP ensemble is configured to represent the physical uncertainty of the weather ahead of time rather than uncertainty as a function of past experience. In practice, this means that the NWP ensembles, especially the multi-scheme approach, can produce outliers, because they are "event driven" and also represent

NWP model uncertainty. This means that they can represent extreme events, even those with return periods of 50 years or more. This is a clear distinction from statistical methods, because even long time-series of historic data contain too few extreme events to have impact in learning algorithms.

3.10.3 Training tools for ensemble forecasting

An example of an ensemble forecasting training tool is the "Ensemble Prediction System (EPS) Training" course created by the Meteorological Service of Canada. This course has three objectives:

(i) introduce participants to ensemble forecasting
(ii) provide basic training on EPS for operational forecasters
(iii) move away from deterministic paradigms towards probabilistic paradigms

The training tool is available for download at: http://collaboration.cmc.ec.gc.ca/cmc/ensemble/Formation-Training/Read-me.html.

Recommendation: when selecting an uncertainty (probabilistic) forecast method for a specific application, it is important to know, whether or not a specific method is suitable for the application or not. There are 3 major branches of uncertainty generating forecasting methods:

1. Statistical methods of probabilistic forecasts
2. Statistically-based ensemble scenarios
3. Physically based ensemble forecasts

We have provided some basic guidance and a graph (Fig. 3.2) summarizing these methods in order to differentiate between the methods, showed the spatial and temporal dependencies of some methods and emphasized that the statistical methods are not suitable for applications that have such dependencies to the uncertainty measure of interest. These are e.g. applications that deal with extremes that may not happen frequently or where the uncertainty estimate is required in each hour of the forecasts rather than over a forecast period of a day or a week.

Additional information on probabilistic methodologies can be found in [1,3].

3.10.4 Applications of uncertainty forecasts in the energy industry

Typical applications in the energy industry, where it is recommended to use uncertainty forecasts, are:

1. **Balancing/trading of wind/solar power:**
   For balancing and trading applications the optimal bid/schedule, from the expected value decision paradigm, is contained in a quantile calculated from the forecasted imbalance costs [16] or a percentile calculated from an ensemble forecasting system [17,18].
   The calibration of uncertainty is a critical requirement for the end-user and has a non-marginal economic impact. Moreover, in electricity markets with high integration levels of wind/solar power, the combination of extreme forecast errors and high imbalance prices is critical and demands for risk modeling techniques and uncertainty forecasts with high accuracy in detecting extreme events (e.g., cut-out wind speed, ramps) [1]. If the portfolio also includes energy storage units, the temporal dependency of forecast uncertainty is a primary requirement [19]. For this use case, the end-user should request ensemble forecasts from physically based methods (see 3.10.2).
2. **Dynamic reserve and ramping reserve requirements:**
   The use of uncertainty forecasts for setting the power system reserve requirements is probably the most well-accepted business case for the energy industry. A critical requirement is minimum deviation from perfect calibration to avoid under- and over-estimation of the risk (i.e., loss of load probability, probability of curtailing renewable energy) [20]. Another criteria in the design of dynamic reserve allocation are the boundaries that need to be defined. The following aspects are crucial boundaries in this respect:
   - **Use the correct type of ensemble data input**
     Physical NWP ensemble: e.g. multi-scheme approach
     Deterministic reserves do not provide uncertainty
     It is the weather uncertainty that generates the errors
   - **Clear definition of the forecast objective**
     Which types of errors are critical
     How to handle outliers
     What type of reserve is the best fit for the end-users objective:
     Typical scenarios are: static, security or dynamic/economic
   - **Definition of the time scales that needs to be forecasted**
     Required ramping capabilities

- **Forecast uncertainty for all weather dependent sources & sinks**
  The uncertainty term should ideally be built upon load+wind+solar
- **Definition of a "noise term" to handle the non-local imbalances**
  Imbalances from interconnections (small system <-> large system)

Allocating reserves dynamically requires probabilistic forecasts, and that the forecast value for the system operator is well-defined. Yet, the following challenges also need to be addressed, when implementing probabilistic forecasts for dynamic reserve requirements and allocation:

(i) communication and visualization of forecast uncertainty and extreme events in TSO dispatch centers

(ii) training of human operators to understand and exploit the probabilistic information, i.e. move from a deterministic/real-time paradigm to probabilistic/predictive operation paradigm.

An example of a dynamic reserve visualization tool is illustrated and described in Appendix C.

3. **Extreme event warnings such as high-speed shut down warnings:**

For risk indices, it is imperative that there is a well-justified and transparent underlying computation of the conditions that may lead to a shut-down event that may impact system security. This should be provided as early in the evolution of the event as feasible.

It is generally accepted that a planned scheduled shut-down at a slightly lower wind speed extends the lifetime of the gearbox system in wind turbines. Therefore, one could argue that there is modest economic loss by executing controlled shutdowns to reduce the ramp-rate in a power system.

The value of such alert systems is realized with early detection of extreme events. This can for example be accomplished by introducing a gradual artificial transition from full generation to no generation at 22.5 m/s. The starting point of such an index will be discussed below. A simple argument for 22.5 m/s is that 2 m/s is the typical forecast accuracy at such high wind speeds.

A "high-speed wind event" can be defined as active, if the hub height wind speed is above 24.5 m/s, while there is no event, if the wind speed is below 22.5 m/s. Table 3.2 shows how such an index may be defined.

The required low level forecast information to raise alerts can be generated in a typical 6-hourly cycle, although it may be coupled with a short-term forecast on a higher frequency dependending on the importance of critical ramps for system security. One of the major challenges for such an alarm system is the strategy of dissemination of the warning information to the user in the control room. If a critical event is discovered about 5 days in advance, the question is how often a warning should be issued in order to avoid too many false alarms or forecast misses. Therefore, threshold values for alert generation should be a function of lead time, time of the day and day of the week.
The more alerts that are generated, the less serious they are taken and the higher the likelihood that a critical event is overlooked. Nevertheless, there are periods where events should create alertness, even though they may not result in a sufficient strong concurrent shutdown.

Table 3.2 Definitions of a high-speed shutdown index for a control area with a high penetration level of wind power and a wind resource with a high variability and wind speeds often exceeding 25 m/s.

wind speed in 100 m	index value
0–22.5 m/s	0.00%
22.5–24.5 m/s	0 – > 100%
24.5 m/s	100.00%

Typical examples could be:

- An alert at a 6-day horizon issued on a Thursday valid for Tuesday morning following a long holiday weekend may be desirable even if the likelihood is low.
- An alert to bring attention to a change of expected ramp rate 6 hours ahead, even though there has already been raised an alert for the event from previous forecasts.

The objective for such an alert should always be to avoid the initiation of costly actions if there is a critical ramp rate in the forecast far enough away that an economic solution can be prepared. As briefly discussed below under *situational awareness*, if a major fraction of the power generation is wind dependent, it would be considered best practice, if the operator is aware of the risk of high-speed shutdown, even if the likelihood is low, but still justifiable. The same applies to the ramp rate caused by a fast moving low pressure system, where the wind speeds at the center of the system may be below the cut-in level. Both event types can simultaneously amplify the ramp down rate and therefore call for a ramp rate based consideration instead of an isolated high-speed shutdown consideration.

4. **Situational awareness:**
   For system operators, but also wind farm operators or traders, information from uncertainty forecasts can be integrated at two levels:
   a. *Visualization and cognition*: provision of alarms and early warnings to human operators about predefined events with impact in the frequency control tasks, e.g. large ramps, wind turbines tripping, large forecast errors. With this information, the human operator can use his/her experience or operating practice to derive a set of control actions (e.g., change current dispatch, activate reserve) that mitigate the effects of renewable energy uncertainty and variability in the system's frequency.
   b. *Technical evaluation of network constraints*: uncertainty forecasts can be integrated in a power flow module, available in commercial energy management systems (EMS), to detect voltage and congestion problems with a certain probability threshold [21]. With this information the human operator can plan preventive actions in advance, e.g. change the market dispatch, or define a cap for market offers in a specific network area/node.

   The end-user should request the following requirements from the forecast provider:
   a. high accuracy in detecting extreme events related to RES uncertainty and variability
   b. capacity to capture temporal and spatial dependency of forecast errors
5. **Flexibility management in smart power grids:**
   The deployment of smart grid technology in form of flexibility management can enable better control and thereby increased generation of distributed energy resources (DER) while maintaining standard quality of supply levels, e.g. by managing storage and demand response. The combination of forecasting systems and optimal power flow tools can be used by transmission and distribution system operators to pre-book flexibility for the next hours in order to handle the technical constraints of their electrical network [22].

   Presently, distribution system operators are starting to explore RES forecasts in the following use cases: (a) forecast grid operating conditions for the next hours; (b) improved scheduling and technical assessment of transformer maintenance plans; (c) contract and activate flexibility from DER to solve technical problems.

In all these cases, a primary requirement is the need to have a spatial-temporal representation of forecast uncertainty, where the temporal component is only relevant, if inter-temporal constraints are required (e.g., operation of storage devices, control of capacitor banks and on load tap changers).

Finally, a current topic of interest is the coordination between the transmission and distribution systems. Different frameworks for information management and exchange are under discussion [23]. It is clear that uncertainty forecasts can be used to provide future information about nodal consumption/injection in the interface between the two networks. For example, the European 7th Framework Project evolvDSO developed the concept of flexibility maps, where RES forecasts are used to quantify the operating point and flexibility range in the TSO-DSO interface [24]. This paves the way to combine information about forecast uncertainty and flexibility, as proposed in [25].

Recommendation: The transition of the energy systems towards a CO_2-free power generation with large-scale integration of renewables on a global basis also requires a restructuring of the power system operation processes. The variable generating units driven by wind and solar resources call for a more dynamic and weather-driven structure for the operating practice.

Probabilistic forecasts can support that dynamic structure and provide the possibility to deal with the uncertainties associated with the non-linear attributes of weather event development as well as extremes that can affect the power system and cause large-scale blackouts. No forecasting solution today should be designed without the uncertainty of weather-driven energy resources in mind. At present, the primary cases of the integration of uncertainty forecasts into the operational processes of energy systems are for the following application types:

1. Balancing/trading of wind/solar power
2. Dynamic reserve and ramping reserve requirements
3. Extreme event warning, e.g. high-speed shut down warnings
4. Situational awareness
5. Flexibility management in smart power grids

The basics of these methodologies have been described in this section. Detailed implementation information about the described probabilistic methodologies can be found in [1,3] and an IEA Wind Task 36 review article "Uncovering wind power forecasting uncertainty sources and their propagation through the whole modeling chain" [4] and on decision making under wind power uncertainty [5,6].

3.10.5 Visualization of forecast uncertainty

Many users have found that the visualization of uncertainty forecasts is a difficult issue. This is especially true for the inexperienced user. While an expert immediately can see the difference between a chart generated with a statistical approach and an ensemble approach as defined in section 3.10.2, a beginner often finds it difficult to differentiate between the results of these two approaches.

The following subsections provide a general overview of alternative approaches for the graphical visualization of uncertainty forecasts.

1. **"Fan Chart"**
   The "fan chart" is a common way of visualizing a set of *forecast intervals* that are aggregated in one plot. Fan chart visualizations as shown in Fig. 3.3 may however provide misleading information to a decision-maker. For example, if the decision-maker interprets each one of the quantiles as a possible evolution of wind power production in time, the user needs to be sure that the visualization tool uses the data that is expected in order to interpret the information correct.
   Differentiation of forecast methods used in the fan chart:
   - **Statistical method**:
     A fan chart generated with a statistical method visualizes the "marginal forecast interval", meaning each interval is only confined to separated forecast lead-times and does not have information about the joint probability distribution across the full set of lead times, or in other words, these intervals are not modeling the inter-temporal dependency structure of forecast uncertainty. These intervals are different for each lead-time. Fig. 3.3 shows an example of a fan chart where the intervals were generated with a statistical model. The lead-time dependence is visible through the relatively equal intervals in size over the entire forecast. In this example, the

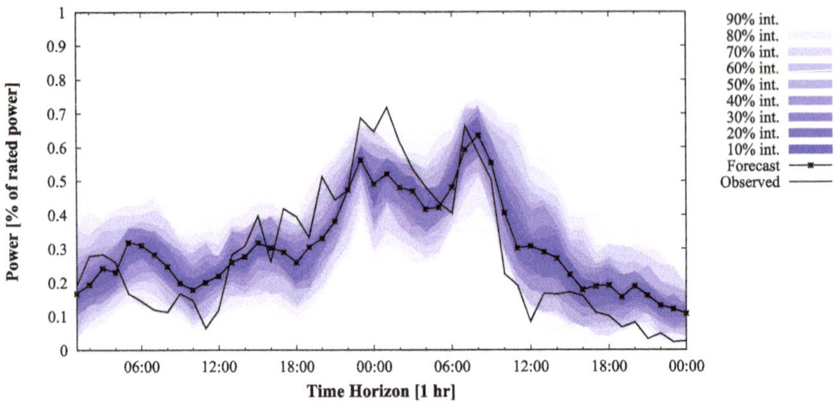

Figure 3.3 Example of a "fan chart" of wind power production at a single wind farm built from marginal forecast intervals of a statistical method.

observations (black solid line) are covered, except for a short period around midnight of the first day.

In that hour there is a probability of around $\alpha = 90\%$ (limited by quantiles 95% and 5%) that the observed value is within approximately $P^L_{t+k} = 0.18$ and $P^H_{t+k} = 0.65$, where H and L are the interval limits at time (t+k).This is the typical interpretation. Looking at the observations, another way to interpret is that there is a 5% likelihood that the observations are within $P^{\tau^L}_{t+k} = 0.63$ and $P^{\tau^H}_{t+k} = 0.65$.

- **Ensemble Method**:

  In Fig. 3.4 we also see forecast intervals for the same wind farm and day. This time, the intervals were based on 300 wind speeds consisting of forecasts from a 75-member multi-scheme NWP-based ensemble prediction system (MSEPS). at 4 different heights. These intervals look very different from the statistically generated intervals. Even though the 90% probability is within approximately $P^L_{t+k} = 0.21$ and $P^H_{t+k} = 0.75$, the 5% probability that the observations is found within the upper quantile has an interval size of 0.25 (range $P^L_{t+k} = 0.50$ and $P^H_{t+k} = 0.75$). That means the interval size is larger by a factor of 10. Compared to the statistical method, this result indicates that the current weather development contains a low probability for a high uncertainty range towards increased production.

  The physics-based multi-scheme approach provides the uncertainty in each time step and quantifies the uncertainty with the knowl-

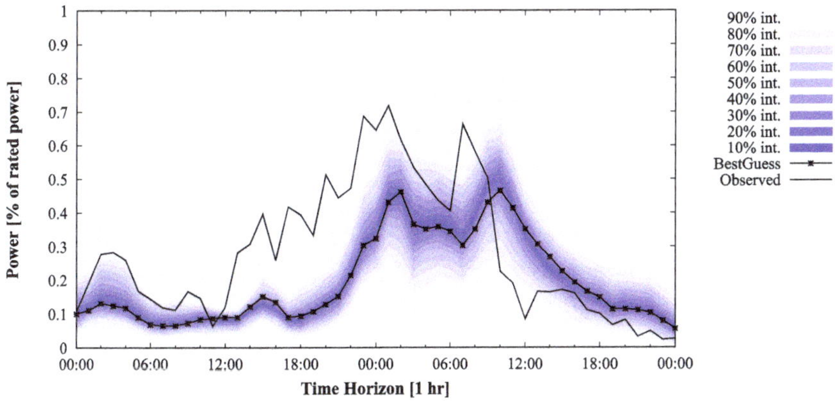

Figure 3.4 Example of a "fan chart" of wind power forecasts at the same time and wind farm as in 3.3, but built by a 75-member multi-scheme NWP ensemble system (MSEPS).

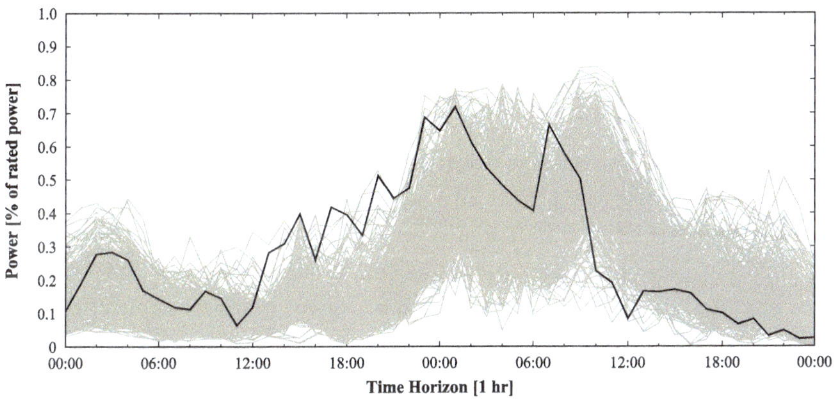

Figure 3.5 Example of a spaghetti plot of 300 wind power forecasts at the same time and wind farm and method as in 3.4.

edge of current meteorological conditions and different physics-based modeling approaches, rather than comparing the situation with past data.

Any application that may be subject to extreme events that may not have happened within the last months or years, should use uncertainty forecasts from this method and make sure that this information is evident in the visualization of the forecasts.

2. **"Spaghetti Plot"**

Fig. 3.5 shows the same wind farm, forecast days and method as in Fig. 3.4, but as individual forecasts in a so-called spaghetti-plot where

each of the 300 wind power forecasts are one line. In this way, it becomes apparent, how individual ensemble forecast "members" can generate outliers.
In comparison to the lead-time dependent approach, the physical approach forms a large outer quantile band and a more condensed inner part, indicating that many of the 75 forecasts are aligned in their atmospheric development, while there are a small number of forecasts that result in higher power generation. The difference here is that the intervals are a result of the NWP ensembles reproducing the physical uncertainty of the current atmospheric processes that generate the power and are fully independent of the lead-time. Here, a large spread can be generated based on a very low likelihood or probability, also if such events have not been observed before (see also section 14.3.3.2 and Fig. 14.5).
An operator or trader has a number of ways to interpret such a forecast. Two likely scenarios could be:

a. ignoring the outer interval and acting upon the highest probability ranges

b. verifying the system upon issues or the market price that could arise, if the low probability of high generation becomes reality

Whether the operator or trader acts upon such a forecast depends on their business practices. Nevertheless, it shows that the information contained in the forecast intervals has a direct practical application.

Take-away from the Visualization of Uncertainty:
The different results illustrate that the successful interpretation of such information depends on an understanding of the algorithm used to generate the uncertainty estimates. The major difference here is that one method is based on current atmospheric conditions (NWP ensemble) and the other relies on an historical dataset of the atmospheric conditions. With the historical method, the intervals of extremes are usually smaller and less pronounced unless there are long time series available that contain a significant number of such extremes to impact the spread in given weather conditions, which is seldom the case.

CHAPTER FOUR

Data communication

Key points

This section provides recommendations for forecast data-related terminology, data description and data formats and exchange protocols.

- The terminology section 4.1 provides definitions for terms commonly used in the description and exchange of data between forecast providers and users.
- The description section 4.2 provides a specification of the mandatory and optional types of data required to train and operate a forecasting system.
- The exchange section 4.3 provides recommended standards for data formats and exchange protocols. The standards are presented for two levels of users:
  - Level 1: basic data format and data exchange for groups with limited IT knowledge and/or experience.
  - Level 2: detailed description of more sophisticated formats and exchange protocols that enable groups with more extensive IT knowledge, experience and resources to achieve higher level of data exchange robustness and efficiency.

Currently, there isn't a best practice or standard for (1) definitions of the various inputs that are used to configure and operate a renewable energy forecasting system, (2) data formats and (3) data exchange protocols. Forecast suppliers and consumers use different terminology and can end up spending many hours on unnecessary communication. This is a problem which ultimately comes at a cost to the forecast supplier, energy forecast purchaser and the operating budget of renewable energy projects. Similarly, there is no standard or recommended best practice for the format of the data used by the forecasting systems and the methods for delivering this data. This also creates additional delays and inefficiencies in the forecast setup process.

Two user groups are targeted in this recommendation. These are referred to as Level 1 and Level 2 users in this document:

Level 1 users: this group typically has limited IT resources or experience. Input documents are geared towards manual input of forecast specifications.

Level 2 users: this user group has a deeper IT knowledge or experience than Level 1 users. Input file format examples and exchange methods presented here may be programmatically adopted for real-time use.

IEA Wind Recommended Practice for the Implementation of Renewable Energy Forecasting Solutions
https://doi.org/10.1016/B978-0-44-318681-3.00014-3

Once adherence to the data exchange standard is attained, the benefits are numerous and tangible. For the supplier of renewable energy forecasts this is:

1. More efficient on-boarding: for Level 1 consumers (i.e., with less experience using forecasts or less IT expertise) standard templates are followed; for more advanced, Level 2 users, the on-boarding process can be mostly automated.
2. Back-and-forth communication time is minimized: Online references to standard documentation reduce communication blockages between forecast supplier and consumer.
3. Greater automation of adding/removing renewable power plants to forecast engine: Adhering to a standard reduces (doesn't eliminate) the need for customized software development.

For the renewable energy forecast consumer, some benefits of adhering to the data exchange interface include:

- A much more efficient process to benchmark different forecast providers
- Easier to add, remove, or switch forecast providers
- Quicker turnaround time in adding or removing forecast projects to an asset portfolio
- No need to develop new processes for different weather-impacted renewable technologies.

This recommended practice can be applied to many types of renewable generation entities. The focus of this specification is forecasting of individual renewable projects. An aggregate or area-level forecast is not specifically addressed in this document, as these configurations are less common. However, aggregations and area forecasts may be treated like a single project or be specifically coded by a unique ID (e.g., "Wind Region 01"). Data field definitions are also provided with the objective of promoting a standard definition for these fields. However, we recognize that there are many factors that make data definition standards more challenging and beyond the scope of this recommendation. For example:

- Industry-specific standards: several industries are involved in the renewable energy industry and each of them have their own data definitions for similar fields. This includes OEMs (original turbine manufacturers), independent engineers (consultants), SCADA software companies, renewable plant developers, utilities, and TSOs or ISOs.
- Geographic location: terminology and translation from one language to another.

Different standardization bodies governing different industries also can present challenges, but for renewable energy forecasting, the International Electrotechnical Commission (IEC) is the generally accepted organization that establishes, promotes, and updates data definition standards.

4.1. Terminology

For clarification, several terms are defined below that appear repeatedly in this section.

Renewable Energy Forecast Customer/Consumer: an institution or corporation that requires a forecast of power from a renewable energy generation facility with a look-ahead time of minutes to days.

Renewable Energy Forecast Provider: an entity that delivers renewable energy forecasts with a look-ahead time of minutes to days. In most cases, the provider is a company whose business includes selling forecasts to customers/consumers.

Renewable Energy Forecast Benchmark: an exercise conducted to determine the features and quality of a renewable energy forecast, such as wind or solar power. The exercise is normally conducted by an institution or their agent and multiple participants, including private industry forecast providers or applied research academics.

Renewable Energy Forecast Trial: an exercise conducted to test the features and quality of a renewable energy forecast, such as wind or solar power. This may include one or more participants and is normally conducted by a private company for commercial purposes. A trial is a subset of a Renewable Energy Forecast Benchmark.

Online measurements: These are observations used for tuning a renewable energy forecast system and adjusting intra-day renewable energy forecasts. Measurements are usually power or energy, since that is the target variable of interest to the consumer. However, other weather variables might be included with online measurements. Online measurements are also referred to as real-time measurements and are transferred between forecast customer and provider on a regular basis.

Offline measurements: These are observations used for tuning a renewable energy forecast system. As opposed to online, offline observations are historical and don't directly impact short term (< 12 hours) forecast horizons. Measurements are usually power or energy since that is the target variable of interest to the consumer. Other weather variables might be used for energy forecast training, monitoring and extreme event identification, especially for a newly operational renewable energy plant.

4.2. Data description

The standard interface is defined on two levels. Ideally, renewable energy forecast customers and renewable energy forecast providers should comply with both level 1 and level 2 of the standard interface, but only complying with level 1 can also provide significant efficiency gains during the setup of a forecasting system.

The two levels are:

Level 1: A high-level description of the information and data required to carry out a successful trial and operation of a specific forecast solution. This level of standardization provides a common terminology that will enable the renewable forecast customer to prepare and organize data facilitating an efficient system configuration process.

Level 2: A detailed specification of both the format and method, which should be used to exchange data between the renewable forecasting provider and the renewable energy forecasting customer. This level of standardization enables an efficient, repeatable and scalable configuration process applicable to trials as well as operational forecast systems. Compliance with level 2 facilitates renewable energy forecast customers to efficiently carry out trials/benchmarks as well as enabling renewable energy forecast providers to participate in trials/benchmarks efficiently and at low costs.

Online/real-time measurements are suited for both intraday and day-ahead forecasting, whereas offline measurements are best for day-ahead forecasting only.

Mandatory and optional data

The metadata tables and definitions below specify some data to be mandatory in order to setup a meaningful forecasting system. Other data is considered optional as those data may improve forecast accuracy, take into account a future operating state of the renewable energy plant, or might be less common requirements of the forecast consumer. All renewable energy forecast consumers should be able to provide the mandatory data and all forecast providers should be able to process mandatory data, whereas optional data depends on specifics to each forecast installation.

Table 4.1 List of the different types of input and output data needed in a forecast setup.

Data	Type of data	Description of the type of data
Master Data	Site information	A specification/description of the Gen. type. A description can contain one or more Gen. type. An entity can be an aggregate of multiple gneration plants. All entities in the same description must have similar data structure as specified in the associated meta data descriptions. If the data structures are not similar, then the entities need to be split up into multiple "entities" and multiple meta data descriptions.
Online Data	Measurements	Observational data from an entity which will be used as input for training models and real-time input data for forecast production in minutes or hours-ahead forecasts. .
	Future Availability	The data about expected future availability of the entities due to maintenance, curtailment or other planned schedules. Used as input to the forecast.
	Forecasts	The output data (results) produced by the forecast system.

4.2.1 LEVEL 1 – data description

Table 4.1 provides an overview of the different data types required by a forecasting system. This data needs to be available to the forecast provider for both training and operating a forecasting system. Table 4.2 provides an overview of the different types of metadata, which describes the attributes of the data types listed in Table 4.1. Tables 4.3 to Table 4.7 contain the data fields and definitions that a forecast solution will require to configure an operational forecast.

It is important to note that "Measurements" data should be made available both as historical data (also referred to as Offline Data) for training of models and as operational or real-time data (also referred to as Online Data) for operational forecasting. If available, the forecast customer should provide a minimum of 3 months of historical "Measurements", but ideally 1–2 years of historical data to capture both seasonal and inter-annual variability.

Metadata, also referred to as Master Data, has a broad definition but generally refers to information that describes the forecast configuration or the data itself. In most cases, it should not change often. The different types of metadata needed for renewable energy forecasts include information about the entities, the measurements, and the forecast configuration. This is detailed in Table 4.2.

The metadata about the renewable energy entity (or power plant) itself is often the first information a forecast supplier will need to initially set up a forecast installation and is, therefore, essential to be accurate and from the forecast consumer. Table 4.3 details the renewable energy entity metadata.

Measurement data for the forecast entity are provided prior to the configuration of the forecast system in order to calibrate the forecast model and thus reduce forecast error. If the renewable energy entity has been in operation for some time, such power observations would typically be available. For new renewable energy entities, where no generation data is yet available, a history of meteorological measurements, e.g. wind speed or irradiance, may be provided to the forecast supplier to help reduce forecast errors until a suitable history of power observations of the forecast target variable is obtained.

Table 4.4 details the specific fields that describe the measurement data required for renewable energy forecast model training. This table should be filled out more than once if the historical measurement data differs in any way from the online (real-time) data being sent to the forecast provider.

Differences may arise due to the type of observation (e.g., SCADA power versus settlement power observations, wind speed from a met tower versus nacelle anemometer average wind speed, etc.).

Most forecast suppliers have the ability to incorporate scheduled changes to the renewable plants' availability in the forecasted output. This comes in the form of reduced capacity due to a reduction in available units (e.g., turbines or inverters) or a generation limit of the power plant (e.g., curtailment or transmission limit).

The important distinction between an "outage" and "limitation" is that an outage is a proportional reduction in the plant's capacity for all wind or solar irradiation conditions. A "limitation" is a maximum capped output (e.g., set point) of the plant based on the available capacity. This information needs to be described as it will routinely be sent from the forecast consumer to the forecast supplier. Table 4.5 details this information.

The forecast "deliverable" is a point time series generated by the forecast software system. This product has characteristics that will vary depending on the consumer's needs. Table 4.6 contains a description of the forecast file metadata. The forecast "deliverable" is the product of many configuration parameters within a forecast software system. Not all forecast software systems have similar built-in features, but Table 4.7 highlight some of the salient details that are important to a forecast system specification regardless of software system implementation details.

Table 4.2 List of different types of meta data needed in a forecast setup.

Type of meta data	Description of the meta data
Entity's characteristics	A description of the renewable energy power plant characteristics. Most of the characteristics don't change often with time.
Measurement specification	A description of the attributes of the observational data sent to the forecasting system. Measurement meta data may be separated into realtime (online) and historical (offline) measurements because these can often be described differently or represent different parameters.
Forecast time series specification	A description of the forecast system product which is the time series output.
Scheduled Availability specification	A description of the forecasted or scheduled availability for the entity.
Forecast system specification	A description of the necessary inputs and outputs that tells the forecasting system how to model the target forecast variable(s). This includes forecast system and output attributes such as units, variables, timing, and temporal resolution.

Table 4.3 Specification of the data required for describing a renewable energy entity. **Entities:** The entity's description can contain data about one or more renewable energy plant(s). An entity can be comprised of an aggregate of plants or, in the case of wind, an aggregate of individual turbines. For each entity the following data needs to be supplied.

Data field	Description	Requirement	Gen. type	Data type
Entity ID	Unique ID (name) used for identifying the entities	Mandatory	Wind,PV	String
Generation Type	Either "Wind" or "Solar"	Mandatory	Wind,PV	String

continued on next page

Table 4.3 *(continued)*

Data field	Description	Requirement	Gen. type	Data type
Latitude	Latitude coordinate of the entity in decimal degrees.	Mandatory	Wind,PV	Float
Longitude	Latitude coordinate of the entity in decimal degrees.	Mandatory	Wind,PV	Float
Capacity	Capacity or rated power of the entity (kW)	Mandatory	Wind,PV	Float
Maximum (Export) Capacity	Maximum export real-power (MW) that may be transferred to the grid	Optional	Wind,PV	Float
Hub height	The average height of the wind turbine hubs (meters)	Mandatory	Wind	Float
Number of turbines	Number of turbines that comprise the entity	Mandatory	Wind	Integer
Wind turbine make and model	Turbine manufacturer and model name	Mandatory	Wind	String
Turbine power curve[a]	Default power curve table of wind speeds and corresponding power capacity factor. Normalized by rated capacity in the range [0, 1]	Optional	Wind	Float
Solar Technology	Description of the PV technology. Fixed-tilt, single axis or dual axis are most common.	Mandatory	PV	String

[a] Turbine power curve table is often appended or delivered separately.

continued on next page

Table 4.3 *(continued)*

Data field	Description	Requirement	Gen. type	Data type
Minimum panel orientation angle	The minimum orientation angle of the PV panels in degrees from north (0 to 359, where east is 90° and west is 270°). If the system is single axis tracking or fixed tilt, then minimum and maximum orientation should be the same.	Mandatory	PV	Integer
Maximum panel orientation angle	The maximum orientation angle of the PV panels in degrees from north (see above).	Mandatory	PV	Integer
Minimum panel inclination angle	The minimum angle of the PV panels in degrees from horizontal (−90°–+90°). If the system is fixed tilt, then minimum and maximum inclination should be the same.	Mandatory	PV	Integer
Maximum panel inclination angle	The maximum angle of the PV panels in degrees from horizontal (see above).	Mandatory	PV	Integer
Panel tested capacity	The total solar panel capacity for the entity (kW) based on standard test conditions (1000W/m^2) at panel temperature of 25°C	Optional	PV	Float
Panel temperature sensitivity	The temperature sensitivity of the PV panels (%/°C)	Optional	PV	Float
Inverter capacity	The capacity (kW) of the inverters	Optional	PV	Float
Inverter efficiency	The inverter efficiency at 95% load	Optional	PV	Float

Table 4.4 Specification of the data required for describing the forecast system input measurements. **Measurements**: The Measurements should be delivered for each entity and contain the information described below. All values must be available with the same granularity, e.g. every 5 minutes and with a fixed update frequency.

Data field	Description	Requirement	Gen. type	Data type
	Time series fields			
Entity ID	Unique ID (name) used for identifying the entities	Mandatory	Wind,PV	String
StartTime	Date and time stamp indicating the start of the observed measurement period.	Mandatory	Wind,PV	String
EndTime	Date and time stamp indicating the end of the observed measurement period.	Mandatory	Wind,PV	String
Power	The power production (kW) when the measurement was observed	Mandatory	Wind,PV	Float
Available capacity	The observed available capacity (kW) of the entity. If parts of the entity are not available (due to maintenance, break downs, etc.), this value is reduced.	Optional	Wind,PV	Float
Limitation level	The limitation (kW) of the entity due to curtailment, set point level, do not exceed limitations or down regulation. This includes non-scheduled changes by grid operator.	Optional	Wind,PV	Float

continued on next page

Table 4.4 (*continued*)

Data field	Description	Requirement	Gen. type	Data type
Wind speed	Wind speed (m/s) from a representative instrument (e.g. anemometer at turbine nacelles or a meteorological tower, LIDAR, SODAR).	Optional	Wind,PV	Float
Wind direction	Wind direction measured in degrees from north (0-359°). East = 90°, South= 180°, West = 270°, North = 0°.	Optional	Wind	Float
Temperature	Air temperature (degrees Celsius)	Optional	Wind,PV	Float
Pressure	Atmospheric air pressure (hectopascals, hPa)	Optional	Wind,PV	Float
Relative Humidity	Relative humidity of the air (%)	Optional	Wind,PV	Float
Precipita-tion	The amount of rain or snow that has fallen on the ground (millimeters, mm)	Optional	Wind,PV	Float
Global Horizontal Irradiance	The total short-wave radiation from the sky falling onto a horizontal surface (W/m^2)	Optional	PV	Float
Global tilted irradiance	The total short-wave radiation from the sky falling onto a tilted surface (W/m^2)	Optional	PV	Float
Direct solar irradiance	The short-wave radiation that has not experienced scattering in the atmosphere (W/m^2). The radiation comes from the disc of the sun.	Optional	PV	Float

continued on next page

Table 4.4 (*continued*)

Data field	Description	Requirement	Gen. type	Data type
Diffuse irradiance	The short-wave radiation from light scattered by the atmosphere excluding from the disc of the sun (W/m^2)	Optional	PV	Float
	Meta data			
Time zone	The time zone of the timestamp in IANA[a] Time Zone (TZ) database format" (e.g, Europe/Barcelona)	Mandatory	Wind,PV	String
Time interval label	Describes what time the measurement point represents. Can be instantaneous, period beginning average (leading), or period ending average (trailing)	Mandatory	Wind,PV	String
Power measurement type	A text description of the power measurement field. It can be, for example: substation meter, SCADA power, active power, potential power, settlement power.	Optional	Wind,PV	String
Wind speed measurement type	Specify if the wind measurement for the entity is from turbine nacelle, average of nacelle, met mast or other.	Optional	Wind,PV	String
Wind speed measurement height	The height of the wind speed measurement in meters.	Optional	Wind,PV	Float

[a] Internet Assigned Numbers Authority.

Table 4.5 Specification of the data required for describing the future availability and curtailments. **Scheduled Availability**: The future availability and curtailments for each entity, should contain the information described below.

Data field	Description	Requirement	Gen. type	Data type
Entity ID	Unique ID (name) used for identifying the entities	Mandatory	Wind,PV	String
StartTime	Date and time stamp indicating the start of the expected unavailability period.	Mandatory	Wind,PV	String
EndTime	Date and time stamp indicating the end of the expected unavailability period.	Mandatory	Wind,PV	String
Daylight Savings Time flag	Flag to indicate whether daylight savings time applies (True or False)	Mandatory	Wind,PV	String
Outage level	The expected available capacity (kW) of the entity. If wind turbines, solar panels or inverters are not available (due to maintenance, break downs or similar) the "Capacity" of the entity is temporarily reduced to available power capacity.	Optional	Wind,PV	Float
Limitation level	The expected available capacity (kW) of the entity due to a limiting factor such as curtailment, setpoint instruction from grid operator or temporary limit on the maximum allowable production.	Optional	Wind,PV	Float

continued on next page

Table 4.5 (*continued*)

Data field	Description	Requirement	Gen. type	Data type
Reason of unavailability	Editable text that gives a reason for the reduction in available capacity (e.g., Maintenance, plant limitation). Often entered by plant manager or remote operations center.	Optional	Wind,PV	String

Table 4.6 Forecast time series specification metadata. **Forecast Time Series**: The attributes of the output forecast time series are described below.

Data field	Description	Requirement	Gen. type	Data type
Plant name ID	Unique ID (name) used for identifying the entities	Mandatory	Wind,PV	String
StartTime	Date and time indicating the beginning of the forecast interval	Mandatory	Wind,PV	String
EndTime	Date and time indicating the ending of the forecast interval	Mandatory	Wind,PV	String
Daylight Savings Time flag	Flag to indicate whether daylight savings time applies (True or False)	Mandatory	Wind,PV	String
Power	The power production forecast (kW) for the period	Mandatory	Wind,PV	Float
Power quantiles	Probabilistic power production forecast corresponding to a specific quantile level	Optional	Wind,PV	Float
Wind speed	Wind speed forecast (m/s)	Optional	Wind,PV	Float
Wind direction	Wind direction forecast in degrees from north (0-359°). East = 90°, South= 180°, West = 270°, North = 0°.	Optional	Wind	Float

continued on next page

Table 4.6 (*continued*)

Data field	Description	Requirement	Gen. type	Data type
Temperature	Air temperature forecast (degrees Celsius)	Optional	Wind,PV	Float
Pressure	Atmospheric air pressure forecast (hectopascals, hPa)	Optional	Wind,PV	Float
Relative Humidity	Relative humidity of the air forecast (%)	Optional	Wind,PV	Float
Precipita-tion	Forecast of the amount of rain or snow that has fallen on the ground (millimeters, mm)	Optional	Wind,PV	Float
Global Horizontal Irradiance	The forecast total short-wave radiation from the sky falling onto a horizontal surface (W/m^2)	Optional	PV	Float
Global tilted irradiance	The forecast total short-wave radiation received on a surface with defined tilt and azimuth, fixed or sun-tracking. This is the sum of the scattered radiation, direct and reflected in (W/m^2)	Optional	PV	Float
Direct solar irradiance	The forecast short-wave radiation part that directly reaches a surface in (W/m^2).	Optional	PV	Float
Diffuse irradiance	The forecast short-wave radiation reaching the Earth's surface after having been scattered from the direct solar beam by molecules or particulates in the atmosphere in (W/m^2)	Optional	PV	Float
Event Forecast	Forecast value of the custom-defined power forecast event (e.g., ramp rate probability, %)	Optional	Wind,PV	Float

Table 4.7 Specification of the data required for describing the Forecast System configuration. **System specification**: This specification describes general aspects (meta data) of the forecast system.

Data field	Description	Requirement	Gen. type	Data type
Entity ID	Unique ID (name) used for identifying the entities	Mandatory	Wind,PV	String
Power unit	Unit of power quantities (MW, KWh)	Mandatory	Wind,PV	String
Time zone	The time zone of the timestamp in IANA[a] Time Zone database format" (e.g, Europe/Barcelona)	Mandatory	Wind,PV	String
Daylight Savings Time flag	Flag to indicate whether daylight savings time applies to forecast file (True or False)	Mandatory	Wind,PV	String
Time stamp format	Format of the date and time stamp (e.g., yyyy-MM-ddTHH:mm:ss).	Mandatory	Wind,PV	String
Forecast interval label	Describes the time the forecast point represents. Can be instantaneous, period beginning average (leading), or period ending average (trailing)	Mandatory	Wind,PV	String
Issue time of day	The time of day that a forecast is issued specified in HH:MM format, e.g. 00:30. For forecast runs issued multiple times within one day (e.g. hourly), this specifies the first issue time of day.	Mandatory	Wind,PV	String
Forecast update frequency	Defines how often the forecast time series is updated (in minutes)	Mandatory	Wind,PV	Integer

[a] Internet Assigned Numbers Authority.

continued on next page

Table 4.7 *(continued)*

Data field	Description	Requirement	Gen. type	Data type
Forecast interval length	The length of time (in minutes) each forecast point represents	Mandatory	Wind,PV	Integer
Measure-ment delay	The expected time delay from when a value is measured until it is available to the forecasting system in minutes	Mandatory	Wind,PV	Integer
Forecast maximum horizon	Horizon (or maximum look-ahead) of the forecast in hours	Mandatory	Wind,PV	Integer
Forecast quantiles /percentiles	Quantile/percentile of the forecast distribution given to the nearest integer. Specify a single or list of quantiles (e.g., P10, P25, P50, P75, P90, P99)	Optional	Wind,PV	String
Forecast weather variable units	Units corresponding to weather forecast variables	Optional	Wind,PV	String
Event forecast	Name and description of custom forecast variable	Optional	Wind,PV	String
Event forecast units	Units of custom forecast event	Wind,PV	String	

4.3. Data format and exchange

4.3.1 LEVEL 1 data format and exchange

Two main considerations in recommending a suitable data format for Level 1 users of forecasts is ease of use for the forecast client and, for the forecast provider, the ability to programmatically read the necessary metadata and measurement data files.

The Comma Separate Value (CSV) format satisfies these conditions and is also an acceptable format for Level 2 users. While Level 2 users can utilize high-level programming languages to generate and process CSV files, Level

1 users can still interact with CSV format through Microsoft Excel or other ASCII-text editors. Another advantage of CSV for Level 1 users is that they can shift to become a Level 2 user, if such IT resources are available or can be procured. It can be done incrementally by keeping the same CSV format or shifting to JSON or XML as described below.

For Level 1 users with limited IT experience or resources, it is recommended that data transfer between forecast consumer and forecast provider be done via *SSH File Transfer Protocol (SFTP)* which is a secure and reliable standard of sharing data. Forecast providers typically will host an SFTP server and issue a unique login credential to the forecast consumer. The forecast consumer can choose among several SFTP applications common in both the Windows and Linux operating system environments. The SFTP application should have the functionality to create batch job configurations such that online measurements can be automatically uploaded between forecast consumer and provider.

Command line SFTP works out-of-the-box with Linux operating system installations. Software applications such as Filezilla that support SFTP can also be installed on a server running Linux. Many file transfer applications built for Windows operating system have SFTP functionality. This includes Filezilla and WinSCP. Most commercial cloud storage systems (e.g., OneDrive, GoogleDrive, Dropbox, AWS) now include SFTP. As API's become more user-friendly and accessible for users without computer programming experience, this recommendation might have to be revised as REST API (along with SFTP) are the Level 2 recommended data exchange methods between forecast provider and consumer.

4.3.2 LEVEL 2 – data format and exchange

Level 2 data exchange is for both providers and consumers of renewable energy forecasts that wish to programmatically exchange data. Thus, the most widely used and extensible tools and formats were selected to allow for more seamless integration. The following three data formats are the most commonly used in the exchange of renewable energy forecasting data and the measurements that feed into forecasting systems:

1. CSV (Comma Separated Value)
2. JSON (JavaScript Object Notation)
3. XML (eXtensible Markup Language)

Each format comes with its own advantages and weaknesses, but all are in ASCII, human-readable form. Examples using representative data are useful for illustrating how metadata, measurement, and forecast data are organized

and may be copied as a template. CSV-format files can be used for both Level 1 and Level 2 users as it has the distinct advantage of being opened and converted in the widely-used Microsoft Excel application. However, for Level 2 users that want to automate processes or configure many forecasts, JSON and XML are much more efficient formats.
Both JSON and XML formats are accompanied by a schema whose main purpose is to enforce consistency and data validity. They also serve as human readable documentation for the forecast system metadata, measurements, and forecast files.

Two widely used modes of data exchange are recommended for Level 2 users. They are:

- SSH File Transfer Protocol (SFTP) [1]
- Web Services based on:
  - Simple Object Access Protocol (SOAP).
    This is a protocol that follows a strict standard to allow communication between the client and the server. It is used to transfer the data. The SOAP protocol was developed so that different programming languages could communicate quickly and with minimal effort. SOAP has SSL(Secure Socket Layer) and WS-security. SOAP uses only XML for exchanging information in its message format.
  - REpresentational State Transfer (REST) Application Programming Interface (API).
    REST is an architectural style that does not follow any strict standard but follows six constraints – Uniform Interface, Client-Server, Stateless, Cacheable, Layered System, Code on Demand. REST has SSL and HTTPS security levels. REST is not restricted to XML and the implementer has the choice of which Media-Type to use (e.g. XML, JSON, Plain-text).

One of the main advantages of programmatically generating metadata and time series measurement and forecast files is the wide number of applications that can be used to exchange this data from forecast provider to forecast consumer and vice-versa. Many commonly used programming languages such as Python, Javascript, R, and Ruby have packages and libraries that make parsing and interacting with JSON and XML formats easier. Additionally, and often overlooked, is that internal applications can rely on

[1] Note, SFTP builds on secure shell protocol (SSH) and adds on file transfer capabilities and should not be mistaken with FTPS, which builds on the file transfer protocol (FTP) and adds on a security and encryption layer.

the same data exchange methods further standardizing code that has to be developed and maintained.

In recommending a data exchange standard, there are several important issues that should be considered:

- International support and usage
- Upfront, transitional and integration resource costs (financial, human)
- Extensibility
- IT Security
- Ease of use

International support and usage can not be overstated. If a method of data exchange becomes obsolete or doesn't have a very large user base, it will not adapt to evolving communication and security standards. Additionally, the number of people familiar with the exchange method is smaller thus putting operational support of automated processes more at risk in case of a disruption in data flows.

The **upfront, transitional and integration costs** all have to do with how much an organization must invest to build, transition, or support the methods of data transfer. If the exchange method is open source and works across operating systems, this is a huge benefit to the organization. If the data exchange methods can be integrated into existing software (e.g., using a simple URL to make requests), this lowers the integration and development costs. Transitional costs associated with adopting the standard or best practice will be a key consideration on whether an organization chooses to incorporate a new data exchange method. These touches upon all the important considerations listed above.

Extensibility is a key issue in choosing an exchange method as society goes through an energy transition away from fossil fuels and towards an energy system with greater electrification, distributed generation and load, and faster internet. Will what works today for sending data back and forth be around in 10 years? This is why we recommend not one data exchange method, but two, since its difficult to predict how computers, electronic devices and communications will change over time. RESTful APIs are quickly becoming the international standard in data communications as it is not constrained to one format (like SOAP is with XML) and doesn't have to be http-based although that is the primary protocol in use today with RESTful APIs.

IT security is crucial in the energy industry as malicious malware usage and cyber attack incidents have grown in number and scale every year. Both SFTP and RESTful API supports secure standard protocols for data

sharing. Secure shell in the case of SFTP and HTTPS using TLS encryption as one example in RESTful APIs. Although these protocols don't eliminate security risks entirely, they reduce the risks of cyber attacks.
Both SFTP and RESTful APIs are supported by most software applications and are **easy to use** since they can be invoked from the most commonly used scripting languages. Ease of use may be the primary factor in deciding whether to adopt a new method to transfer data for the purpose of renewable energy forecasting.

A forecast provider can develop a web application to accept any of the recommended formats. There are many tools and applications which then allow the forecast consumer to verify or view the metadata, measurements and forecasts in a web browser. A good example of this can be seen in the US Department of Energy Solar Forecast Arbiter (SFA) project [26].

This project developed an open-source RESTful API that uses JSON formatted messages. Forecast site metadata, measurements, and forecast time series are exchanged through POST and GET commands. Once the data is uploaded via the API, a dashboard has been built that allows the forecast provider and consumer to visualize, download, and create verification reports.

4.4. Sample formatted template files and schemas

The following sample formatted template files and accompanying schema files have been developed in CSV, JSON, and XML format for download and are accessible via the open access companion page of this book (https://www.elsevier.com/books-and-journals/book-companion/9780443186813):

- *availability_specification_wind.schema*
- *measurement_specification_wind.schema*
- *meta_data_wind*
- *forecast_specification_wind.schema*
- *measurements_wind*
- *forecast_wind*
- *meta_data_specification_wind.schema*

CHAPTER FIVE

Concluding remarks

While every forecasting solution contains customized processes and practices, there are a number of attributes and components that all forecasting solutions have in common. For any industry, it is important to establish standards and standardize practices in order to streamline processes, but also ensure security of supply with a healthy competition structure.

This document provides an overview of state-of-the-art practices that have been carefully collected by experts in the area and reviewed by professionals and experts in an appropriate number of countries with significant experience in renewable energy forecasting. The recommendations are to encourage both end-users and forecast service providers to bring focus to areas of practice that are common to all solutions. The document will be updated as the industry moves towards new technologies and processes.

The key element of this recommended practice is to provide basic elements of decision support and thereby encourage end-users to analyze their own situation and use this analysis to design and request a forecasting solution that fits their own purpose, rather than applying a "doing what everybody else is doing" strategy.

This document is also intended to serve forecast service providers new to the market or those wanting to evolve to a new level of service and support as a guideline to state-of-the-art practices that should be incorporated into business processes.

IEA Wind Recommended Practice for the Implementation of Renewable Energy Forecasting Solutions
https://doi.org/10.1016/B978-0-44-318681-3.00015-5

PART TWO

Designing and executing forecasting benchmarks and trials

Editors (1) and Authors (2):
Dr. Corinna Möhrlen, WEPROG, DK, DE[1,2]
Dr. John W. Zack, MESO Inc., USA[1,2]
Dr. Gregor Giebel, Technical University of Denmark, DK[1]

Contributing Authors:
Dr. Craig Collier, Energy Forecasting Solutions, USA
Dr. Aidan Tuohy, EPRI, USA
Dr. Jakob W. Messner, MeteoServe Wetterdienst, AT
Dr. Jeffrey Lerner, ENFOR, DK
Dr. Jethro Browell, University of Glasgow, UK
Dr. Justin Sharp, Sharply Focused, USA
Mikkel Westenholz, ENFOR, DK

CHAPTER SIX

Designing and executing benchmarks and trials

6.1. Before you start reading

This is the **second part** of the IEA Wind recommended practice for the implementation of renewable energy forecasting solutions.

This **second part**, *Design and execution of benchmarks and trials*, addresses the design, execution and analysis of customized forecasting benchmarks and trials. The **first part**, *Forecast solution selection process*, is focused on the design of a customized process to select an optimal forecast solution for a user's specific situation and application. The **third part**, *Forecast solution evaluation* presents methods and guidelines for the meaningful evaluation of alternative forecasts, operational and non-operational forecasts and entire forecast solutions. The **fourth part**, *Meteorological and power data requirements for real-time forecasting applications* provides guidance for the selection, deployment and maintenance of meteorological sensors, power measurements and associated data quality control relevant to real-time forecasting.

If your main interest is (1) selecting a forecasting solution, (3) verifying the quality of forecast solutions, or (4) setting up meteorological sensors or power measurements for real-time wind or solar power forecasting, please move on to part 1, part 3 or part 4 of this recommended practice guideline to obtain recommendations on these specific issues, respectively.

It is recommended to use the table of contents actively to find the topics that are most relevant for you.

6.2. Background and introduction

The effectiveness of forecasts in reducing the variability management costs of power generation from wind and solar plants is dependent upon both the accuracy of the forecasts and the ability to effectively use the forecast information in the user's decision-making process. Therefore, there is considerable motivation for stakeholders to try to obtain the most effective forecast information as input to their respective decision tools.

IEA Wind Recommended Practice for the Implementation of Renewable Energy Forecasting Solutions
https://doi.org/10.1016/B978-0-44-318681-3.00017-9

This document is intended to provide guidance to stakeholders on a primary mechanism that has been used extensively in the past to assess the accuracy of potential forecasting solutions: benchmarks and trials.

This guideline focuses on the key elements to carry out a successful trial or benchmark and on typical pitfalls. It will also provide recommendations as to when it is beneficial or too risky or expensive in terms of resources to carry out a trial or benchmark.

6.3. Definitions

The two main terms and concepts "trial and benchmark" that are used in this recommended practice shall be defined in the following. Note, the focus has been on forecasting processes in the power industry and the definition may not have a completely general character to be applied to other areas of business. Additionally, it should be noted that "forecasting trials and benchmarks" will be abbreviated with "t/b" throughout this document for simplicity.

6.3.1 Renewable energy forecast benchmark

A "renewable energy forecast benchmark" is defined as an exercise conducted to determine the features and quality of a renewable energy forecast such as wind or solar power. The exercise is normally conducted by an institution or their agent and multiple participants, including private industry forecast providers or applied research academics.

6.3.2 Renewable energy forecast trial

A "renewable energy forecast trial" is defined as an exercise conducted to test the features and quality of a renewable energy forecast, such as wind or solar power. This may include one or more participants and is normally conducted by a private company for commercial purposes. A trial is a subset of a renewable energy forecast benchmark.

6.4. Objectives

The guidelines and best practices recommendations are based on years of industry experience and intended to achieve maximum benefit and efficiency for all parties involved in such benchmark or trial exercises. The entity conducting a trial or benchmark taking the recommendations provided in this guideline into consideration will have the following benefits:

1. Effective assessment of which of a set of alternative forecast solutions and forecast service providers (FSP) best fits a user's need, specific situation and operational setup
2. Short-term internal cost savings, by running an efficient t/b
3. Long term cost savings of forecast services, by following the trial standards and thereby help reduce the costs for all involved parties.

The discussion of the process of obtaining the best possible forecasting solution, uses a number of terms and concepts. Several of the key terms and concepts are defined in the following subsections.

It should be noted that these definitions are kept as general as possible with respect to forecasting processes in the power industry and may not be sufficiently generalized for application in other areas of business.

CHAPTER SEVEN

Initial considerations

Key points

This section is targeted to the decision and following task of engaging a forecast service provider (FSP) and how to navigate through the vast amount of information. Before a decision is made, it is recommended to go through the benefits (Table 7.1) and drawbacks (Table 7.2) for specific portfolios and applications and their associated limitations and determine, if the effort is warranted. A "cheat sheet" checklist is provided at then end of the chapter (section 7.5) for those that decided for a benchmark or trial.

7.1. Deciding whether to conduct a trial or benchmark

The most important initial consideration when planning a forecasting trial or benchmark (t/b) is the formulation of a clear specification of the desired outcome.

The following tables provide information about the benefits and drawbacks of conducting a t/b as a key part of the selection process. Before a decision is made to conduct a t/b, it is recommended to consider the information in these tables to determine if the effort is warranted.

A possibly attractive alternative approach for a forecast user that wishes to evaluate a set of forecast solutions for their ability to meet the user's needs is to engage an independent trial administrator. An experienced and knowledgeable administrator can act as a neutral third party and advocate for both the vendors and the end-users in the design and execution of a t/b and the evaluation and interpretation of the results. Such an arrangement builds trust in the process among all parties.

An effective administrator can take the requirements from the user and ensure they are realistically incorporated into the trial design. There obviously is a cost to engage such an administrator, but this approach may be more cost-effective for the user and generate more reliable information for the user's decision-making process.

7.2. Benefits of trials and benchmarks

Table 7.1 shows typical situations in which a trial or benchmark is likely to be beneficial for the end-user.

IEA Wind Recommended Practice for the Implementation of Renewable Energy Forecasting Solutions
https://doi.org/10.1016/B978-0-44-318681-3.00018-0

Table 7.1 Decision support table for situations in which trials/benchmarks are likely to be beneficial for the selection of a forecast solution.

Situation	Benefit
Real-time trial for an entire portfolio	High cost, but information gain is great and representative; provides the best estimate of the error level and which solution/FSP is best for the target application
Real-time trial for a selected number of sites	Lower cost, but still a substantial information gain, if sites are well selected; provides a reasonable estimate of the error level and a good indication of which solution/FSP fits best for the target applications
Blind forecast without historic measurements	Test to get an indication of the accuracy of forecasts from an FSP in the startup phase of a project, where no historical data are available. Excludes statistical methods, which need historical data. An inexpensive way to get an indication of forecast accuracy for larger portfolios (> 500MW), where measurement data handling is complex. NOTE: There is an inherent risk that the result may be unrepresentative beacuse FSPs may use different methods for blind forecasting than they do for forecasting with measurement data. See also Table 7.2 for limitations of this approach
Retrospective benchmark with historic data for a specific time period and different from a supplied training data set	Low cost: In multi-FSP systems, the error level of an additional FSP is secondary, while the correlation with other FSPs determines, whether the additional FSP improves the overall error of a multi-FSP composite forecast

7.3. Limitations with trials and benchmarks

Table 7.2 shows typical situations in which a t/b is likely to deliver limited or no benefits for the end-user.

Table 7.2 Decision support table for situations in which a t/b is likely to provide limited value to the end-user and therefore a t/b is not recommended.

Situation	**Limitation**	**Recommendation**
Finding the best service provider for large portfolio (> 1000MW) distributed over a large area	Trial for entire portfolio is expensive for client and FSP in terms of time and resources.	Limiting scope of trial limits representativeness of results for entire portfolio. RFI and RFP in which FSP's methods are evaluated and the use of an incentive scheme in the contract terms provides more security of performance than a limited trial.
Finding best service provider for a medium sized portfolio (500MW< X < 1000MW) over a limited area	Trial for entire portfolio is expensive for client and service provider in terms of time and resources.	Limiting scope of trial limits representativeness of results for entire portfolio. RFP in which FSP's methods are evaluated. Design of a system that enables an easy change of FSP and use of an incentive scheme is more a more cost effective approach than a trial.
Finding best service provider for a small sized portfolio (< 500MW)	Trial for entire portfolio usually requires significant staff resources for about 6 months.	Trial is feasible, but expensive. Difficult to achieve significance on target variable in comparison to required costs and expenses – trial costs makes solution more expensive. Less expensive to setup an incentive scheme and a system in which the FSPs can be changed relatively easily.
Finding best service provider for micro portfolio (< 100MW) or single plants	Cost of a trial with many parties can easily be higher than the cost of a 1-year forecasting contract.	Time for a trial can delay operational forecast utilization by up to 1 year! Select FSP based on an evaluation of methods and experience.
Design a system that enables an easy change of FSP and use an incentive scheme for FSP performance	Power marketing	Best score difficult to define, as sale of energy is also dependent on market conditions and a statistical forecast performance score such as RMSE or MAE does not reflect the best marketing strategy More efficient and timely to perform back test of historical forecasts combined with historical prices, or make a strategic choice with an performance incentive.

continued on next page

Table 7.2 *(continued)*

Situation	Limitation	Recommendation
Market share of FSP in a specific power market is high	FSP monopolies in a specific power market mean that forecast errors are correlated and hence increase balancing costs.	Ask about the market share of a provider and do not choose one with a share > 30% as the only provider!
Blind forecasting, i.e. no historic measurement data available	Without measurements the value of a trial is very limited due to the significant improvement from statistically training forecasts and the importance of real-time data for intra-day forecasts	Evaluation can only be meaningfully done for day-ahead or longer forecasts. It is only suitable to get an indication of the accuracy of a forecast method or overall area average error levels. See also Table 7.1 forecast.
Test of methods for forecasting with and without historic training data	Results are limited to testing general quality on e.g. upstart phase of new projects, where no historical data exist. Works only for physical methods or transfer learning methods. Other statistical methods need historical data. See also Table 7.1.	For single sites, the benefits of training are so large (>50% of error reduction at times) that the result cannot be compared. For larger portfolios it can provide an indication of quality – works only for physical conversion methods and transfer learning functions (e.g. [27])!

7.4. Time lines and forecast periods in a trial or benchmark

Time lines and forecast periods need to be set strictly in a trial or benchmark in order to achieve a fair, transparent and representative exercise.

The following time lines should be considered:

1. Start and stop dates of the t/b must be fixed
2. Start and stop dates must be the same for all FSPs
3. Pre-trial setup and test dates for IT infrastructure (including any required security protocols) for trial must be specified and enforced
4. Delivery times of forecasts must be set and enforced
5. Forecasts for periods with missing forecasts from one FSP must be excluded for all FSPs.

7.5. 1-Page "cheat sheet" checklist

Fig. 7.1 shows a checklist to help trial organizers save time, apply best practices, and avoid common pitfalls when designing and executing forecast trials. It has been compiled by leading forecast vendors and researchers with many years of experience.

Forecast Trial Checklist

--Preparation--

- ☐ Determine outcomes / objectives
- ☐ Consult expert with experience
- ☐ Establish timeline and winning criteria
- ☐ Decide on live or retrospective trial
- ☐ If live trial with datafeed, begin datafeed setup
- ☐ Gather metadata (use IEA checklist spreadsheet)
- ☐ Determine if adequately resourced to carry out
- ☐ Obtain historical data
- ☐ Invite forecast service providers
- ☐ Distribute historical and meta-data
- ☐ Finalize datafeed configuration (if applicable)
- ☐ Allow two weeks Q&A prior to start
- ☐ Begin

--During Trial--

- ☐ Develop validation report
- ☐ Check interim results
- ☐ Provide interim results (if no live data being provided)
- ☐ End

--Post Trial--

- ☐ Provide final results
- ☐ Notify winner(s)
- ☐ Contract with winner(s)
- ☐ Start Service

Figure 7.1 "Cheat sheet" checklist.

CHAPTER EIGHT

Conducting a benchmark or trial

Key points

Deterministic trials have become an established way to test different forecast vendors or test the compatibility and benefits of combining various forecast methods in the forecast solution selection process. Such trials are complicated and the required resources to conduct a fair, transparent and representative trial are often underestimated. In order to generate meaningful results for foreacst solution selection, such trials need to follow a specific structure, which is characterized by three phases:

- Phase 1: Preparation (section 8.1)
- Phase 2: During Trial (section 8.2)
- Phase 3: Post Trial (section 8.3)

These three primary phases of a trial are described in detail in this chapter.

8.1. Phase 1: preparation

The time required for the pre-trial preparation is significant and should not be underestimated to ensure a successful outcome. If the operator of the trial has no experience in renewable energy forecasting or running a t/b, it is recommended that an experienced individual, organization or forecast provider be contacted to obtain feedback on what can reasonably be accomplished given the target time line and objectives. Part 1 of this recommended practice contains a decision support path that may be useful for determining the proper course of action.

8.1.1 Key considerations in the preparation phase

Once the objectives of the t/b are known (see Section 6.2 and 6.4), there are some key decisions to be made that will play a major role in determining the complexity of the trial. They are:

1. **Choice of forecast horizon:**
   Are forecast horizons less than 6 hours operationally important? If the answer is "no", establishing a live data feed may not be necessary. Although there are advantages of running a trial with a live data feed, it is one of the most time consuming aspects of trial and its preparation.

IEA Wind Recommended Practice for the Implementation of Renewable Energy Forecasting Solutions
https://doi.org/10.1016/B978-0-44-318681-3.00019-2

Are forecast lead times greater than "day-ahead" operationally important? If the answer is "no", this will reduce the volumes of data that need to be processed, saving time and resources.

If many lead times are of operational importance, consider that the performance of different providers will likely vary across lead times, and different lead times, e.g. hour-ahead, day-ahead and week-ahead, should be evaluated separately, which often results in significant variations in relative FSP performance by lead-time.

2. **Weather conditions for the exercise:**

   Will the benchmark take place during periods of more difficult to predict weather conditions that reflect the organization's difficulties in handling renewable generation, e.g. windy or cloudy periods? The answer here should be "yes" to insure the sample size of harder-to-forecast events is sufficient. If the answer is "no", the trial operator should strongly consider doing a retrospective forecast (also known as "back-cast") that includes the types of conditions that are critical for the user's application.

3. **Historical data/observations for the exercise:**

   For locations in which there are significant seasonal differences in weather conditions and the associated renewable generation levels and variability, it is best to provide 12 months or more of historical data from the target generation facilities to the FSPs for the purpose of training their forecast models. However, if it is not feasible to make this amount of data available or if the target location does not exhibit much seasonal variation, most FSPs can typically train their forecast models reasonably well with 3–6 months of on-site historical observations.

   It should be noted that advanced machine learning methods often exhibit significantly greater performance improvement over less sophisticated methods as the training sample size increases. Thus, FSPs that employ the latest and most advanced machine learning prediction tools may not be able to demonstrate the ultimate value of their approaches, if only short historical data sets are provided. If 6–12 months of data are not available, the trial operator might consider another location or conduct a longer trial on the order of 4–6 months to monitor forecast improvements over time as more data becomes available to the FSPs to improve the quality of the training of their prediction models.

   In general it is recommended that the t/b operator should provide a data set of the typical length that is available for the target application of the t/b. If more historical data is available for a t/b than in the typical real-world application, care should be taken in the evaluation of methods, as e.g. machine learning methods might outperform e.g. physical methods in the trial, but perform worse in the real-world application and vice versa due to the benefits and drawbacks associated with the length of available data sets.

4. **Representativeness:**
   Is the benchmark location representative from a climatology perspective of the scope of locations for which the operator will ultimately require operational renewable forecast services? That is, the trial operator should select a location that is needed for subsequent real-world forecasting or a location with a similar climatology.
   Operators should also be aware of the randomness of forecast performance on single locations, if a large area with many sites is the target.
   It should also be noted, that if different vendors provide forecasts for only one single site, that forecast performance has a certain random quality over shorter periods of weeks or months due to the non-linear behavior of weather conditions and associated variable performance of NWP and power conversion models (see e.g. [28] and the Reference Material accompanying this book[1] for an example demonstrating this challenge). Additionally, forecast performance exhibits a significant "aggregation effect". That is, the magnitude and patterns of forecast errors vary substantially depending on the size and composition of the forecast target entity. Thus, the characteristics of forecast errors for an individual turbine, a single wind park and a portfolio of wind parks will typically be quite different, and the forecast evaluator should be very careful when inferring forecast performance characteristics from one scale of aggregation (e.g. a single wind park) to a different scale (e.g. a geographically diverse portfolio of wind parks over a large area) (see also part 3 of this recommended practice for more details on evaluation methods).
5. **Metrics:**
   Are the metrics that will be used to evaluate the forecasts representative of the sensitivity of the user's application to forecast error? There are a wide variety of well-documented error metrics that penalize forecast errors differently. For example, root mean squared error penalizes large errors more than small errors and considers phase, but not amplitude! It is important to choose a set of metrics, that reflects the value

[1] Reference material is available at the companion website accompanying this book (https://www.elsevier.com/books-and-journals/book-companion/9780443186813).

of an improved forecast to the user's application and can discriminate between different forecast solutions. Please refer to part 3, chapter 14 and Appendix F for details on metric selection.

8.1.2 Metadata gathering in the preparation phase

Details of the forecast trial, such as location and capacity of the target generator, are required by all FSPs and comprise the trial's "metadata". Appendix A "Metadata Checklist" provides the information that is typically needed by FSPs for participation in a trial and is designed to be used as a spreadsheet form that is completed during the preparation phase of a typical t/b. This should also include the desired format (filename and content) of the forecasts to be compared. The best way to communicate the forecast file format to multiple FSPs is to provide an example file. Additional information on data and IT communication can be found in part 1, chapter 4.

8.1.3 Historical data gathering in the preparation phase

On-site observations of power production and the renewable resource (e.g., irradiance or wind speed at hub height) are critical for helping the FSPs statistically "train" their forecast models and thus reduce error and bias in the forecasts. Good quality data is critical. "Good quality" means that the data does not, for example, contain many gaps or unrepresentative values. Curtailed power data should be accompanied by plant availability or a curtailment flag.

Time intervals of the data should be regular and there should be a clear documentation of the units, how the observations were averaged, the time zone of the data, and whether there's a shift in time due to daylight savings time. Appendix D of this document has a concise list of the necessary historical data attributes required to efficiently start a t/b.

8.1.4 IT/data considerations in the preparation phase

Most organizations have constraints on the amount of IT resources available for a t/b. Therefore, it is best to plan ahead or keep the sending and receiving of data very simple. The primary IT issue is typically the selection and setup of data formats and communication protocols that will be used for the t/b operator to send data to the FSPs and for the FSPs to send forecasts to a platform designated by the t/b operator. Additional information on data and IT communication can be found in part 1, chapter 4.

Data formats:

There are many possibilities for data formats, which range from a simple text file with comma separated value (CSV) to more sophisticated XML or openAPI formats. See Appendix E for example formats in csv and xml.

Similarly, there are a wide range of communication protocols that can be used. These range from the relatively simple SSH File Transfer Protocol (SFTP) to the more standard web service (HTTPS) and sophisticated API structures. The more sophisticated structures have advantages and there are many IT companies and resources that use and support these structures today, but they almost unavoidably increase the complexity of the setup. (See part 1, chapter 4 and section 4.3 for recommendations and Appendix E for a sample forecasting file structure).

Unless adequate IT resources or knowledge are available for all participants (especially the operator) it is recommended that simple data formats and communication resources be employed for a t/b. This typically means the use of the CSV data format and an SFTP or HTTPS data communications protocol.

Live trial considerations:

If a live trial is planned (most common), but real-time data will not be made available to the FSPs, then a place for each FSP to send forecast files will need to be setup. One of the metrics that is often used to evaluate an FSP is the timeliness of forecast delivery. In this case, it is important that a mechanism to verify the time of delivery be established and updating of forecasts after the delivery time be denied. If real-time data is provided by the t/b conductor, it is typically easiest to create a common password-protected file server directory from which FSPs can download the data via a protocol such as SFTP. Another approach is to use SFTP to push data files to each FSP. This typically requires more effort, especially for the t/b operator.

Historical data can be provided to FSPs in the same data format via the same communication protocol. However, it often requires a SCADA engineer or expert on third party software to extract the historical data from the SCADA (or other) data archive.

Legal Agreements:

Another often-overlooked data-related issue is the legal agreements required to disseminate data from possibly multiple data provider entities (e.g. the wind facility owners/operators) to multiple data user entities (e.g. the FSPs in the t/b). This may be relatively simple in cases in which the user (such as a generator fleet operator) owns all the data and is willing to make it available for the t/b with few restrictions. However, it is a very complex and time consuming process in cases in which the user (e.g. a system operator) does not own the data and merely serves as a conduit from the multiple data owners with different data dissemination restrictions to the data users.

In such cases, the process of formulating and executing the required legal documents (such as non-disclosure agreements (NDAs)) can cause substantial delays in the initiation of a t/b and perhaps even change its scope.

8.1.5 Communication in the preparation phase

Transparency:
Anonymizing the FSPs for all communication is considered a best practice as it ensures transparency of the available information, promotes competition and entry from smaller FSPs trying to become more established in the industry. Communication via email therefore should always be consistent with blind copies to all FSPs.
Consistency:
Consistent in this context means always sending and sharing emails with the same group of FSP users. Common information sharing engenders and the perception of fairness in the t/b process. In the preparation phase, it is not uncommon that the FSPs will have questions that could affect how the trial is conducted.

For this reason, it is recommended to have a 2-week question and answer period before the official start date to allow FSP participants to ask questions that then can be answered in a living document that contains all questions and answers up to the present time. All participants should be notified whenever this document is updated.
Frequency:
The importance of frequent and clear communication cannot be overstated when conducting a t/b. Not only will the t/b operator receive the most accurate forecasts, it will make it much easier the next time a t/b is executed to engage the state-of-the-art in forecasting technologies and features.

8.1.6 Test run in the preparation phase

It is recommended to allocate a minimum of one-week for a test period before the official start date of the t/b to identify and remove any technical issues that could invalidate forecast results. This helps to improve the likelihood that all results can be included in the final validation calculations without the need for omitting the first part of the t/b.

8.2. Phase 2: During benchmark/trial

Verification & Validation Report preparation:
Often the forecast provider that is most valuable fora user's application is one that can show steady improvement over time. Providing an interim validation report will not only prepare the trial operator for the final validation report but will give important feedback to the FSPs – not only throughout the t/b, but also in daily operations.
Validation Strategy:
Part 3, chapter 11 of this recommended practice provides information about validation and verification that incentivices the FSP to make improvements, where they are most beneficial to fulfill the end-users requirements.
Verification strategy:
Draxl et al. [29], emphasizes that verification of validation code is an essential part of a validation. In the case of a t/b, it is recommended that the verification strategy and the input data for the validation is shared with the FSP. In that way, the verification code is tested as recommended by Draxl et al. [29] and there is transparency on the results. If the FSPs result differs from the end-user's result, the errors can be detected and solved. Appendix G lists a number of code examples that can be used to initiate a structured verification setup.

8.2.1 Communication during the b/t

In a well-designed t/b, most of the communication between the trial operator and FSPs should be during the pre-trial period. However, issues often arise, especially during a live trial with a real-time data feed. It may be helpful to all t/b participants to establish an open forum during the first part of the live t/b period (e.g. the first 2 weeks) to provide a way to effectively and uniformly resolve all issues early in the t/b period However, it is strongly recommended that if any attributes of the t/b are changed at any point during the live part of the t/b, the changes should be communicated to all participants immediately as they might require action on the FSP's part.

Examples include changing the forecast validation metric, specification of periods of unreported outages that should be omitted for future model trainings, and changes in the location of the data feed or forecast file destination. It should be emphasized that all communications related to the t/b should be distributed to all FSPs without exception. Additional communication with individual FSPs (including forecast incumbents) can be interpreted as bias on the part of the operator of the t/b and in some cases may actually bias the t/b result due to information that impacts forecast design, production or delivery not being equally available to all FSPs.

8.2.2 Forecast validation and reporting during the b/t

Forecast validation reports are often compiled during the t/b. With forecast data coming in at regular intervals, the t/b operator has real data to feed into the validation report. If the t/b has a duration of several months (i.e., > 3 months), it is recommended that the t/b operator provide at least one interim report to FSPs that includes anonymized results for all FSPs.

This benefits the t/b operator as errors in the evaluation process or the report generation can be flagged earlier and ways to make the report generation more efficient can be realized. The interim report benefits the FSPs as course-corrections can be made during the t/b to improve the forecasts. If there are several FSPs participating, efficiencies can be realized by automating part or most of the validation metrics calculation, especially as the forecast file format should be the same from all FSPs.

8.3. Phase 3: Post trial or benchmark

The post trial phase is an important aspect of the t/b, because FSP selection will likely occur during this phase based on the criteria set out at the start of the t/b (see part 1, section 3.8 and part 3, section 15.3).

8.3.1 Communication at the end of the b/t

If the t/b operator hasn't already done so, an email should be sent within a week before the end date of the t/b to alert FSPs that the end of the t/b is near and to communicate the timeline for sharing results and re-iterate the specifications of the FSP selection process.

8.3.2 Forecast validation & reporting after the b/t

If an interim report was provided during the t/b, then the final report can either be an updated version of the interim report expressing the bulk metrics or an appended month-by-month forecast validation results. For transparency and to promote further forecast improvements, it is recommended that the t/b operator shares the anonymized forecast results from each FSP at the time-interval frequency that forecasts were being made at (e.g., hourly). This will help FSPs discover where forecasts are similar or different from the competition, which may spawn improved methodologies. Detailed information on the validation can be found in part 3.

CHAPTER NINE

Considerations for probabilistic benchmarks and trials

Key points

Testing, verification and validation of probabilistic forecast solutions need to be handled fundamentally different from deterministic solutions.
The latter can be aggregated, combined and compared and has in the past been mostly used to foster improvements on "typical error" statistical metrics.
Probabilistic forecasts theoretically can be used as deterministic forecasts as well, for example a mean, a percentile or quantile forecast with a specific target. In that case, the deterministic evaluation can be applied as described in sections 8.1, 8.2 and 8.3.
When dealing with uncertainties in the forecast process chain, probabilistic forecasts have value beyond a deterministic forecast and hence, the evaluation is different (see section 9.1). Such forecasts serve a different purpose and can be compared, and also – aggregated or combined - but not in a straight forward or easy way!
Instead, it is recommended to apply "Event evaluation" (see section 9.2) and develop "Cost-Loss Functions" that measure the sensitivity of a user's application to the forecast error, e.g. whether the observations are within the forecasted uncertainty spread or uncertainty measures such as quantiles or percentiles (see section 15.1.4.1).
In t/b with probabilistic solutions, the verification should be done by method (see examples in Table 15.3) and – in most cases – with event based verification metrics (see section 9.2).

Probabilistic forecast solutions distinctly different attributes than deterministic forecast solutions. Therefore, their evaluation also needs specific requirements and attention.

The three phases (Preparation – During Benchmark/Trial – Post Benchmark/Trial) described in chapter 8 contain considerations that are equally valid for probabilistic forecast solutions and are recommended to be studied thoroughly before starting a t/b process. The following sections provide specific additional recommendations for each of the three t/b phases for a t/b that intends to evaluate probabilistic forecast solutions.

9.1. Preparation phase challenges for probabilistic b/t

In the preparation phase of a b/t it is crucial to understand that a number of processes that are often applied in a deterministic b/t are not possible or not recommended for probabilistic forecasts.

https://doi.org/10.1016/B978-0-44-318681-3.00020-9

The most common processes performed by the conductor of a b/t are averaging forecasts and/or aggregating locations to test which combination of forecasts (if any) may be better than the best performing single forecast.

This is neither a good idea with probabilistic forecasts nor recommended. In some cases it can even lead to wrong results (e.g. aggregating quantiles over locations) – as it undermines to some extent the fundamental purpose of probabilistic forecasts, which is to provide a realistic estimate of the variations in the uncertainty of the forecast. Also, mean forecasts smooth out outliers instead of providing a warning or pinpointing a bad forecast.

In contrast to deterministic forecasting, the evaluation scores of probabilistic forecasts typically do not benefit from aggregation or averaging. In fact, in most cases, it is scientifically not correct to do so. For example, if percentiles are built at multiple locations, aggregating the percentiles and averaging them would lead to a wrong result. In this case, one can only use the raw data of each ensemble member at each location and calculate the percentiles of the aggregated values.

Also, if quantiles have been built from ensemble forecasts from one provider and generated with a statistical approach from another provider, adding quantiles and averaging them would lead to physically wrong results, because the principles underlying the quantile computations and therefore the uncertainty interpretations are fundamentally different. Statistical approaches for example lack the temporal component and the spacial-temporal methods lack the ability to identify extremes. In that context, probabilistic forecasts are most useful as a tool to deal with weather and forecast uncertainties chosen from a method that fits the target application. More details on the different approaches and their attributes are presented in section 3.10 and in Bessa et al. [30].

To summarize, evaluating the usefulness and applicability of a probabilistic forecast to provide specific information about the risk of occurrence of a certain event, cannot be handled in the same way as deterministic forecasts. Hence, the t/b also needs to follow probabilistic verification rules and methods. More information on structuring verification and finding the best t/b target can be found in part 3, chapter 14.3 and in Appendix F and F.1.

9.2. Evaluation challenges for probabilistic b/t

Many evaluation metrics are useful scientific instruments for the development of forecasts, but often are not useful to define the value of a forecast for the end-user. Therefore, it is recommended that the user follow a "forecast value concept, in which ... forecasts only have value, if a user takes action as a result of a forecast, and that action saves the user money", that was introduced by Mylne [31]. The concept also considers the ability of the end-user to be able to discriminate uncertainty and spread from forecast scenarios and ensembles, e.g. should I be more or less confident in today's forecast than yesterday's in my decision-making?

In this context, it is important to know how forecasts will be applied in order to find appropriate scoring rules. There is a lot of literature describing statistical metrics and recommendations provided in Part 3, chapter 14.3.

The following list provides recommendations and examples of appropriate metrics for typical applications in the context of a t/b that is intended to evaluate one or multiple forecast suppliers. As described in the key considerations in section 8.1.1 and Part 3 of this recommended practice, it is usually a good idea to develop a framework of several types of metrics and then construct a composite overall evaluation score by weighting the individual metrics according to the perception or quantitative knowledge about the relevance of each one to the user's application.

The most common and useful scores for probabilistic forecasts used in typical renewable energy applications are explained in detail in part 3 in section 14.3. A brief summary of the most useful metrics to a wide range of end-users is:

- **Brier Scores** is the "MAE of probabilistic forecasts" and evaluates categorical forecasts of binary events (see [32–34]).
- **The Continuous Ranked Probability Score (CRPS) and Energy Score** can be interpreted as the integral of the Brier score over an infinite number of predictand classes of infinitesimal width and with possible threshold values for the parameter under consideration. For a deterministic forecast system, the CRPS reduces to the mean absolute error (see [35–38]).
- **Relative Operating Characteristics (ROC)** measures the skill of a forecast in predicting an event in terms of hit rates and false alarm rates (see [39–41]).
- **Rank-, Talagrand or PIT[1] histograms** measure the extent to which the spread covers the forecast uncertainty and can reveal BIAS in the probabilistic forecast. A rank histogram does not evaluate resolution – also associated with *sharpness* and *calibration* –, and must be used in

[1] Probability integral transform.

conjunction with other forecast tools such as the ROC, Brier scores, or ranked probability scores to generate a more complete picture of the quality of a probabilistic forecast [42–44].

- **Reliability (Calibration) Diagram** illustrates the amount of agreement between the predicted probabilities of an event and their observed frequencies. This provides insight into how well calibrated a probabilistic forecast is. It is a good complementary metric to the Brier scores (see section 4.3.1 in Part 3 or [32]) and the Relative Operating Characteristics (ROC) curve (see section 14.3.4, Fig. 14.6 or [39,41]).
- **Categorical event analysis** in form of e.g. contingency tables or critical success index (CSI) shows how well a forecast performs for the prediction of a targeted event and provides insight into what type of errors are being made. With the four categories of hits, misses, false alarm, and correct negatives, it is possible for an end-user to easily associate costs and benefits to a forecast outcome and thereby evaluate its value.

Table 15.3 in Part 3, section 15.1.4.1 shows the most common application examples and corresponding recommended evaluation metrics. Details about how to compute or construct the recommended metrics and diagrams can also be found in section 14.3, section 15.1 and metrics and example code for evaluation, verification and validation can be found in Appendix F and G, respectively.

CHAPTER TEN

Best practice recommendations for benchmarks/trials

Although there are many different ways that a t/b may be conducted, there are some common elements of a successful t/b that provide the t/b operator with the best forecast solution and the participants with useful knowledge of where their forecast ranks among the competition. This chapter provides a summary of the best practices for the design and execution of a t/b and also a list of common pitfalls to avoid.

10.1. Best practice for b/t

1. A clear purpose for the t/b exercise
2. Pre-defined, explicit accuracy metrics & solution selection criteria[1]
3. A well-defined time line (start/end dates, selection announcement, contract award)
4. Anonymized forecast results. Ask FSP's approval to share results. This helps FSPs find ways to improve their forecast accuracy and see their shortcomings
5. Question & answer period before t/b period begins (1–2 weeks)
6. Sufficient time allocated for testing the transfer of data between participant(s) and operator
7. Prompt communication to all participants regarding any t/b design or protocol changes and/or answers to questions raised by one or more FSP participants
8. Consistent forecast file format requested of all – provide example file to all (e.g. Appendix E)
9. Consistent data formats (both observations and forecast files) ideally as close to (if not identical to) what the t/b operator needs, once contract is executed (see Chapter 4)
10. Provide the same historical and project metadata to all participants (see also 4.2)

[1] See guideline for forecast evaluation and code examples in Part 3 and reference material of this book's companion website https://www.elsevier.com/books-and-journals/book-companion/9780443186813.

IEA Wind Recommended Practice for the Implementation of Renewable Energy Forecasting Solutions
https://doi.org/10.1016/B978-0-44-318681-3.00021-0

11. Allocation of sufficient resources by the t/b conductor to furnish data and perform validation.

10.2. Pitfalls to avoid

This section provides a list of mistakes that are commonly made in the design, setup and execution of a t/b and recommendations on how to avoid them. The consequences of errors and omissions in a t/b are often underestimated. However, if results are not representative, the resources that have been employed in a t/b can effectively be wasted. Some of these common pitfalls can be expensive to the t/b operator because they result in placing the operator in a position of making a decision without having truly objective and representative information to base it on.

1. Poor Communication:
   All FSPs should receive the same information. Answers to questions should be shared with all FSPs. Fairness, and perception of fairness, are important when running and evaluating the results of a t/b.
2. Unreliable Validation Results:
   Don't compare forecasts from two different power plants or from different time periods. Forecast performance will vary depending on location and specific time periods. Only forecasts for the same period and location/power plant/portfolio should be compared.
3. Examples of Bad Design:
   a. A trial with 1 month length during a low-wind month
   b. No on-site observations shared with FSPs
   c. Hour-ahead forecasts based on once a day data update
   d. Data only processed in batches or at the end of a real-time t/b – this is an invitation for cheating to the FSPs. In most cases, there will be some that use the opportunity to do so.
4. Examples of Missing or Non-communicated Data
   a. daylight savings time changes are not specified
   b. no specification of whether the data time stamp represents interval beginning or ending
   c. plant capacity of historical data differs from present capacity
   d. data about curtailment and maintenance outages not provided.
5. Possibility of Cheating:
   In any type of competition, cheating is a reality. If precautions are not taken, results may be biased and decisions may be based upon incorrect

results. It is recommended that the possibility of cheating be seriously considered and the t/b be designed to minimize this possibility.

Typical situations, where cheating has been observed are:

a. Historic period: A t/b conducted for a period of time for which (some) FSPs have been given data or have data from previous activities. Recommendation: separate historical data from t/b period and ensure all have the same data available or run forward in time.

b. Uneven data availability: if there is one or more incumbent FSP with a longer history of data, this should be taken into consideration in the evaluation, as such an FSP may not be able or willing to modify forecast models for the purpose of being "comparable" in a t/b. Recommendation: see limitations in Table 7.2 and part 3 of this recommended practice.

c. Missing forecasts: FSP leave out "difficult situations" as missing forecasts are often not penalized. However, missing data may bias "average" forecast metrics, potentially resulting in the formulation of incorrect conclusions. Recommendation: exclude dates from the evaluation if forecasts are not available for all FSPs (i.e. if one or more FSPs have not provides forecasts).

d. Forecast renewal: If delivered forecasts from a FSP as part of a live trial are not downloaded, moved or copied in accordance with the operational process being simulated, and certainly before the time period being forecast, FSPs can potentially renew forecasts with higher accuracy due to fresher information being available. Recommendation: Such an omission should not be underestimated and care taken for the evaluation.

PART THREE

Forecast solution evaluation

Editors (1) and Authors (2):
Dr. Corinna Möhrlen, WEPROG, DK, DE[1,2]
Dr. John W. Zack, MESO Inc., USA[1,2]
Dr. Gregor Giebel, Technical University of Denmark, DK[1]

Contributing Authors:
Dr. Jakob W. Messner, MeteoServe Wetterdienst, AT
Dr. Jethro Browell, University of Glasgow, UK

Contributions:
Dr. Craig Collier, Energy Forecasting Solutions, USA
Dr. Aidan Tuohy, EPRI, USA
Dr. Stephan Vogt, Fraunhofer Institute IEE, DE

CHAPTER ELEVEN

Forecast solution evaluation

11.1. Before you start reading

This is the **third part** of this IEA Wind recommended practice for the implementation of renewable energy forecasting solutions.

In this **third part**, *Forecast solution evaluation* methods and guidelines for the meaningful evaluation of alternative forecasts, operational and non-operational forecasts and entire forecast solutions are presented. In the **first part**, *Forecast solution selection process*, the design of a customized process to select an optimal forecast solution for a user's specific situation and application is addressed. In the **second part**, *Design and execution of benchmarks and trials*, the design, execution and analysis of customized forecasting benchmarks and trials is addressed. In the **fourth part**, *Meteorological and power data requirements for real-time forecasting applications* guidance for the selection, deployment and maintenance of meteorological sensors, power measurements and associated data quality control relevant to real-time forecasting is provided.

If your main interest is in (1) selecting a forecasting solution, (2) testing or evaluating different forecasting solutions, or (4) setting up meteorological sensors or power measurements for real-time wind or solar power forecasting, please move on to part 1, part 2 or part 4 of this recommended practice guideline to obtain recommendations on any of these specific issues, respectively.

It is recommended that the table of contents be actively used to find the most relevant topics.

11.2. Background and introduction

The evaluation of forecasts and forecast solutions is an essential task for any forecast provider as well as end-user of forecasts. It is important, because economically significant and business-relevant decisions are often based on evaluation results. Therefore, it is crucial to allocate significant attention to the design and execution of forecast evaluations to ensure that the results are significant, representative and relevant. Additionally, forecast skill and quality has to be understood and designed in the framework of

IEA Wind Recommended Practice for the Implementation of Renewable Energy Forecasting Solutions
https://doi.org/10.1016/B978-0-44-318681-3.00023-4

forecast value in order to evaluate the quality of a forecast on the value it creates in the decision processes.

In this part, we focus on a number of conceptual processes to introduce a framework for evaluation of wind and solar energy forecasting applications in the power industry. For this purpose, we adopted concepts from state-of-the-art publications (e.g. [35–37,45–54]) specifically developed for wind and solar forecasting evaluation for use in typical industry acpplications. The concept's origin will be referenced accordingly. The focus areas in this part of the recommended practices guideline can be summarised to:

1. **Impact of forecast accuracy on application**
   First, it's often difficult to define the impact of forecast accuracy on the performance of an application metric, because forecasts are just one of many inputs. Second, trials or benchmarks often last longer than anticipated or are too short to generate trustworthy results. Thus, the end-user is often under pressure to wrap up the evaluation quickly or to produce meaningful results with too little data. As a consequence, average absolute or squared errors are employed due to their simplicity and widespread use, even though they seldom effectively assess the value of a forecast solution for the user's specific applications.
2. **Cost-Loss relationship of forecasts**
   A forecast that performs best in one metric is not necessarily the best in terms of other metrics. In other words, there is no universally best evaluation metric. Using metrics that do not effectively represent the relationship between forecast errors and the resulting cost in the forecast user's application, can lead to misleading conclusions and non-optimal (possibly poor) decisions. Knowing the cost-loss relationship of their applications and to be able to select an appropriate evaluation metric accordingly is important. This becomes especially important as forecasting products are becoming more complex and the interconnection between errors and their associated costs more proportional. Apart from more meaningful evaluation results, knowledge of the cost-loss relationship also helps the forecast service provider to develop customized forecast solutions that are optimized for the intended application.

Evaluation of forecast solutions is a complex task, and it is usually not easy nor recommended for the evaluation process to be simplified. As a general recommendation, such a process needs to follow an evaluation paradigm that assigns an appropriate level of attention to three core principles of an evaluation process:

1. **representativeness**
2. **significance**
3. **relevance**

The setup of an evaluation process that satisfactorily addresses these three principles is the focus of this part of the recommended practice guideline.

The outline of this part of the guideline is as follows. In chapter 12 these three main principles are outlined and the general concept of evaluation uncertainty is explained as this should be the foundation for the design and execution of an evaluation project. In chapter 13, the uncertainty of measurement data collection and reporting is explained as a basic issue of evaluation and verification tasks. If forecasts are evaluated against data that have inherited errors, results may still show some significance, but may no longer be considered relevant and representative. In chapter 14 metrics for evaluation and verification will be conceptualized and categorized in order to provide an issue-oriented guideline for the selection of metrics in a evaluation framework. The last chapter 22 introduces the concept of developing an evaluation framework. It provides practical information on how to maximize the value of operational forecasts and how to conduct an evaluation for benchmarks, trials and new forecasting techniques. Lastly, recommendations are made for a number of practical use cases for power industry specific applications.

CHAPTER TWELVE

Overview of evaluation uncertainty

Key points

All performance evaluations of potential or ongoing forecast solutions have a degree of uncertainty, which is associated with the three attributes of the performance evaluation process: (1) representativeness, (2) significance and (3) relevance.
A carefully designed and implemented evaluation process that considers the key issues in each of these three attributes can minimize the uncertainty and yield the most meaningful results.
A disregard of these issues is likely to lead to uncertainty that is so high that the conclusions of the evaluation process are meaningless and therefore decisions based on the results are basically random.

Uncertainty is an inherent characteristic of the forecast evaluation process. The objective of the design and execution of a forecast evaluation procedure is to minimize the uncertainty and thereby reduce its impact on the decisions association with forecast selection or optimization. In order to minimize forecast evaluation uncertainty it is useful to understand the sources of uncertainty within the evaluation process.

The sources of forecast evaluation uncertainty can be linked to three key attributes of the evaluation process: **(1) representativeness (2) significance** and **(3) relevance**. If any one of these are not satisfactorily addressed, than an evaluation will not provide meaningful information to the forecast solution selection process and the resources employed in the trial or benchmark will essentially have been wasted. Unfortunately, it may not be obvious to the conductor of a forecast evaluation or the user of the information produced by an evaluation process whether or not these three attributes have been satisfactorily addressed. This section presents an overview of the key issues associated with each attribute. Subsequent sections of this document will provide guidance on how to maximize the likelihood that each will be satisfactorily addressed.

12.1. Representativeness

Representativeness refers to the relationship between the results of a forecast performance evaluation and the performance that is ultimately

IEA Wind Recommended Practice for the Implementation of Renewable Energy Forecasting Solutions
https://doi.org/10.1016/B978-0-44-318681-3.00024-6

obtained in the operational use of a forecast solution. It essentially addresses the question of whether or not the results of the evaluation are likely to be a good predictor of the actual forecast performance that will be achieved for an operational application. These are many factors that influence the ability of the evaluation results to be a good predictor of future operational performance.

Four of the most crucial factors are:

1. size and composition of the evaluation sample,
2. quality of the data from the forecast target sites,
3. the formulation and enforcement of rules governing the submission of forecasts (sometimes referred to as "fairness"),
4. availability of a complete and consistent set of evaluation procedure information to all evaluation participants (sometimes referred to as "transparency").

12.1.1 Size and composition of the evaluation sample

The size and composition of the evaluation sample are the most important representativeness factors. Both the size and composition of the sample is a key factor in determining the extent to which the results are influenced by random variations (i.e. noise) compared to true differences in forecast skill. The following considerations are recommended in order to ensure representative evaluation samples:

- **Data set representation and composition:**
  The selected data set should be representative of the application and all forecast solutions under consideration should be evaluated with exactly the same data sets. Results from different locations, seasons, lead times etc. are in general not comparable. The composition should be constructed so that all significant modes of variation of the forecast variable (e.g. wind or solar power production) are included in the evaluation sample. For example, if there is a high wind season and a low wind season, then both should have a representative number of cases in the evaluation sample. Or, in the case of solar power forecasts, there should be representative samples of both clear and cloudy weather periods. However, if this is not practical, then there should at least be a representative sample of the most important weather modes for the application.
- **Data set length:**
  The size of the evaluation sample is one of the most important representativeness and significance factors. The size of the sample is a key

factor in determining to what extent results are influenced by random variation, or noise, compared to true differences in predictive performance. The use of a small sample increases the probability that any conclusions reached from the evaluation will be due to noise (random and unrepresentative events) in the sample. For example, the occurrence of very unusual weather events for a few days in a short sample may dominate the evaluation results.

That leads to the question of how large of a sample is adequate? A commonly used sample size guideline when gathering data for statistical analysis is 30. If all the sample points are independent, then a sample of 30 provides a reasonably adequate minimization of the probability that sampling noise will meaningfully impact the conclusions. But the key phrase is that the sample data points must be independent (uncorrelated) for this guideline to be valid. However, weather processes are typically highly correlated over time periods of 3 to 4 days. This means that an adequate sample from a continuous evaluation period should be 3 to 4 times larger than 30 or in other words, 90 to 120 days [55] (see also 15.1.2, 14.1.4 and 15.1).

- **Data set consistency:**

  For a fair evaluation of a forecast, whether against alternative forecasts, measurements or reference forecasts such as persistence, it is very important to use the same data set to derive the evaluation results. If an individual forecast is not available for a specific time, this time has to be disregarded for all the other forecasts. If this is not done the evaluation results may be significantly skewed. For example, if forecasts from a specific source are missing for days that are particularly difficult to predict, they would exhibit better overall performance than other forecasts that are likely to have high errors for these difficult days. This also applies for curtailment data. It is important to evaluate a forecast against the weather-related performance and remove all non-weather-related impacts that are out of the forecasters control. Especially, if forecasts are evaluated against a persistence forecast, e.g. in minute- or hour-scale forecasts, where models are adapted to measurements that may contain curtailment or data failures due to turbine unavailability or communication issues. In such cases, the corresponding persistence need to be computed accordingly. If this is not done, the forecast performance of the persistence will be overestimated and the performance of the forecast underestimated.

12.1.2 Data quality

The quality of the data used in the forecast evaluation process can be a major source of uncertainty. The data from the forecast target location is typically used for three purposes: (1) training data for the statistical components of each forecast system, (2) real-time input data to forecast production processes, which is especially important for very short-term forecast time horizons (minutes to a few hours ahead) and (3) forecast outcome data (i.e. the actual value used to compute forecast errors) for the evaluation of the forecast performance. If the data have many quality issues, then the representativeness of all three of these applications is compromised. The quality issues may include: (1) out of range or locked values, (2) biased values due to issues with measurement devices or location of measurement, (3) badly or not at all calibrated instruments and (4) power production data that are unrepresentative of meteorological conditions because of undocumented generation outages or curtailments. If a substantial amount of data with these issues is used in the evaluation process for any of the three purposes, the results will likely not be representative of the true skill of the forecasting solutions that are being evaluated.

12.1.3 Forecast submission control

A third important factor is the formulation and enforcement of rules for the submission of forecasts to be used the evaluation process. This is sometimes noted as a "fairness" issue and it is indeed an issue of fairness to the forecast providers who are typically competing to demonstrate the skill of their system and thereby obtain an award of a contract for their services. However, from the user's perspective, it is a representativeness issue. If it is possible for some forecasting solution providers to provide forecasts with unrepresentative skill then the conclusions of the entire evaluation process are questionable. A couple of examples can illustrate this point. One example is a situation in which there is no enforcement of the forecast delivery time. In this case it would be possible for a forecast provider to deliver forecasts at a later time (perhaps overwriting a forecast that was delivered at the required time) and use later data to add skill to their forecast or even wait until the outcome for the forecast period is known. Although one might think that such explicit cheating is not likely to occur in this type of technical evaluation, experience has indicated that it is not that uncommon, if the forecast delivery protocol enables its occurrence.

A second example illustrates how the results might be manipulated without explicit cheating by taking advantage of loopholes in the rules.

In this example the issue is that the evaluation protocol does not specify any penalty for missing a forecast delivery and the evaluation metrics are simply computed on whatever forecasts are submitted by each provider. As a forecast provider it is not difficult to estimate the "difficulty" of each forecast period and to simply not deliver any forecasts during periods that are likely to be difficult and therefore prone to large errors. This is an excellent way to improve forecast performance scores. Of course, it makes the results unrepresentative of what is actually needed by the user. Often it is good performance during the difficult forecast periods that is most valuable to a user.

12.1.4 Process information dissemination

A fourth key factor is the availability of a complete and consistent set of information about the forecast evaluation process to all participants. Incomplete or inconsistent information distribution can occur in many ways. For example, one participant may ask a question and the reply is only provided to the participant who submitted the inquiry. This can contribute to apparent differences in forecast skill that are not associated with true differences in the skills of the solution. This of course results in unrepresentative evaluation of the true differences in forecast skill among the solutions.

12.2. Significance

Significance refers to the ability to differentiate between performance differences that are due to noise (quasi-random processes) in the evaluation process and those that are due to meaningful differences in skill among forecast solutions. Performance differences that stem from noise have basically no meaning and will not represent the performance differences that a user will experience in a long-term operational application of alternative solutions. *Real* performance differences on the other hand should be stable and should not change if an evaluation process is repeated, e.g. one year later. A certain degree of noise is inevitable in every evaluation task but both, minimization of noise and awareness of the uncertainty it causes are crucial in order to make reliable decisions based on the evaluation results.

As mentioned above, repeatability is a good practical indication of significance in evaluation results. The highest potential for achieving repeatability is the use of a representative evaluation sample. This means the sample should include as many potential weather events, seasons, and perhaps forecast locations as possible. Otherwise, there is a high probability that the results will be different for features that are not well represented in the evaluation sample. Thus, significance is highly related to representativeness and very much depends on the evaluation sample size and composition.

12.2.1 Quantification of uncertainty

In addition to noise minimization through the use of representative evaluation data sets, it is also very useful to quantify the significance (i.e. the uncertainty) of the evaluation results. Quantification of the uncertainty is important for decision making. For example, if a number of forecast solutions are evaluated with a specified metric, but their differences are much smaller than the uncertainty in the result due to e.g. measurement uncertainty, the meaning of their ranking is actually very limited and should not be used for important decisions.

12.2.1.1 Method 1: repeating the evaluation task

The simplest approach to estimate evaluation uncertainty would be to repeat the evaluation task several times on different data sets. This approach is often effective, because the typical variation or uncertainty of the evaluation results is mostly attributable to their dependence on the evaluation data set and therefore results often vary among different evaluation data sets. However, since evaluation data sets are usually very limited, this is often not a feasible approach.

12.2.1.2 Method 2: bootstrap resampling

A simple alternative method is to simulate different data sets, through the use of a bootstrap resampling process. In this approach an evaluation data set of the same length as the original data set is drawn from the original data set with a certain percentage "N" being replaced with random numbers and the evaluation results are derived on this set. By repeating this "N" times, "N" different evaluation results become available and their range can be seen as the evaluation uncertainty. Alternatively, parametric testing can also provide information on the significance of evaluation results. Typically two sample paired t-tests applied on the sets of error measures for each evaluation sample provide a good estimate of the significance of the results. Diebold et al. [56] proposed a variation of this t-test to account for temporal correlations in the data and can therefore provide a more accurate significance quantification. Messner et al. [55] also describes different parametric testing or bootstrap resampling approaches that can be employed to quantify the evaluation uncertainty.

If it is found, that the forecast that is identified as the "best" from an evaluation process does not exhibit significantly better performance than some of the other alternative forecasts, the final selection of forecast solutions should only consider differences among forecast solutions that are significant. For example, if there is a group of forecast solutions that are at the top of the metric-based performance ranking list, but there are no significant differences in performance among them, the selection process should treat them as equivalent in terms of forecast accuracy and the differentiation among them should be based on other factors.

12.3. Relevance

Relevance refers to the degree of alignment between the evaluation metrics used for an evaluation and the true sensitivity of a user's application(s) to forecast error. If these two items are not well aligned then even though an evaluation process is representative and the results show significant differences among solutions, the evaluation results may not be a relevant basis for selecting the best solution for the application. There are a number of issues related to the relevance factor.

1. **Best Performance Metric**
   First, the selection of the best metric may be complex and difficult. The ideal approach is to formulate a cost function that transforms forecast error to the application-related consequences of those errors. This could be a monetary implication or it might be another type of consequence (for example a reliability metric for grid operations). However, if it is not feasible to do this, another approach is to use a matrix of performance metrics that measure a range of forecast performance attributes.
2. **Multiple Performance Metrics**
   If there is a range of forecast performance attributes that are relevant to a user's application, it most likely will not be possible to optimize a single forecast to achieve optimal performance for all of the relevant metrics. In that case, the best solution is to obtain multiple forecasts with each being optimized for a specific application and its associated metric.
3. **Multiple Forecast Solutions**
   Another type of issue arises when the user intends to employ multiple (N) forecast solutions and create a composite forecast from the information provided by each individual forecast. In this case it may

be tempting to select the best N performing forecasts in the evaluation according to the metric or metrics identified as most relevant by the user. However, that is not the best way to get the most relevant answer for the multiple provider scenario. In that case the desired answer is to select the N forecasts that provide the best composite forecast for the target metric(s). This may not be the set of N forecasts that individually perform the best. It is the set of forecasts that best complement each other. For example, the two best forecasts according to a metric such as the RMSE may be highly correlated and provide essentially the same information. In that case, a forecast solution with a higher (worse) RMSE may be less correlated with the lowest RMSE forecast and therefore be a better complement to that forecast.

CHAPTER THIRTEEN

Measurement data processing and control

Key points

- Measurements from the forecast target facilities are crucial for the forecast production and evaluation process and therefore much attention should be given to how data is collected, communicated and quality controlled.
- Collection and reporting of measurement data requires strict rules and formats, as well as IT communication and cybersecurity standards in order to maximize its value in the forecasting process; information about standards and methods for collecting and reporting data is provided in Chapter 4 of Part 1 of this RP.
- An effective quality control process is essential since bad data can seriously degrade forecast performance; standard quality maintenance and control procedures have been documented and some are noted in this section.

In any evaluation, the measurements or observations are alpha and omega for trustworthy results. For this reason, this section is dedicated to the importance of data collection, verification and the identification of the measurement uncertainty. In the evaluation of renewable power forecasts, power data is considered most important; but also meteorological measurements are often provided to the forecast providers as input to improve their forecast models. Furthermore, failure of generation assets (unscheduled outages), service periods of generation assets (scheduled outages), curtailment and other disturbances in the power measurements can have significant impact on the results of an evaluation. The following section deals with these aspects and provides recommendations for a correct handling of such data in the evaluation phase.

13.1. Uncertainty of instrumentation signals and measurements

All data are derived from different measurement devices and depending on the quality of these devices the measurements can deviate from the reality to a certain degree. In fact, measurement errors can never be avoided completely and can potentially affect the representativeness or significance of evaluation results. Therefore, it is crucial to establish and maintain spe-

IEA Wind Recommended Practice for the Implementation of Renewable Energy Forecasting Solutions
https://doi.org/10.1016/B978-0-44-318681-3.00025-8

cific quality requirements for the measurement devices to obtain data of good quality and thus keep the measurement uncertainty to a low level. This will not only improve the significance and representativeness of the evaluation results, but also assure an optimum quality of forecasts that use the measurements as input.

For power data, the measurement quality is usually ensured by existing grid code standards that are verified in the commissioning phase and are serviced as part of the turbine's SCADA system maintenance.

Recommendations on minimum technical requirements beyond the scope of this recommended practice guideline. For anyone intending to collect and process bankable wind measurements, the following standards and guidelines provide a basis for the adaptation of those measurements for real-time operational applications:

1. the International Electrotechnical Commission (IEC)
2. the International Energy Agency (IEA)
3. the International Network for Harmonized and Recognized Wind Energy Measurement (MEASNET)
4. United States Environmental Protection Agency (EPA)

If these requirements are fulfilled, the measurement error is usually negligible compared to other sources of uncertainty in the evaluation procedure.

13.2. Measurement data reporting and collection

Once wind farms are operational and the production data are measured it is important to collect, store and report them properly, which requires strict rules and formats, as well as IT communication standards. Standard protocols for collecting and reporting power data are usually enforced by jurisdictional grid codes.

There are however a number of aspects that are not covered in the grid codes that are essential for the evaluation of forecasting tools. This section discusses the main aspects to be considered for any measurement data collection and archiving. In the following, the description is limited to the purpose of evaluation of forecasts in a real-time operational framework or a forecast test framework.

13.2.1 Non-weather related production reductions

Raw power production data contains a number of non-weather related reductions that need consideration in the collection or archiving of measurement data, such as

- failure of turbines in a wind park (availability)
- scheduled and non-scheduled maintenance
- curtailment
- reductions due to environmental constraints (noise, birds, ...)

The so-called "Net to Grid" signal is often disturbed by such technical constraints that are usually not part of the wind power forecasting task. Therefore, to evaluate the actual forecast quality, such events have to be filtered in the evaluation. Especially in the case of curtailment, the forecast user needs to decide whether the target parameter is the real power production or available power. If it is the latter, data with curtailment should be removed from the evaluation data set, because errors are not meaningful for the forecast performance, unless the curtailments are predicted as well. Ideally, direct signals from the turbines on their available active power are used to filter such data for evaluation and verification purposes, even if the signals are provided retrospectively.

- To obtain *relevant* results, remove events from the evaluation data set that are affected by non-weather related production constraints unless these are to be predicted as well.

13.2.2 Aggregation of measurement data in time and space

Often, temporally or spatially aggregated data (averages, sums) are more useful in power applications than instantaneous signals. The aggregation level of the data should always be communicated to the forecast provider to assure optimum forecast performance for the intended application. This also applies in the absence of any aggregation over time, for example, it should be explicitly specified, if hourly values are provided that are not hourly averages of higher resolution data, but instantaneous values taken at the start of the hour. Furthermore, it is strongly recommended that the measurement data should be aggregated according to the intended applications before comparing, analyzing and verifying forecasts. Otherwise, the evaluation results might not be relevant for the forecast user.

When aggregating measurement data over parks, regions, control zones or other aggregation levels, it is important to consider non-weather related events as discussed in Section 13.2.1.

In particular:

- Non-reporting generation units
- IT communication failures or corrupt signals

have to be identified and reported, and the aggregated data should be normalized accordingly. Such failures are impossible to predict by the forecast vendor and should therefore not be part of the evaluation process. Instead, it is recommended to follow these general guidelines:

- for *relevant* results, average the measurement data over a time frame that is consistent with the intended application.
- for *representative* results, non-weather related events should be identified and the aggregated signals normalized accordingly.

13.3. Measurement data processing and archiving

In any real-time environment, measurements should be delivered as is, but flagged, if they are considered wrong (1) at the logger level and (2) after a quality control before employing measurements in a forecast process.

The optimal data archival structure is dependent on the plans for the further processing of the data. In most cases, it is useful to archive data in a database. There are many types of database structures available today. Such structural decisions are out of the scope of this guideline. Nevertheless, there are general considerations when planning and designing a database for operational data. For example, a data point may get "stuck" on a set value. Monitoring of the incoming data is therefore an important feature to ensure correct measurement data, where this is possible.

While measurements are available only at one specific time, forecast data have overlapping time periods and need to be separated from measurement data. At the design level, it is necessary to consider the following aspects:

1. single or multiple time points per measurement signal in database
2. flagging at each data point and
    a. possibility to overwrite corrupt data in database
    b. possibility to add correct data point in database
    c. knowledge of time averaging level of data signal
3. single or multiple measurement points per wind farm
4. ability to expand and upscale the database: expansion with increasing number of measurement points/production units
5. importance of access to historical data

The database dimensions and setup of tables should take such decisions and requirements into consideration.

13.4. Quality assurance and quality control

Quality of data is a crucial parameter for any real-time forecasting system. If the data that real-time forecasts are based on are corrupt or misleading, the result can be worse than not having measurements or observations at all. Therefore, any real-time system using measurements needs a quality control mechanism to discard bad data. However, reasons for bad, corrupt or misleading data signals are almost unlimited, which means that specific limits, operating ranges and validity checks need to be established when dealing with observational data. Is it also worth mentioning that as well as the quality, the latency of the data, i.e. the lag between the measurement time and when the data is available for forecast use, is critical for live applications. This will affect what time lags can practically be used in any forecast model.

While all this is critical in real-time environments, the quality of measurement data in the verification phase is equally important. For example, if a wind power forecast is verified against observations from a wind farm and a maintenance schedule or a curtailment from the system operator is not filtered out or marked in the data time series, then the result may be bad for the wrong reason. Trustworthiness in data can only be a result of control and maintenance of both the hardware and the corresponding software and data archiving. Part 4, section 21.4 outlines the most important parts of quality control and quality assurance for both historic and real-time data, screening techniques and black/and whitelisting methodologies that should be carried out regularly in real-time environments and prior to verification or evaluation exercises.

Recommendation:
For *relevant* evaluation results, the data has to be of high quality, and faulty or corrupt data has to be detected, flagged and disregarded for the evaluation process. A detailed description of quality assurance and control processes can be found in part 4, section 21.4.

CHAPTER FOURTEEN

Assessment of forecast performance

Key points

- All performance evaluations of potential or ongoing forecast solutions have a degree of uncertainty.
- The evaluation uncertainty is associated with three attributes of the performance evaluation process:
  1. representativeness
  2. significance
  3. relevance.
- A carefully designed and implemented evaluation process that considers the key issues in each of these three attributes can minimize the uncertainty and yield the most meaningful results.
- A disregard of these issues is likely to lead to uncertainty and/or decisions based on unrepresentative information.

The relevance of different aspects of forecast performance depends on the user's application. For instance, one user may be concerned with the size of *typical* forecast errors, while another may only be concerned with the size and frequency of particularly large errors.

There are a wide range of error metrics and verification methods available to forecast users, but their relationship to different attributes is not always clear.

This chapter deals with the issues around evaluating specific attributes of forecast performance, including metric selection and the verification and the use of some specific metrics in forecast optimization.

14.1. Forecast attributes at metric selection

Forecast users may be interested in either a single attribute, or a range of forecast performance attributes. When evaluating forecasts to either track performance changes or discriminate between different forecasts, it is important to consider those attributes relevant to the intended use of the forecasts. Where a forecast is used in multiple applications, there is no guarantee that these attributes will be aligned and it may be necessary to

IEA Wind Recommended Practice for the Implementation of Renewable Energy Forecasting Solutions
https://doi.org/10.1016/B978-0-44-318681-3.00026-X

compromise or procure multiple forecast products. Selecting an appropriate metric, or set of metrics, is a key requirement in order to produce an evaluation of forecast performance that is relevant to the forecast's end use.

Quantitative evaluation methods are usually the core of the evaluation framework, since they allow an evaluator to objectively rank different forecast solutions. Typical choices of quantitative metrics are the (root) mean squared error, the mean absolute error or the quantile score (see [53] for details) for continuous forecasts and various quantities derived from contingency tables for categorical or binary forecasts (see 15.1.3.1).

As emphasized in Section 15.1.5, the selection of metrics should be informed by the forecast user's intended use, and if a forecast is intended to be used for multiple applications, different basic metrics should be applied and merged into a weighted sum. A range of forecast attributes and their relation to different evaluation metrics are discussed in the following subsections.

14.1.1 "Typical" error metrics

The most common error metrics used in renewable power forecast applications summarize 'typical' errors by averaging the absolute or squared value of errors, often normalized by installed capacity. Such metrics are simple to produce and give a high-level view of forecast performance. They give equal weighting to all errors in the sample, which may be appropriate if the forecast is used to inform decisions at any time, as opposed to only when a particular event is predicted.

In energy trading, for example, the forecast is used to inform decisions for every trading period and the cost implication of a forecast error is usually proportional to the error. In this case, the absolute value of the error is directly related to the forecast's end-use, so mean squared error would not be as informative as mean absolute error.

However, average error metrics hide some information which may be of interest. For example, a forecast with mostly small errors and occasional large errors could return a similar "typical error" score to one with all moderate errors. In some cases this may not be an issue, but some users may prefer to experience fewer large errors even if that also means fewer small errors.

Examples of typical error metrics are discussed in section 15.1, in section 15.1.2 and provided in Appendix F.

14.1.2 Outlier/extreme error

Another important attribute is the prevalence of large errors. Some applications are primarily sensitive to large errors, such as managing reserve energy or other risk management. Calculating metrics based on large errors is more challenging than for 'typical' errors, as large errors are more affected by specific situations. It is recommended that different root causes of large errors should be considered separately, and also that positive and negative errors are treated separately.

For example, large errors at a single wind farm during a period of high wind speed may be caused by high speed shut down, but are unlikely if the wind speed is only just above rated. If considering aggregated production from multiple wind farms, large errors may be caused by wind speed forecast errors in the vicinity of large areas of concentrated capacity.

14.1.3 Empirical error distribution

The empirical distribution of past forecast errors gives a detailed picture of the frequency of different size errors. It can be useful to examine the distribution of errors for specific situations, such as when power was forecast to be $70 \pm 2\%$, as the shape of the distribution will depend on power level, particularly for individual wind farms.

14.1.4 Binary or multi-criteria events

Some attributes of forecast performance relate to the prediction of events such as ramps (of a particular rate and duration) which may span multiple lead-times and spatial scales. Furthermore, events typically have multiple attributes, such as timing and magnitude. Different attributes may be of more or less interest depending on the use case for the forecast. In these cases, average error metrics may not be representative of the desired forecast attribute.

For example, ramp rate may be of most importance to one user, whereas the timing or ramp magnitude may be of more importance to another. This effect is illustrated in Fig. 14.1. Timing or *phase* errors are penalized heavily by mean absolute error so the forecast that best predicted both the ramp rate and magnitude appears worse by this measure. A similar principle applies to events such as the duration of high or low power periods. In general, "typical error" metrics favor 'smooth' forecasts rather than those that capture the precise shape of specific events.

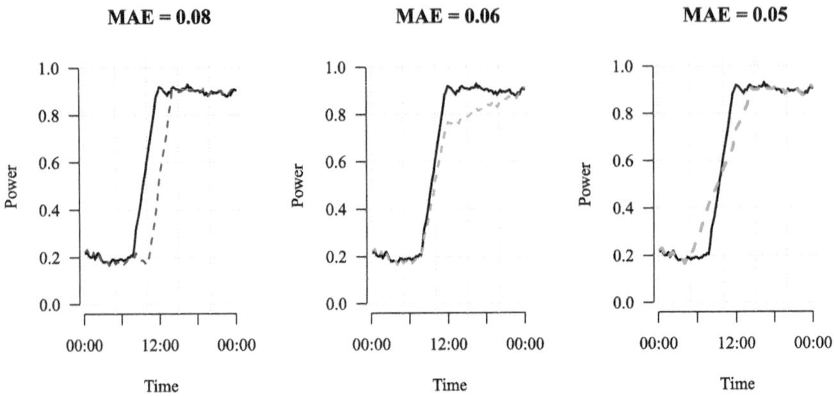

Figure 14.1 Examples of different types of ramp forecast error. Actual power is shown as solid black lines, forecasts are colored dashed lines. From left to right: phase or timing error, amplitude error and ramp rate error. The mean absolute error (MAE) for each forecast is shown above the plots. Despite being the only forecast that correctly predicts the ramp rate and duration, the forecast with a phase error has the largest MAE.

Contingency tables provide a framework for quantifying the prediction of categorical events, which can be defined to match the user's decision making process. For example, the user may define a particular ramp event with some tolerance for phase and amplitude error and then evaluate the performance of a particular forecast solution at predicting such events. There are four possibilities for each predicted and/or actual event: a true positive (hit), true negative (correct negative), false positive (false alarm) or false negative (miss). From these, a range of metrics can be calculated and used for comparison with other forecast systems. Furthermore, if the cost implications of decisions based on the forecast are known (or can be estimated) then the relative value of forecasting systems may be calculated.

Examples on how to verify outliers can be found in section 15.1, and 15.4.2.1.

14.2. Prediction intervals and predictive distributions

Prediction intervals may be supplied to provide situational awareness or to information or quantitative risk management. These intervals predict an upper and lower bound which the observation will fall between with some probability. It is therefore an important attribute that observations do in fact fall between the interval with the prescribed frequency. This property is call 'reliability' and can be evaluated by simply counting the frequency of observations within and outside the interval. A more accurate forecasts with a narrower interval are said to be 'sharp' and provides greater confidence than a wide interval, but must be reliable in order to inform risk-based decision making. Therefore, prediction intervals should be evaluated following the principal of *sharpness subject to reliability*.

A predictive distribution is a smooth probability density function for the future value. It provides full information about probability of all possible value ranges rather than a single interval. In this case the principal of *sharpness subject to reliability* still applies, but sharpness and reliability needs to be evaluated for a range of probability levels.

In quantitative decision-making under uncertainty, the optimal decision is often a *quantile*, i.e. the value that is forecast to be exceeded with some probability. For example, if the cost of taking precautionary action is C to protect against an uncertain adverse effect with potential loss L, then the precautionary action should be take in the probability of the adverse effect happening is greater than the cost-loss ratio C/L.

In applications of wind power forecasting, the adverse event could be exposure to imbalance costs, or holding insufficient energy reserves. In most cases, the values of C and L will be changing continuously and the decision maker will be aiming to select a future value of energy production which will be achieved with some probability $p = C/L$. Therefore, it is necessary to have access to the full predictive distribution in order to make an appropriate decision. Where the cost-loss ratio is known, the relative economic value of different forecasting systems can be calculated.

14.3. Probabilistic forecast assessment methods

Probabilistic forecast evaluation is a complex topic. There are a number of classical metrics, just like for deterministic forecasts. However, the evaluation of probabilistic forecasts places greater importance on an end-user's knowledge of a cost function that provides a good indication of how well the forecast performance has met the requirements of the user's application. (see also 15.1.5).

The considerations from chapter 12 on the performance evaluation and its inherent uncertainty are even more important here. The three attributes *(1) representativeness, (2) significance* and *(3) relevance* are equally important to consider when setting up evaluation or benchmarking of probabilistic forecasts.

For probabilistic forecast evaluation, another set of three attributes is often mentioned: (1) reliability, (2) sharpness and (3) resolution. These attributes are associated with specific metrics and verification scores or scoring rules.

- **Reliability (Calibration)** – can be measured in the Brier Score 14.3.1, *reliability diagram* 14.3.3.2, *rank histogram* 14.3.3.1 or the CRPS 14.3.2.1 and refers to the statistical consistency between the distributional forecasts and the observations and is a joint property of the predictions and the observed values [37].
- **Sharpness** – is a forecast attribute and property: the ability of the forecast to predict extreme probability values (i.e. near 0% or 100%) and is essentially a representation of the estimated forecast uncertainty. Its opposite is often a climatology or a persistence forecast. Forecast probabilities should be well distributed, or the spread be "refined", i.e. in large spread forecasts have the potential to cover a broad range of conditions. A narrow spread indicates a lack of refinement (see e.g. [57], [50] pp. 256ff). In the reliability diagram the sharpness can be identified in relation to a perfect calibration (see Fig. 14.5).
- **Resolution** – can be measured as a de-composite of the Brier Scores 14.3.1 and refers to how well the forecast is capable of separating events according to whether they occur or do not occur.

In some cases, it might also be best to only use a graphical inspection of how well observations lie within forecast intervals. This can then be extended to an interval evaluation to provide objective values to the visual impression from the graph. This is similar to the "dichotomous event evaluation" described in 15.1.3.1 for predefined events. These scores can also be used for probabilistic/uncertainty forecasts, if the application is about how well the probabilistic forecasts or forecast intervals have captured the observations. In fact, a number of typical probabilistic scores are based on graphical evaluation due to their non-binary character, such as the reliability diagram, the relative operating characteristics (ROC) curve, and the rank histogram. In the same way, as for deterministic forecasts, the verification is dependent on the desired attribute a forecast is supposed to fulfill, and often, more than one metric is required to achieve proper evaluations.

It is therefore important to follow the recommendations in the "best practice recommendations" Chapter 22 on how to build up an evaluation platform that reflects the purpose of the forecasts and provides an incentive to the forecast provider to match these criteria with the appropriate methods.

Therefore, the following description of metrics only provides a set of possible tools that can be used for the evaluation of probabilistic forecasts and the user must select the most appropriate set depending on the characteristics of the user's application and objectives of the forecast evaluation.

14.3.1 Brier scores

The Brier score [32] is probably the most prominent and widely-used probabilistic forecast performance metric. It is a useful measure for a general assessment of the performance of probabilistic forecasts. However, the formulation of the basic Brier makes it suitable only for the evaluation of probabilistic forecasts of binary forecasts (i.e. occurrence or non-occurrence of a defined event).

The Brier Score (BS) is the equivalent of the mean-squared error (MSE) for probabilistic forecasts with the same limitations as for deterministic forecasts. That means, the Brier Score is sensitive to the climatological frequency of events in the sense that the rarer an event, the easier it is to get a good BS without having any real skill. The BS is defined as,

$$BS = \frac{1}{N} \cdot \sum_{i=1}^{N} (p_i - o_i)^2 \tag{14.1}$$

where p_i is the *forecast probability* at time i, o is the observation at time i, and N is the number of forecasts. The forecast probabilities range in value between 0 and 1, the observed values are either 0, if the event does not occur, or 1, if the event occurs.

Eq. (14.1) is bound mathematically to values between 0 and 1. A lower Brier score, similar to the MSE, indicates greater accuracy. The maximum squared error is 1, because all squared errors will lie between 0 and 1. A *perfect accuracy* is reflected in the Brier score with 0, i.e. there is no difference between frequencies of an event and someone's probabilistic predictions for those events. The opposite, i.e. a Brier score of 1, reflects perfect inaccuracy, which means that there are probabilities of 0 given to events that occur and probabilities of 1 to events that do not occur.

In order to gain further insight into the behavior of the Brier score, it can be decomposed algebraically into three components:

$$BS = CAL - RES + UNC \tag{14.2}$$

where, the CAL is the Calibration and is also sometimes referred to as the "reliability", RES is the resolution and UNC is the uncertainty.

In [51], these three components can be explained in a way that is easy to understand and relate to applications:

- *CAL* is a squared function of forecasted probability (f_p) and the mean probability ($\overline{x_p}$) and measures whether the forecasted values consistently represent the frequencies with which events occur (i.e., is the forecasted probability too large or too small on average?). For example, does the event occur 30% of the time when a forecast of 0.30 is issued? Specifically, CAL measures the difference between the actual frequency of occurrence and the forecast prediction. This is also referred to as the "reliability" of a probabilistic forecast.
- *RES* is a squared function of ($\overline{x_p}$) and ($\overline{x}$) and measures how much the frequency of event occurrence varies among the forecasts. It measures the ability of the forecast to distinguish between event and non-event. For example, if the average frequency of event occurrence across all forecasts is 0.50, the relative frequency of occurrence ($\overline{x_p}$) should be much smaller for events, when the forecast is 0.10 (low likelihood of event) and much larger when the forecast probability is 0.90 (high likelihood of event). Higher RES scores indicate more skill and therefore appears in Eq. (14.1) with a negative sign. In the worst case, when the same probability (for example, the climatological probability) is always forecasted, the resolution is zero.
- *UNC* is a function of ($\overline{x}$) only and does not specifically measure how well the forecasts predict the event. Instead, UNC is an important measure of the difficulty of the forecasting situation. Large values of UNC (e.g., when the event is very rare) indicate that the forecasting situation is more difficult. It is inappropriate to compare forecasts for systems with significantly different UNC values.

In [51] a very useful list of specific questions that the Brier score answers have been listed:

1. ***Brier Score (BS)*** answers how accurate the probability forecasts are in general.
2. ***Calibration (CAL)*** answers how well does the conditional relative frequency of occurrence of the event match a situation?
3. ***Resolution (RES)*** answers how well does the forecast separate events according to whether they occur or don't occur.
4. ***Uncertainty (UNC)*** answers how difficult/uncertain is the forecast situation.

14.3.2 Ranked probability (skill) score (RP(S)s)

The Ranked Probability Score (RPS) and Ranked probability Skill Score [58] (RPSS) is widely used for multi-category probability forecasts that have a magnitude order to them (such as generation forecasts). The RPS is the multi-category extension of the Brier score, and the "Skill" part refers to a comparison of the RPS of a specified forecast to the RPS of a reference forecast (such as climatological probabilities).

In other words, the RPS measures the cumulative, squared error between categorical forecast probabilities and the observed categorical probabilities, and the RPSS measures the error relative to a reference (or standard baseline) forecast (climatology, persistence or other reference forecast). The observed categorical probabilities are 100% in the observed category, and 0% in all other categories [58,59].

$$RPS = \frac{1}{M-1} \cdot \sum_{m=1}^{M} \left(\sum_{k=1}^{m} p_k \sum_{k=1}^{m} o_k \right)^2 \tag{14.3}$$

where M is the number of forecast categories, p_k is the predicted probability in forecast category k, and o_k is an indicator (0=no, 1=yes) for the observation in category k.

The higher the RPS, the poorer the forecast. RPS=0 means that the probability given to the category that was observed was 100%. The RPSS is based on the RPS for the forecast compared to the RPS For a reference forecast such as one that simply gives climatological probabilities.

RPSS > 0 when RPS for actual forecast is smaller (i.e. better) than RPS for the reference forecast.

$$RPSS = 1 - \frac{RPS_{forecast}}{RPS_{observation}} \tag{14.4}$$

The RPSS is made worse by three main factors [60]:

(1) Mean probability biases.

(2) Conditional probability biases (including amplitude biases).

(3) The lack of correlation between forecast probabilities and observed outcomes.

(1) and (2) are calibration factors and (3) involves discrimination. The tercile category system can be seen as a two category system if the two tercile boundaries are considered one at a time: below normal vs. not below normal above normal vs. not below normal.

14.3.2.1 The continuous ranked probability skill and energy score

As described above in 14.3.1, the Brier Score (BS) is useful for binary events (e.g. critical ramp/not critical ramp). When analyzing discrete multiple-category events (e.g. below critical/critical/above critical ramping) the Ranked Probability Score (RPS) (see 14.3.2) is preferably used. In the continuous case, where there are an infinite number of predictand classes of infinitesimal width, the RPS is extended to the Continuous Ranked Probability Score (CRPS) [49]. Alternatively, it can be interpreted as the integral of the Brier score over all possible threshold values for the parameter under consideration. For a deterministic forecast system, the CRPS reduces to the mean absolute error [35].

For an ensemble prediction system, the CRPS can be decomposed into a reliability part and a resolution/uncertainty part, in a similar way to the decomposition of the Brier score. The reliability part of the CRPS is closely connected to the rank histogram of the ensemble (see section 14.3.3.1), while the resolution/uncertainty part can be related to the average spread within the ensemble and the behavior of its outliers [35]. It also expresses how much improvement can be gained with probability forecasts

Hersbach [35] explains the relationship between CRPS and Brier Score and how the CRPS can be reduced to the mean absolute error (MAE) of a deterministic forecast in the following way:
if we consider the parameter of interest being denoted by x. For instance, x could be the 100 m wind speed or power output. Suppose that the forecast by an ensemble system is given by $r(x)$ and that x_a is the value that actually occurred. Then the continuous ranked probability score expressing some kind of distance between the probabilistic forecast r and truth x_a, is defined as

$$CRPS = CRPS(P, x_a) = \int_{-\infty}^{\infty} (P(x) - P_a(x)]^2)dx \tag{14.5}$$

Here, P and P_a are cumulative distributions:

$$P(x) = \int_{-\infty}^{\infty} P_y(y)dy \tag{14.6}$$

and

$$P_a(x) = H \cdot (x - x_a), \tag{14.7}$$

where H is the well-known Heaviside function, defined to

$$H(x) = \begin{cases} 0 & \text{for x} < 0 \\ 1 & \text{for } x \geq 0 \end{cases} \tag{14.8}$$

So, $P(x)$ is the forecasted probability that x_a will be smaller than x. Obviously, for any cumulative distribution, $P(x) \in [0, 1]$ $P(-\infty) = 0$, and $P(\infty) = 1$. This is also true for parameters that are only defined on a subdomain of $\mathbb{R}$. In that case $r(x) = 0$, P is constant outside the domain of definition. The CRPS measures the difference in the cumulative distributions of the forecasts and outcomes (observations).

Its minimal value of zero is only achieved for $P = P_a$, that is, in the case of a perfect deterministic forecast.

In this definition, the CRPS has the dimension of the parameter x (which enters via the integration over dx). In practice, the CRPS is averaged over an area and a number of cases:

$$CRPS = \sum_k CRPS(P_k, x_k^a) \tag{14.9}$$

where k labels the considered grid points and cases.

This is where the CRPS can be seen as the limit of a ranked probability score with an infinite number of classes, each with zero width and it is not difficult to see that if $k = i$ and $p_k = P_k(x_t)$ and $O_k = P_k^a(x_t)$ the CRPS is directly connected to the Brier score by

$$CRPS = \int_{-\infty}^{\infty} BS(x_t)\, dx \tag{14.10}$$

For a deterministic forecast, that is, $x = x_d$ without any specified uncertainty, $P(x) = H(x - x_d)$. In that case, the integrand of Eq. (14.5) is either zero or one. The non-zero contributions are found in the region where $P(x)$ and $P_a(x)$ differ, which is the interval between x_d and x_a. As a result,

$$\overline{CRPS} = \sum_k |x_d^a - x_a^b| \tag{14.11}$$

which is the mean absolute error (MAE).

Although the CRPS is widely used (see e.g. [36,48,54]), in most real-world applications, it is no longer appropriate, when assessing multivariate forecasts.[1] To assess probabilistic forecasts of a multivariate quantity, Gneiting et al. [48] therefore proposes the use of the so called "energy score",

[1] A forecast is multivariate, when it consists of multiple variables, which typically refer to multiple time-steps, multiple sites or multiple parameters.

which is a direct generalization of the CPRS (14.5), to which the energy score reduces in dimension $d = 1$. Gneiting and Raftery [37] showed its propriety and noted a number of generalizations. If $P = P_{ens}$ is an ensemble forecast of size m, the evaluation of the energy score is straightforward, i.e., the predictive distribution P_{ens} places point mass 1/m on the ensemble members $x1, \ldots, x_m \in R_d$, and the "energy score" is defined as:

$$ES(P_{ens}, x) = \frac{1}{m}\sum_{j=1}^{m} \| x_j - x \| - \frac{1}{2m^2}\sum_{i=1}^{m}\sum_{j=1} m \| x_i - x_j \| \tag{14.12}$$

If $P = \delta\mu$ is the point measure in $\mu \in R_d$, that is, a deterministic forecast, the energy score reduces to

$$ES(\delta\mu, x) = \| \mu - x \| \tag{14.13}$$

Thus, the energy score provides a direct way of comparing deterministic forecasts, discrete ensemble forecasts and density forecasts using a single metric that is proper[2] If such closed form expressions for the expectations in (14.13) are unavailable, as is often the case for density forecasts, it is recommended to employ Monte Carlo methods [48].

14.3.2.2 Logarithmic and variogram scoring rules

In addition to CRPS, other recently investigated scoring rules for probabilistic forecasts in the energy sector are the Logarithmic Score (LogS) and Variogram Score (VarS). Details of these scores, examples of basic calculations and suggestions for software implementations can be found in Bjerregård, Møller and Madsen [54], where the authors also distinguish forecasting evaluation for energy systems between univariate and multivariate forecasts.

A forecast is considered multivariate, when it consists of multiple variables, which typically refer to multiple time-steps, multiple sites or multiple parameters. Obviously, for multivariate and multi time-step forecasts the errors typically show some inertia or auto-correlation,[3] and a proper modeling of these auto-correlation is important for many applications, such as use of battery facilities associated with wind farms.

[2] Defined here according to [48]: A proper scoring rule is designed such that it does not provide any incentive to the forecaster to digress from the true beliefs of the forecaster's best judgment.

[3] Representation of the degree of similarity between a given time series and a lagged version of itself over successive time intervals.

Also, with these more sophisticated metrics, it has become clear and can be considered a common understanding [48,54] that no scoring rule performs optimally in all aspects. A proper evaluation of multivariate forecasts is mainly of interest when the auto-correlation structure of the forecast is assumed to be important, i.e. a high degree of similarity between a given time series and a lagged version of itself over successive time intervals. Such multivariate forecasts can be evaluated using the VarS score [54]. However, in energy systems it is often crucial to have well-calibrated univariate forecasts, and these have to be evaluated by applying the univariate LogS or CRPS score.

14.3.3 Reliability measures

There are a number of reliability measures that assess the same attribute: the agreement between forecasted probabilities and observed frequencies.

The differences and similarities among these metrics and diagrams are explained and discussed in the following sections, so that the use and benefits of combining some of these measures become clear.

It is also worth noting that the CAL term in the Brier Score (BS) is basically a quantification of what is seen in these diagrams.

14.3.3.1 Rank histogram

Rank histograms measure the consistency and reliability and assume that the observation is statistically indistinguishable from the ensemble members.

The rank histograms are developed by ranking the N ensemble members from lowest to highest and identifying the rank of observation with respect to the forecasts (see Fig. 14.2). Fig. 14.3 show typical distributions and their characteristics with respect to their skill.

Hamill [43] summarized the rank histogram as "a tool for evaluating the reliability of ensemble forecasts. Errors in the mean and spread of the ensemble can be diagnosed with the rank histogram. Uncritical use of rank histograms, however, can lead to misinterpretations of the qualities of that ensemble". The following are a number of potential problems that should be considered when evaluating rank histograms that Hamill [43] pointed out:

- A flat rank histogram does not necessarily indicate reliability of the ensemble. A flat rank histogram can still be generated from ensembles with different conditional biases, or by non-random sampling of a different probability distribution than that from which the truth is drawn".

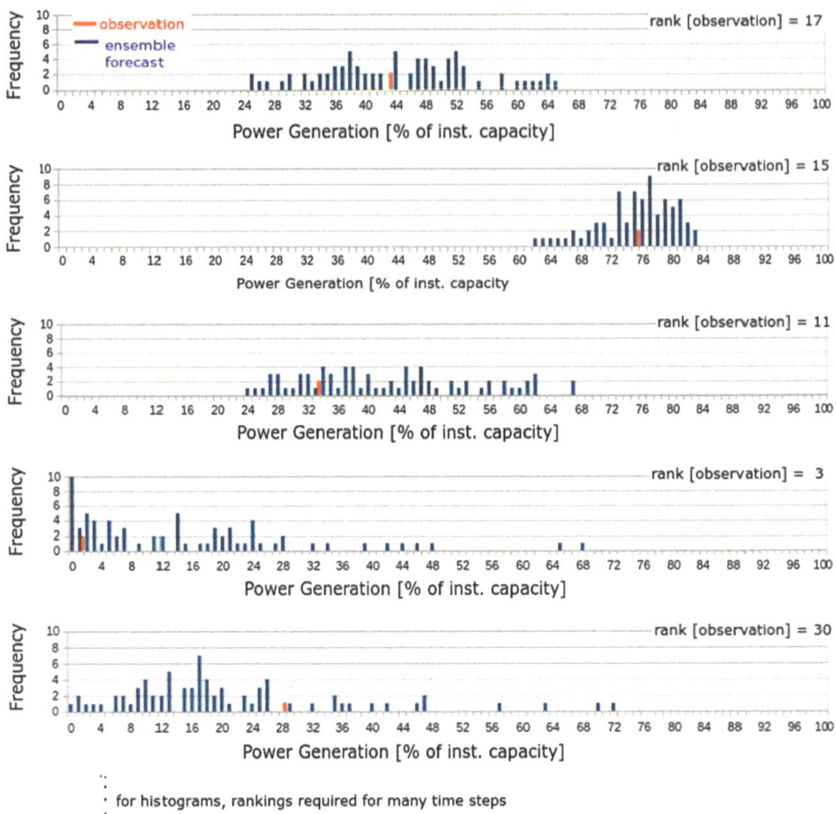

Figure 14.2 Schematic of how to generate a rank histogram from 75 ensemble forecasts and observations. The frequency is higher than 1 if more than one ensemble forecast was within this power generation value. To generate a histogram, a ranking in each of many time steps is required.

- A flat rank histogram may also indicate that the ensemble is correctly specifying the variance at a grid point, but covariances may still be misspecified. This can be checked somewhat by generating rank histograms for differences between values at different grid points or by using other diagnostics such as the minimal spanning tree.
- A U-shaped rank histogram, commonly understood as indicating a lack of variability in the ensemble, can also be a sign of conditional biases. If possible, rank histograms for subpopulations should be generated to determine if the shape varies from one to the next; this can provide some perspective on whether the U shape indicates conditional biases or under-variability.

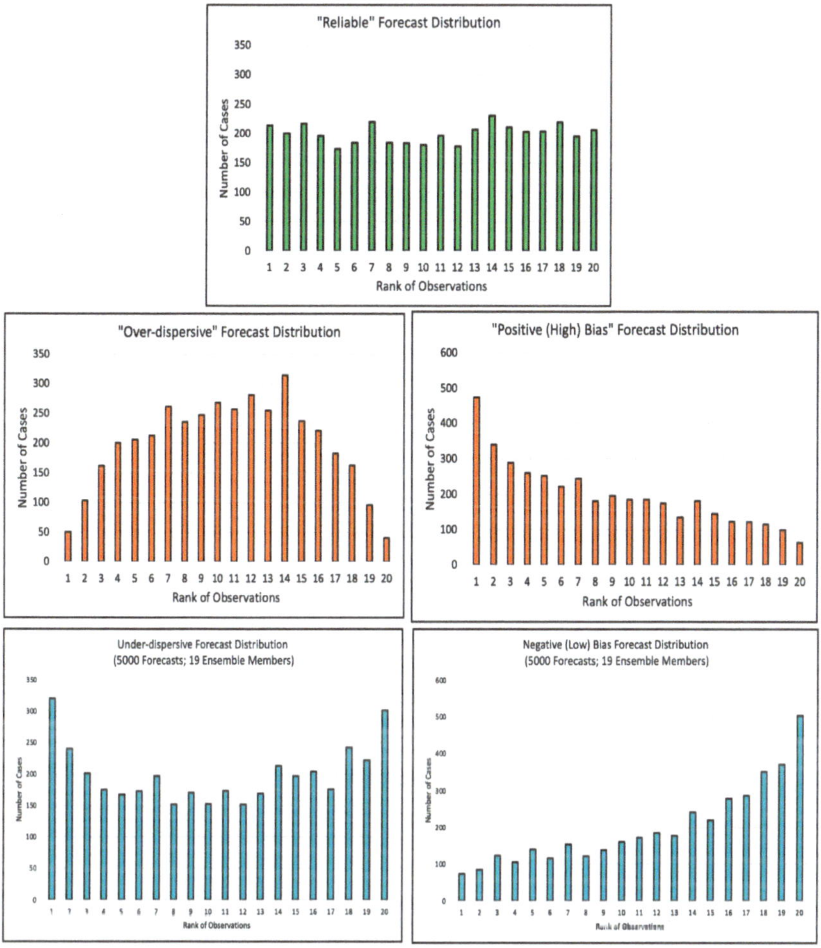

Figure 14.3 Examples of rank histograms with different attributes, generated from 4000 synthetic generated forecasts of 19 ensemble members. The top graph shows a well calibrated ensemble, which the red histograms show ensemble forecast that are over-dispersive (left) or with a positive BIAS (right) and the blue graphs show ensemble forecasts that are under-dispersive (left) and with a negative BIAS (right).

- Imperfect observations are commonly used for the verification value in generating the rank histogram. Observational errors, if not accounted for, may affect the shape of the rank histogram; the larger the error, the more U-shaped the rank histogram will appear, even if the ensemble is reliable. If observational error characteristics are known, this can be dealt with by adding random noise to each ensemble member, consistent with the observational error statistics.

- If a statistical hypothesis test is to be performed to test for uniformity, then samples used to populate the rank histogram must be located far enough away from each other in time and space to be considered independent.

14.3.3.2 Reliability (calibration) diagram

The reliability (calibration) diagrams tell how well predicted probabilities of an event correspond to their observed frequencies and provide insight into how well calibrated a probabilistic forecast is and is a complementary tool to the Brier scores (14.3.1) and the Relative Operating Characteristics (ROC) curve (14.3.4).

The reliability diagram plots the observed frequency against the forecast probability, where the range of forecast probabilities is divided into K bins (for example, 0–5%, 5–15%, 15–25%, etc.). The sample size in each bin is often included as a histogram or values beside the data points [61].

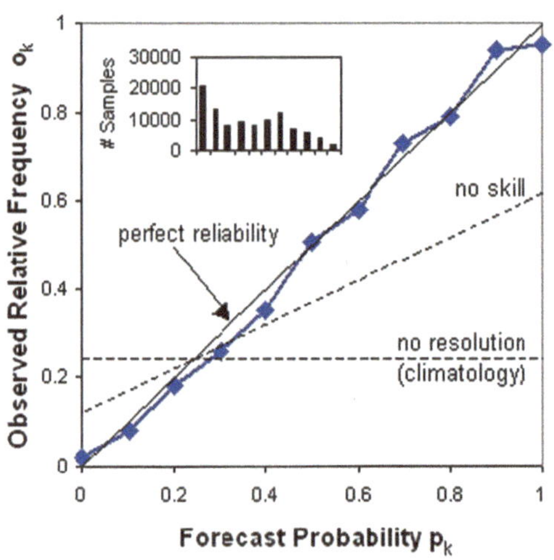

Figure 14.4 Connection between rank histograms and reliability diagrams. Figure from [61], created by Beth Ebert, Bureau of Meteorology, Australia under the Creative Commons Attribution 4.0 International license [62].

The characteristics of the reliability are indicated by the proximity of the plotted curve to the diagonal. The deviation from the diagonal gives the conditional bias. If the curve lies below the line, this indicates overforecasting (probabilities too high); points above the line indicate underforecasting (probabilities too low). The flatter the curve in the reliability diagram, the less resolution it has. A forecast of climatology does not dis-

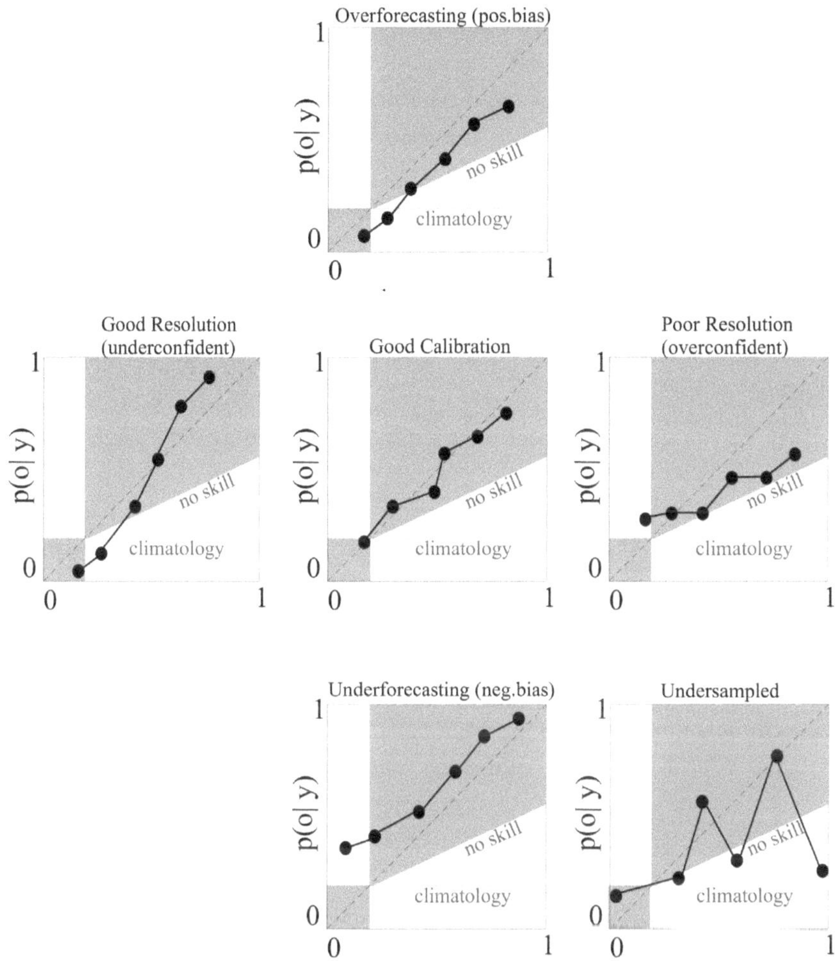

Figure 14.5 Examples of reliability diagrams. The left upper and lower figure correspond to the histograms for over- and under-dispersive distributions in Fig. 14.3. The horizontal line indicates no resolution (climatology), the unity line is perfect reliability, the gray line separates no resolution from no skill. Reproduced with modifications from Wilks [63] with permission from Elsevier.

criminate at all between events and non-events, and thus has no resolution. Points between the "no skill" line and the diagonal contribute positively to the Brier skill score. The frequency of forecasts in each probability bin (shown in the histogram) shows the sharpness of the forecast [61]. Fig. 14.4 show this principle and Fig. 14.5 show typical examples of reliability diagrams for various forecast flaws.

The reliability diagram is conditioned on the forecasts (i.e., given that an event was predicted, what was the outcome?), and can be expected to give information on the real meaning of the forecast. It is a good partner to the ROC, which is conditioned on the observations. Some users may find a reliability table (table of observed relative frequency associated with each forecast probability) easier to understand than a reliability diagram.

14.3.4 Event discrimination ability: relative operating characteristic (ROC)

This metric assesses a probabilistic forecast's ability to predict the occurrence/non-occurrence of events and can be used to compare forecasts, ratings of risk (e.g. low, medium, high) or probabilities of event occurrence [39].

The *ROC* diagram depicts the performance of forecasts at different probability thresholds. One important aspect of the ROC is that it ignores calibration of the forecasts, i.e. the relationship between estimated probability and relative frequency [39,40]. That means, a poorly calibrated forecast will not be penalized by the ROC. Thus, it is important to pair the ROC evaluation with an evaluation of forecast calibration, such as the calibration diagram described in the previous section.

The ROC is based on computing two categorical statistics (see 15.1):

1. True Positive Rate (TPR) also known as the Probability of Detection (POD), Hit Rate (HR), recall or sensitivity.
2. False Positive Rate (FPR) also known as the False Alarm Rate (FAR).

The ROC curve is created by plotting the true positive rate (TPR) versus the false positive rate (FPR) over a range of thresholds. The false-positive rate can also be calculated as (1−*specificity*) [40,41].

Fig. 14.6 depicts examples of ROC curves. The orange line represents a forecasting system with little skill, the green depicts moderate (better) skill and the blue line a forecasting system with relatively high skill.

As shown in Fig. 14.6, when the ROC curve falls below the diagonal line the forecasts are random classifiers, or in other words have no skill according to this metric. The blue line shows a good, or better forecast skill, where the curve is pushed up towards in the upper left corner (TPR = 1.0). The area under the ROC curve provides a useful measure of forecast skill [41].

It can also be thought of as a plot of the power as a function of the Type I Error of the decision rule (when the performance is calculated from

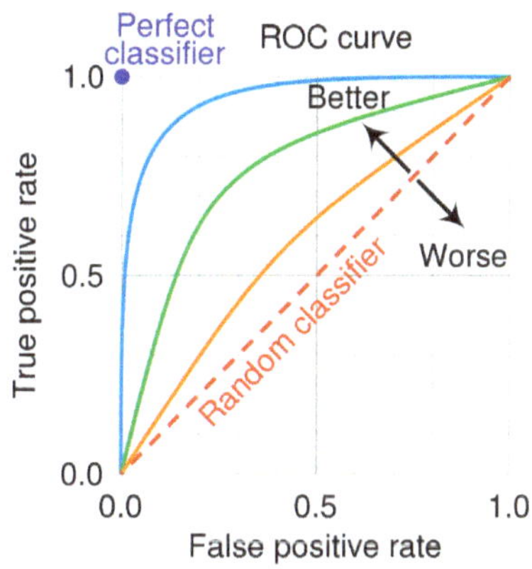

Figure 14.6 Example of a "Relative Operating Curve" (ROC) curve – image by Martin Thoma from Wikipedia [41] under the Creative Commons Attribution 4.0 International license [62].

just a sample of the population, it can be thought of as estimators of these quantities).

The ROC curve is thus the sensitivity or recall as a function of fall-out.

In general, if the probability distributions for both detection and false alarm are known, the ROC curve can be generated by plotting the cumulative distribution function (area under the probability distribution from $-\infty$ to the discrimination threshold) of the detection probability in the y-axis versus the cumulative distribution function of the false-alarm probability on the x-axis [41].

14.3.5 Uncertainty in forecasts: Rény entropy

General forecast metrics such as MAE and RMSE do not measure the uncertainty of the forecast and are only considered unbiased, if the error distribution is Gaussian, which is seldom the case. In order to define this, and compare it with uncertainty forecasts, it is recommended to use the Rény entropy, defined as the variation of wind or solar forecast errors in a specified time period [51].

The Rényi entropy is defined as:

$$H_\alpha(X) = \frac{1}{1-\alpha} log_2 \sum_{i=1}^{n} p_i^\alpha$$

where α (where $\alpha > 0$ and $\alpha \neq 1$) is the order of the Rényi entropy, which enables the creation of a spectrum of Rényi entropies with p_i being the probability density of the i discrete section of the distribution. Large values of α favor higher probability events, while smaller values of α weigh all instances more evenly. The value of α is specified by the metric user.

14.4. Metric-based forecast optimization

Once the most important attributes of a forecasting system and an evaluation metric or matrix have been specified, it may be possible to optimize the forecasting system to have desirable properties. Many forecasting solutions are optimized (also referred to as "tuned") for specific performance criteria either at the post-processing stage (conversion of weather forecasts to power forecasts) or even in the numerical weather models themselves. For example, many statistical post-processing techniques allow the user to specify whether to minimize (root) mean squared error or mean absolute error. The former is implicit in *ordinary least squares*, a widely used method for estimating the parameters of linear models or methods that are based on maximum likelihood estimation assuming Gaussian (or 'Normally') distributed errors. The latter has no closed form solution for estimating linear models, and requires the application of numerical methods to solve.

It is recommended that the desired properties of a forecasting solution be considered from the outset and communicated to those responsible for the solution's development and implementation [4].

14.5. Post-processing of ensemble forecasts

The output from ensemble forecasts is often post-processed to statistically adjust the attributes of the probabilistic forecasts derived from the ensemble members (e.g. remove bias, calibrate the probabilities etc.) and also to calculate derived forecast variables (e.g. the power production) that are not part of the raw ensemble variable set.

Although post-processing is not an evaluation method, verification methods are used to "process" or "calibrate" an ensemble and thereby can be an essential part of applying an ensemble forecast for specific tasks. In [64] statistical post-processing of ensemble forecasts are discussed in a comprehensive way with useful information and guidelines on how to carry out post-processing in support of renewable energy applications, how to post-process long-range forecasts from months to decades and how to evaluate the post-processed ensemble data. One chapter [53] provides guidelines and software code in the R programming language in order to assist developers, researchers and end-users to implement post-processing. The code project is publicly available and is recommended as a useful implementation of state-of-the-art methodologies. It also includes examples for the verification of probabilistic and ensemble forecasts as discussed in this chapter.

The following verification example verification methods are provided in [65]:

- scatter plots
- rank histogram (see 14.3.3.1)
- spread skill relationship.

CHAPTER FIFTEEN

Best practice recommendations for forecast evaluation

Key points

The recommendations in this section are based on the idea that the verification framework or scoring rules chosen to evaluate forecasts shall assist end-users and forecast providers in the determination of which aspects of the forecast should be the focus of forecast improvement efforts. To achieve this, the following set of principles shall be considered:

- Verification is subjective
  it is important to understand the limitations of a chosen metric
- Every verification has an inherent uncertainty
  due to its dependence on the evaluation data set
- Evaluation should contain a set of metrics or scoring rules (framework)
  in order to measure a range of forecast performance attributes
- Evaluation should reflect a "cost function"
  i.e. the metric combinations should provide an estimate of the value of the solution

Example code for evaluation, verification and validation can be found in Appendix G.

In this chapter, the principles developed in the previous chapters are brought to the application level. This means that the somewhat theoretical considerations from the previous chapters are now applied to real-world problems. In chapter 12, the concept of forecast evaluation uncertainty was introduced with the three attributes "representative", "significant" and "relevant" to help users understand the major sources of the evaluation uncertainty and thereby provide guidance on how to minimize it. The following chapter 13, introduced the concept of measurement uncertainty with the associated uncertainty in the evaluation process and how to minimize the errors in the evaluation due to this type of uncertainty. In the previous chapter 14 the performance assessment was described in general terms with examples that are relevant for all types of evaluation in the power sector.

IEA Wind Recommended Practice for the Implementation of Renewable Energy Forecasting Solutions
https://doi.org/10.1016/B978-0-44-318681-3.00027-1

15.1. Developing an evaluation framework

Key points

The construction of a comprehensive evaluation framework is an alternative to a one-metric forecast evaluation approach and can be an effective way to mitigate the "relevance" issues associated with the tuning (optimization) of forecasts to target metrics that are not optimal indicators of value for an end user's application.

Example code for evaluation, verification and validation can be found in Appendix G.

The "typical forecasting task" considered in this section is defined as forecasts generated to fulfill operational obligations in electric system operation or the trading and balancing of renewable energy in power markets. There are certainly many other tasks and applications of weather and power forecasts in the energy industry that can also benefit from the following best practice recommendations. However, the primary target for the following recommendations is the evaluation of forecasts for these particular applications. In this section we define the evaluation framework and its components and considerations. Section 15.2 deals with the evaluation to maximize value from operational forecasts, section 15.3 with the evaluation of trials and benchmarks and in the use cases section 15.4 there are example evaluations for energy trading and balancing, power ramps and reserve allocation.

15.1.1 Scoring rules for comparison of forecast types

Over the past decade, a common practice in industry had been to request 'some' forecast, and then evaluate the forecaster(s) by using 'some' (set of) scoring function(s), which is not a very meaningful endeavor [66]. In various studies that address the issue of the fair and appropriate evaluation of forecasts (e.g. [66–70]), it is argued that effective forecasting depends on 'guidance' or 'directives' that should be supplied to the forecaster. It is noted that the forecaster(s) should receive two of the three directives:

1. disclosure of the scoring function a priori
2. request of a specific functional of the forecaster's predictive distribution, such as the mean or a quantile
3. the forecaster is rewarded for skilled forecasts and no advantage is permitted to an unskilled strategy.

When designing an evaluation framework, the following guidelines should therefore be considered:

Scoring Rules as Summary Measure ("cost/loss functions")

Scoring rules for the evaluation of deterministic or probabilistic forecasts can be defined as summary measures by which a numerical score based on the predictive distribution and the event or value that materializes (i.e. the outcome) is assigned [48]. In this sense, scoring rules are negatively oriented penalties that a forecaster wishes to minimize and are often also referred to as "loss functions".

Proper Scoring Rules

A scoring rule also needs to be proper which means that a forecaster maximizes the expected score for an observation drawn from the distribution F, if the forecaster issues the probabilistic forecast F, rather than $G \neq F$. In prediction problems, proper scoring rules encourage the forecaster to make careful assessments and to be honest. In estimation problems, strictly proper scoring rules provide attractive loss and utility functions that can be tailored to the problem at hand [37], [66].

Significance in Evaluation

In recent years, where the possibilities for more profound evaluations, also due to more available open source software (see Appendix G), have become possible, a common understanding has been established (e.g. [37], [49], [48], [50], [54]) that no single scoring rule performs optimally in all aspects. The end-user therefore needs to determine which aspects of the forecast should be the focus of forecast improvement efforts over time.

If there is more than one aspect to consider, or even contradicting aspects due to the use of one forecast for different applications, a framework will:

1. assist in identifying contradicting forecast performance objectives
2. allow giving weight to different forecast aspects for an overall evaluation.

With the energy score described in section 14.3.5, it is also possible to directly compare deterministic forecasts, discrete ensemble forecasts and density forecasts using a single metric that is proper.

15.1.2 Forecast and forecast error analysis

In this discussion, forecast errors are defined as forecast minus observation (*fc – obs*). Errors in forecasting are inevitable. The primary objective is, of course, to minimize the magnitude of the error. However, a secondary objective may be to shape the error distribution in ways that are beneficial to a specific application. A direct and deep analysis of the prediction errors can provide considerable insight into the characteristics of forecast performance as well as information that can allow users to differentiate situations in which forecasts are likely to be trustworthy from those that are likely to produce large errors.

The construction of a frequency distribution of errors (also referred to as density functions or probability density functions) is an effective way to obtain insight about forecast error patterns. These are created by sorting errors and visualizing their distribution as e.g.,

- (probability) density function/curve
- histogram (frequency bars) (see sec. 15.1.3.3 and 14.3.3.1)
- box plot (see sec. 15.1.3.2).

All of these chart types show the same basic information but with different degrees of detail. Density curves provide the most detail since they depict the full probability density function of the forecast errors. Histograms provide an intermediate level of detail by showing the frequency of a specified number of error categories. Box plots condense this information into several quantiles (see 15.1.3.2). Errors of a well calibrated forecast model should always be scattered around zero. A frequency distribution that has a center, that is shifted from zero indicates a systematic error (also known as a bias).

For power forecasts one will often see positively skewed error distributions, which are due to the shape of the power curve which has flat parts below the cut-in wind speed and at wind speeds that produce the rated power production. The skewed distribution is often the result of the fact that forecasts close to zero cannot have large negative errors. The inverse is true for forecasts of near rated power (i.e. large positive errors cannot occur) but forecasts of rated power are often less frequent than near zero forecasts and hence have less impact on the error distribution.

15.1.3 Choice of deterministic verification methods

As noted previously, there is not a single best metric that can be effectively used for all applications. The definition of "best metric" highly depends on the user's intended application and should be based on a quantification of the sensitivity of a user's application to forecast error. For example, if a user has to pay a penalty for forecast errors that are proportional to the squared error, a mean squared error metric is well suited as an error metric for that application.

However, if the penalty is proportional to the absolute error, a mean absolute error metric would be a better choice. If the user is interested in predictions of specific events such as high wind shutdown or large wind ramps, the mean squared or absolute error metrics are not good choices, because they do not provide any information about the ability of a forecast to predict these events due to their averaging characteristics. In this case, an event-based metric should be employed. An example of this type of metric is the critical success index (CSI), which measures the ratio of correct event forecasts to the total number of forecasted and observed events.

"Loss function":

In order to get forecast performance information that is relevant for a user's application, it is crucial to carefully select the evaluation metrics and ideally they should be based on the so-called "loss function" for the user's application. The "loss function" is also often referred to as a "cost function", especially when related to costs that can be associated with specific forecast errors. Conceptually, a well-formulated "loss" or "cost" function measures the sensitivity of a user's application to forecast error. If one forecast is used for different applications with different loss functions, a set of metrics should be derived. If a single metric is desired, then a composite metric can be constructed by weighting the individual application-based metrics by the relative importance. More details on how to develop such loss functions and evaluation matrices can be found in 15.1.5.

15.1.3.1 Dichotomous event evaluation

One may quantify desirable qualities of a forecast by considering a range of dichotomous (yes/no) events, such as high-speed shut-down or ramps. A forecast might imply that "yes, a large ramp will happen" and trigger the user to take action, but the ability of a forecasting system to make such predictions is not clear from the average error metrics. Therefore, one should employ a quantitative verification approach to assess this ability by analyzing the number of correct positive, false positive, correct negative and false negative predictions of particular events [69], [59]. Table 15.1 provides an example table to carry out such categorical evaluations.

Recommendation for applications with (Extreme) Event Analyzes:

Categorical statistics can be computed from such a yes/no contingency table. The list below is an excerpt of a comprehensive list of categorical statistical tests published by the Joint World Weather Research Program (WWRP) and Working Group Numerical Experimentation on Forecast

Table 15.1 Example of a dichotomous evaluation table.

		Observations	
		YES	**NO**
Forecast	YES	a correct event forecast	b false alarm
	NO	c surprise events	d no events

Verification (WGNE) and provides the most commonly used metrics and their characteristics that are relevant for forecast applications in the power industry. Details, equations, a more comprehensive explanation on their use as well as references can be found (online) in [59]. It is recommended to apply these categorical statistics in particular for applications, where standard "typical error" metrics do not provide a measure of the true skill of a forecast to predict a specific event. In renewable power forecasting applications this is particularly important for extreme event analysis, ramp events, and high-speed wind turbine shutdown forecasting, etc. In such applications, it is important to distinguish between *quality of a forecast* (the degree of agreement between the forecasted and observed conditions according to some objective or subjective criteria) and *value of a forecast* (the degree to which the forecast information helps a user to achieve an application objective such as improved decision-making). Wilks [71] and Richardson [72] present concepts for the value versus skill for deterministic and probabilistic forecast evaluation of that type, respectively. See Table 15.2.

15.1.3.2 Analyzing forecast error spread with box and wiskers plots

The box-and-whiskers plot is a visualization tool to analyze forecast performance in terms of the error spread when comparing forecasts with different attributes such as forecast time horizons, vendors, methodologies. Fig. 15.1 shows the principle of a box and whiskers plot. This type of charts can be used to illustrate the spread of forecast performance in each hour of the day-ahead horizon. It can also show that some forecasts in some hours have very low errors compared to the average error in that hour, as well as occasionally very high errors. In section 15.2.4.1, a use case for the application of box plots is demonstrated to verify significance of results.

Table 15.2 Concepts for categorical statistics that distinguish value versus skill for deterministic and probabilistic forecast evaluation according to Wilks [71] and Richardson [72].

Attribute	Answers the Question	Range	Perfect Score
Accuracy	Overall, what fraction of the forecasts were correct? Limitation: misleading as heavily influenced by "no events"	$0-1$	1
Bias score	How did the forecast frequency of "yes" events compare to the observed frequency of "yes" events? Limitation: measured only relative frequency	$0-1$	1
Probability of detection (POD)	What fraction of the observed "yes" events were correctly forecast? (important component for ROC) Limitation: ignores false alarms, is sensitive to climatological frequency of events	$0-1$	1
False alarm ratio (FAR)	What fraction of the predicted "yes" events actually did not occur (i.e., were false alarms)? Limitation: ignores misses, is sensitive to climatological frequency of events	$0-1$	0
Probability of false detection (POFD)	What fraction of the observed "no" events were incorrectly forecast as "yes"? (important component for ROC) Limitation: ignores misses	$0-1$	0
Success ratio	What fraction of the forecast "yes" events were correctly observed? (plotted against POD in categorical performance diagram) Limitation: ignores misses	$0-1$	1
Relative value curve (versus skill) for deterministic forecast	For a cost/loss ratio C/L for taking action based on a forecast, what is the relative improvement in economic value between climatological and perfect information? Limitation: not comparable, cost/loss ratio is different for different users	$-1-1$	1

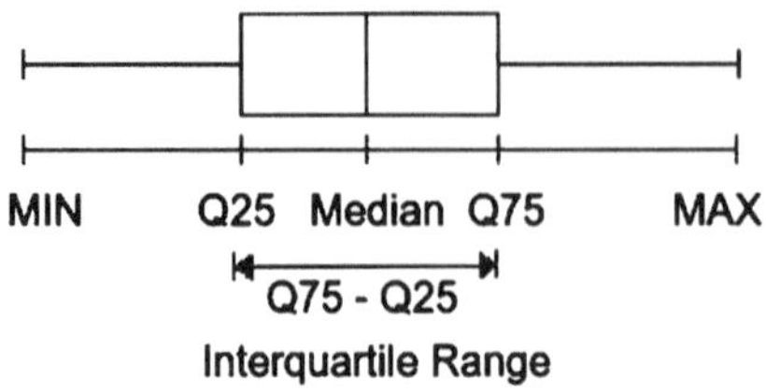

Figure 15.1 Principle of a box-and whiskers plot. The plot displays a five-number summary of a set of data, which is the minimum, first quartile, median, third quartile, and maximum. In a box plot, a box from the first quartile to the third quartile is drawn to indicate the interquartile range. A vertical line goes through the box at the median.

15.1.3.3 Visualizing the error frequency distribution with histograms

Histograms allow one to (1) quantify the frequency of occurrence of errors below or above a specified level or (2) visualize the forecast error distribution for specified error ranges. In case (1) a graphical or tabular presentation can be directly used to derive a metric that indicates that errors are less than x% of the installed capacity in y% of the time. In this way, histograms function as a metric providing the percentage of time that errors are within a specified margin [47]. In case (2) the error distribution of a forecast can be derived from the graphical or tabular presentation of the histogram information. This enables an easy identification of the frequencies of large errors and provides the possibility to analyze and possibly modify the forecast system to minimize these errors. In summary, histograms visualize two main attributes:

- Robustness of a forecast
- Large Errors in an error distribution

In [47] an example can be found for the way histograms help to interpret statistical results and error distributions. In their example, they directly determined that a 1 hour-ahead prediction contained errors less than 7.5% of the available capacity in 68% of the time, while a 24 hour-ahead prediction showed errors of that size only in 24% of the time. For large errors, they determined from the histogram that the same 1 hour-ahead prediction's largest errors were 17.5% of available capacity in only 3% of the time.

Fig. 15.2 provides two example histograms with typical frequency distribution of errors for a 2-hour forecast horizon (left) and a day-ahead horizon (right) as described in [47].

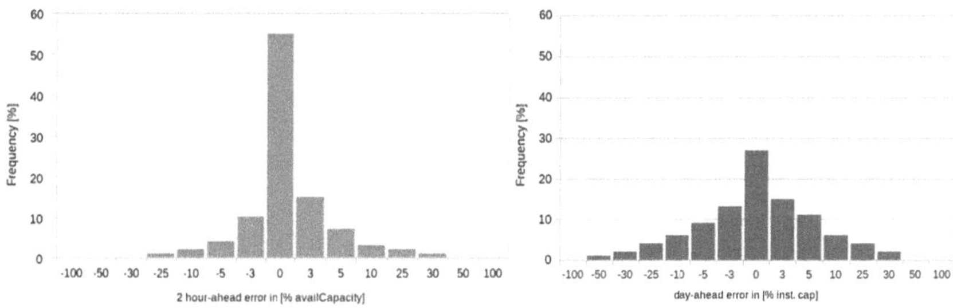

Figure 15.2 Examples of two histograms showing typical frequency distribution of errors for a 2-hour forecast horizon (left) and a day-ahead horizon (right).

Recommendation: If the application requires that specified error sizes should occur less than a certain, specified percentage of the time, a histogram analysis should be used to directly identify, whether or not a forecast's performance fulfills the specified criteria.

15.1.4 Specific probabilistic forecast verification

As in the case of the verification of deterministic forecasts, it is recommended that multiple verification scores be employed for the evaluation of probabilistic forecasts. A well-chosen set of probabilistic forecast evaluation metrics will provide an indication of several key aspects of forecast skill and value, and thus provide a more comprehensive representation of forecast performance than a single metric.

This also holds for more complex metrics such as the "Logarithmic Scores" (LogS) or "Variogram Scores" (VarS) (see section 14.3 and 14.3.2.2), when the so-called auto-correlation structure[1] of multivariate[2] forecasts is assumed to be important, or in energy systems, where it may be crucial to have well-calibrated univariate forecasts. These can then, for example, be evaluated by applying the univariate *LogS* or CRPS score to all the marginal densities, and depending on whether the shapes of the tails are considered important, a *LogS* could additionally be used or if not, a CRPS may additionally be more appropriate [54].

In the optimal case, the verification framework or scoring rules assist users and forecast providers in the determination of which aspects of the forecast should be the focus of forecast improvement efforts.

[1] Representation of the degree of similarity between a given time series and a lagged version of itself over successive time intervals.

[2] Consisting of multiple variables, which typically refer to multiple time-steps, multiple sites or multiple parameters.

An evaluation of probabilistic forecasts should ideally be made of three components:

1. a metric that measures overall quality (discrimination and calibration together), such as the Brier Score (BS) or Ranked Probability Score (RPS)
2. a metric that measures discrimination alone, such as the ROC
3. a metric or chart that provides an indication of the reliability (calibration) such as the ranked histogram, reliability diagram or CAL component of the Brier Score.

This combination of metrics will provide a broad perspective on forecast performance and can also assist in the identification of forecast performance issues. For example, when discrimination is good, but calibration (biases) issues are degrading the overall quality, a reliability diagram can reveal the nature of the calibration problems [73]. The next subsection provides some guidance on the choice of metrics for specific applications.

Details about how to compute or construct each of these metrics and diagrams can be found in section 14.3 and example code for evaluation, verification and validation can be found in Appendix G.

15.1.4.1 Choice of application for benchmarking probabilistic forecasts

Table 15.3 shows the most common application examples and corresponding recommended evaluation metrics. Note, that in Table 15.3, a number of scoring rules are used that are not directly measurable and are part of other scoring rules. These are explained in detail in section 14.3 and Appendix F and are briefly translated, explained and referenced in the following list:

- Sharpness – is a forecast attribute and property: the ability of the forecast to predict extreme probability values (i.e. near 0% or 100%) and is essentially a representation of the estimated forecast uncertainty. Its opposite is often a climatology or a persistence forecast. Forecast probabilities should be well distributed, or the spread be "refined", i.e. in large spread forecasts have the potential to cover a broad range of conditions. A narrow spread indicates a lack of refinement (see e.g. [57], [50] p.256ff). In the reliability diagram the sharpness can be identified in relation to a perfect calibration (see Fig. 14.5).
- Reliability – can be measured in the Brier Scores (see section 14.3.1 in Part 3 or [32]), the *Reliability diagram* and the *Relative Operating Characteristics (ROC) curve* [39] and answers the question on how well the

predicted probabilities of an event correspond to their observed frequencies [52].

- Calibration – can be measured in the Brier Score [32], *reliability diagram*, *rank histogram* or the CRPS 14.3.2.1 and refers to the statistical consistency between the distributional forecasts and the observations and is a joint property of the predictions and the observed values [37].
- Quantile scores – is a Brier Score [32]) for quantiles derived from a probabilistic forecast (e.g. [74]).

The "uncertainty method" numbers in Table 15.3 are taken from Fig. 3.2 in Part 1 of this Recommended Practice, which describes the standard methods of uncertainty forecast generation and are defined as follows:

1. **Statistical Methods to generate probabilistic Forecasts:**
   These methods generate probabilistic forecasts by applying statistical methods to a deterministic forecast by modeling the dependency of forecast errors in space or time.
   These include, but are not limited to, probability density functions (PDF), multi-dimensional distributions, kernel density estimation [75], space-time structures from analog ensembles (see e.g. [12])
2. **Spacial-temporal Statistical Scenario Forecasts**:
   These methods also generate forecasts by applying statistical methods to a deterministic forecast and modeling the dependency of forecast errors in space *and* time, i.e. a temporal and spacial dimension is modeled.
   These methods include conditional quantiles or PDFs [30], Schaake filters [76], and multi-variate predictive distribution based on (Gaussian, vine, etc.) copulas ([13,14])
3. **Physically based Ensemble Forecasts**:
   a. Physics-based ensembles – alternate formulations of model physics are employed using different physics schemes in one model (multi-scheme approach) or multiple models (multi-model approach)
   b. Initialisation of data-based ensembles – input data for a specific forecast is perturbed within the range of measurement uncertainty.

The most significant difference between the statistical methods (1) and (2) and the physics-based ensembles is that there is no physical dependency in the statistical approaches. Therefore, they are limited to representations of conditions or events contained in the historical sample that is used to statistically derive the probability distributions. In contrast, physics-based ensemble approaches are not limited to an historical precedent since they can represent any event that is physically possible.

Table 15.3 Relationship between end-user applications and recommended evaluation metrics. The Uncertainty methods are defined in section 15.1.4.1 as (1) Statistical method, (2) Spatial-temporal Statistically-based Scenario method, (3a) Physical Ensembles with multiple members, (3b) Physical Ensemble from perturbation of a deterministic forecast. The decision tasks and end-user requirements are typical for today's application and our recommendations. The evaluation metrics are recommended scores that should be combined and selected according to section Part 3 section 15.1. References are samples, not exhaustive.

Decision-Making Task	Uncertainty Method(s)	Evaluation Metric	End-User Requirements	Reference
Extreme Events (System Operation and Market bidding)	3a, 3b	Event analysis[a], Brier scores, Rank/PIT histograms, ROC, Reliability diagram, extended CRPS, Spread-Skill(Error) Relationship	High Sharpness → uncertainty forecasts needs to be spacial and temporal Uncertainty must be model generated → independent of historic data Verification with multiple test required [43,57,77]: • Distribution verification → aims to quantify general fitness to observations • Realizations verification → assess improvement over climate statistics	[39,43, 66,77,78]
(Ramping) Reserve (System Operation, Market bidding)	2, 3a	Categorial event analysis, Brier Scores, ROC, (C)RPS, Reliability diagram	High Sharpness → low reserve requirements High calibration → Adequate estimation of tails quantiles leads to accurate risk quantification Resolution → dynamic reserve requirement according to power system operating conditions	[14,79, 80]
Unit commitment (UC) and economic dispatch (ED)(System Operator)	2, 3a, 3b	Categorial event analysis, Brier Score, rank histogram, energy score	Hich Calibration → cost savings; Uncertainty adequacy dependent on ensemble method; High skill for event detection → ramping (up and down) detection skill	[78,81]

[a] Contingency table, Critical Success Index (CSI).

continued on next page

Table 15.3 *(continued)*

Decision-Making Task	Uncertainty Method(s)	Evaluation Metric	End-User Requirements	Reference
Market bidding (Market Player)	1, 2, 3a	Categorial event analysis, Brier Scores, ROC, Reliability diagram, CRPS	Maximize profit, minimize costs (cost-loss evaluation); Low sharpness → low uncertainty (reduced imbalance cost)	[17,18, 31,80,82]
Virtual power plant operation (Market Player)	2, 3a, 3b	(i) Calibration, sharpness, quantile score and CRPS (ii) Log Score, p-variogram score, energy score, value score	(i) Perfect calibration → perfect reserve reliability estimation; High sharpness → high reserve margin (ii) temporal or spatial dependence structure → proper forecast uncertainty	[31,37, 48,80]
Predictive grid management (System Operator)	3a	Event analysis, ROC, energy score, reliability diagram	High calibration → reduction of false alarms; High sharpness → low operating costs; low computational requirements	[31,37, 48]
Maintenance scheduling (Wind Farm Operator/ Market Player)	1, 3a	Calibration and sharpness; Cost-loss model under uncertainty, ROC	High Sharpness on event detection for low wind speed periods; High calibration → risk cost minimization	[37]
Long-term portfolio planning (Market Players, System Operator, Wind Farm Operator)	1, 3a, 3b	Calibration/rank, reliability and sharpness diagrams, RPSS, CRPS, Brier skill score, value score	Calibration → trustworthiness; Reliability → resolution and skill versus climatology; Sharpness → aligns predictive distributions	[31,32, 37,72]

15.1.5 Establishing a cost function or evaluation matrix

Due to the complexity of the task and the fact that the objectives of forecast users are not the same, the following section is an introduction to the concept of an evaluation framework in which structured procedures for the evaluation and verification of forecasts are established. The structure may be shortened and adapted depending on the size of the forecasting system and the importance in the overall business processes.

Best practice in this context is to follow a procedure, where the evaluation/verification reflects the importance of forecasts in the role of the business processes and provides incentives for the forecast service provider to generate forecasts that fit the specified purpose.

As a minimum requirement when establishing such an evaluation framework, the following set of procedures should be considered:

1. **Definition of the forecast framework**

   It is important to exactly define the forecast applications, the key time frames and a ranking of the relative importance of each application.

   In many cases, the value of a forecast can also simply be broken down and defined in terms of "money saved" as the most relevant verification score [31]. In many applications and for many end-users the consideration of forecast uncertainty in their decision-making can also increase the value of a forecast, especially when measured in savings. For most forecast users, two basic guidelines are:

   a. Effective (point) forecasting can only be achieved, if the scoring function(s) are specified a priori, or, if the forecaster(s) receive a directive in the form of a statistical function or metrics associated with the decision target (see e.g. [66] for example framework development)

   b. Probability forecasts have greater value than the deterministic forecasts from a higher resolution model [31]. The definition of the forecast's target (or value) is therefore essential; even a target such as "saved money" can be used to define appropriate scoring rules and evaluation metrics.

2. **Base performance evaluation on a clearly defined set of forecasts**

   The base performance should contain "typical error" metrics in order to monitor an overall performance level.

   - time frame: minimum 3 months, ideally 1 year
   - "typical error" metrics: nMAE, nRMSE, BIAS

3. **Quality assessment of the evaluation sample data**
   The detection of missing or erroneous data and a clear strategy how to deal with such missing data needs to be made at the outset of any evaluation period to ensure that verification and forecasting is fair and transparent.
4. **Specific Performance evaluation on a set of error metrics**
   - Visual Inspection
   - Use of more specific metrics:
     a. deterministic: SDE, SDBIAS, StDev, VAR, CORR
     b. probabilistic: Brier Score, ROC curve, Probability Interval Forecast Evaluation (14.3)
   - Use of histogram or boxplot for evaluation of outliers
   - Use of contingency tables for specific event analysis
   - Use of improvement scores relative to a relevant reference forecast for comparisons

Note, details on the framework and evaluation metrics can be found in [47] and [53], specific metrics and explanation of metrics can be found in [83], [84] for deterministic forecasts and for probabilistic forecast metrics in [31,35–37,45–51,53,54,59]. Significant tests can be found e.g. in [85].

15.1.5.1 Evaluation matrix

Establishing an evaluation matrix is complex, but can be straightforward if the principles of forecast uncertainty and choice of appropriate metrics are incorporated into the evaluation strategy.

Best practice for the establishment is to go through the various steps outlined in section 15.1.5 to choose the components for the evaluation framework. The core concept is to use this framework to define a formal structure and then add multiplication factors to weight each of the selected individual metrics according to their relative importance.

The matrix can be setup in a spreadsheet environment with macros or within a database environment, where all data is available and metrics may even be directly computed though the database software. The key point of the matrix is that the forecast performance results can be collected, multiplied with an "importance factor", normalized and transferred into the summary table to visualize the scores. For example the scores can be visualized with a bar chart that indicates the performance in a scale from e.g. 0 to 1 or 0 to 100 as shown in 15.3. Such a evaluation matrix provides important information in a comprehensive way and can be applied for comparisons of forecast solutions and for the analysis of the potential for forecast improvement.

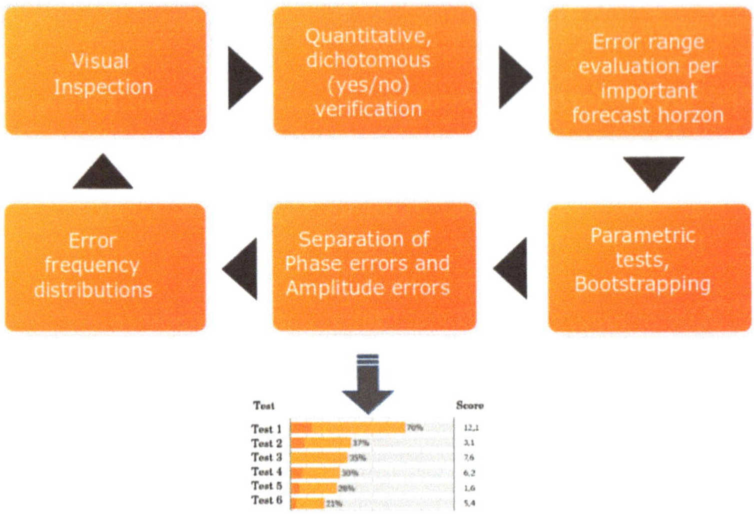

Figure 15.3 Example of an evaluation matrix that verifies forecasts with 6 test metrics and displays the scores for a holistic overview of the forecast performance.

As an example, the framework developed by Gneiting, 2011 [66] can be recommended. He further developed the perspectives of Murphy and Daan [86] and Engelberg et al. [70].

It was noted that *there has been little recognition that the common practice of requesting 'some' point forecast, and then evaluating the forecasters by using 'some' (set of) scoring function(s), is not a meaningful endeavor.*

It is therefore argued that *effective point forecasting depends on 'guidance' or 'directives', which can be given in one of two complementary ways: (1) by disclosing the scoring function ex ante to the forecaster, or (2) by requesting a specific functional of the forecaster's predictive distribution, such as the mean or a quantile.*

15.2. Operational forecast value maximization

Key points

- Once operational forecasts have been established it is important to monitor the quality of generation facility data supplied to the forecast system(s) and used for forecast evaluation; often attention to this diminishes after a benchmark is completed (see section 15.2.1, 12.1.2, 13.3, 13.4)
- Ongoing "deep analysis" of forecast performance and effective provider and user communication is critical for maintaining and refining forecast performance (see section 15.1)
- Focus should be on maximizing forecast value for the application and not on maximizing performance of standard metrics; this may include identifying or refining the "cost" function for a user's application and/or working with the provider to optimize forecasts for the application(s) (see section 15.1.5 and e.g. [31,66])
- A plan should be developed to motivate and reward providers to continually refine forecast methods and adapt new approaches from the latest research; this may include financial incentive schemes (see section 15.2.5)
- Maintaining forecast performance at a state-of-the-art level is an important objective for any end-user, but especially for those with complex IT infrastructure systems or multiple suppliers of forecasts that are bound to statistically consistent forecasts over a period of time for highest performance.

This Section outlines how analysis, diagnostics and evaluation of improvements need to be structured in order to ensure sustained improvement and maximization of forecast value over time without radical changes in existing infrastructures and the typical pitfalls associated with such evaluations.

Operational forecasts should be evaluated in the context of their end-use. Different use cases will have different cost functions, some of which may be complex or virtually impossible to define. Organizations evaluate operational forecasts for a variety of reasons and on a wide range of scales, from individual wind farms to entire fleets, and from short lead times to horizons spanning several days.

Simple evaluation metrics such as MAE or RMSE can be used to get an overview of general forecast performance and to provide an indication of forecast performance for decisions with (symmetric) linear or quadratic loss functions, respectively. However, in most cases, the true cost of wind power forecast errors will be more complex and depend on externalities.

Systematic evaluation of operational forecasts is however an important business function for forecast users. Whether this is monitoring the quality of the forecasts produced in-house or procured from vendors, regular evaluation supports continuous improvement in forecast performance and end-use. This section provides a guide to the best practices in evaluation of operational forecasts. It begins by reviewing common motivations for continuous and periodic evaluation of operational forecasts, and then discusses different evaluation paradigms for specific use-cases.

15.2.1 Performance monitoring

Continuous monitoring of forecast performance is considered best practice because it develops an understanding of forecast capability and identifies issues with raw forecast data or its processing. While failure of forecasting systems is extremely rare, weather models, IT systems, and the forecast target (e.g. individual wind farm, portfolio of wind farms, national wind output) are constantly evolving. This has the potential to introduce new and unforeseen sources of error.

15.2.1.1 Importance of performance monitoring for different time periods

Short Periods (monthly): While error metrics or contingency tables calculated over short periods do not provide reliable measures of overall performance they can provide an indication of problems with a forecasting system and large errors should be logged and investigated. Abrupt changes in forecast performance can result from errors in data processing, such as incorrect availability information during maintenance.

Long Periods (> 6 months): Changes in performance over longer time scales may be a result of changes to a supplier's numerical weather model(s) or changes in the behavior of wind power plant as they age. Slow changes may be more difficult to detect, but over time can accumulate significant biases which should also be investigated.

For both cases, it is necessary to dis-aggregate forecast metrics to identify some sources of error. Important factors to consider when dis-aggregating errors are to include lead-time, time of day, power level and weather type.

Regular reporting and tracking of forecast performance over relevant periods can help foster an understanding of forecast capability across business functions and support staff and process development.

Recommendation:

- Forecasts performance should be monitored continuously to quickly identify technical problems
- Large errors should be investigated and recorded for future analysis
- Error metrics should be dis-aggregated by appropriate factors, e.g. lead-time, power level
- Regular reporting for error metrics supports forecast users' interpretation of forecast information

15.2.2 Forecast diagnostics and continuous improvement

Forecast evaluation is the first stage in identifying areas for potential improvement in forecasting systems. Periodically evaluating operational forecast performance and its impact on wider business functions can be a valuable exercise. For example, changes in the way forecasts are used, or the importance of different lead-times or variables may be a cause to change the way forecasts are produced or communicated internally.

In an operational environment, where the IT infrastructure is complex and the amount of resources required to change a forecast service provider is high relative to the likely gain in forecast performance that would be produced by such a change. Improvements in forecast skill over time in such real-time environments are difficult to measure. The improvement of forecasts may have a steep curve in the first years, or when constant changes in the system become less frequent.

However, over time, forecast performance has a limit and the rate of improvement will be reduced. This needs to be taken into account as much as the ability of a forecast solution to develop over time to maintain a state of the art character.

Nevertheless, in most cases, where a single or multiple operational forecasts are produced or supplied, regular benchmarking can add value as different services are upgraded over time or exhibit different performance characteristics.

Recommendation:

- Evaluation underpins forecast improvement and insights should be shared between forecaster(s) and end-user
- Evaluation and improvement should be driven by end-use and business value

See also Table 15.4, which is a guideline for the evaluation of forecasts and diagnostics for such improvement monitoring (see also 15.2.5).

15.2.3 Maximization of forecast value

Forecast value can be maximized by continuously monitoring and evaluating operational processes of both forecasts and measurement quality. Additionally, the use of forecasts and the interaction with other business processes should also be taken into consideration if they can impact the quality of the forecasts or the correctness and trustworthiness of the evaluation.

The use of a single metric such as a mean absolute or root mean squared error for forecast evaluation may be a way to start a process and can be helpful in identifying errors in the system that can cause unwanted costs. This is a valid and useful approach. However, it is recommended that such simplified methods be used only for monitoring purposes and not as the primary verification tool (see also chapter 12, especially sections 12.2, 12.3 and 15.1).

Recommendation: The following aspects should be taken into consideration when identifying a "loss function" or "cost function" in the selection process of performance metrics for operational forecasts. Details on some metrics can be found in the Appendix F, a comprehensive database for metrics can be accessed online [59] together with the concepts of the metrics and valuable combinations of metrics, which have also been described in more detail in section 15.1.

- **Evaluation should contain a selection of metrics, such as:**
  - One metric alone is not indicative of overall forecast performance
  - Use de-compositions of errors to identify the origin of errors. e.g. look at bias and variance alongside MAE or RMSE.
  - Selected metrics should reflect the costs of errors or security constraints to the greatest extent possible based on the user's knowledge of the application's characteristics
  - Box plots, histograms and scatter plots reveal additional important information compared to a "typical error" metric

- **Evaluation metric combinations can provide a representative approximation of a "cost function" by using:**
  - subjective evaluation through visual inspection
  - quantitative, dichotomous (yes/no) verification of critical events such as high-speed shut-down or ramps with e.g. contingency tables
  - error ranges per important forecast horizon
  - error ranges per hour of day or forecast hour
  - error frequency distributions in ranges that have different costs levels
  - separation of phase errors and amplitude errors according to their impact
  - parametric tests, bootstrapping can be used to look at individual error measures before averaging

15.2.4 Maintaining state-of-the-art performance

If expensive long-term solutions have been established it can be challenging for an end-user to ensure that state-of-the-art performance is maintained. This can be due to the stiffness of the established IT solution (see also Part 1 of this recommended practice), but also due to the fact that there is no monitoring of the performance.

Recommendation: It is recommended that performance monitoring takes place, where those forecasts that are relevant for the business processes are compared against a suitable and objective measure.

The most common measures are climatology values, persistence values or comparison to previous periods, such as the previous calendar year. Such techniques can provide motivation and can be used with a reward scheme for the forecast provider to improve forecasts with time and improved knowledge of the specific challenges and needs of the end-user's forecast problem. (see Table 15.4)

15.2.4.1 Significance test for new developments

Most forecast vendors and researchers are always seeking improvements by developing or refining existing forecast methods or investigating new technology or techniques to add value for specific forecasting applications. Whenever a new development is ready for testing, the researchers or technical staff are confronted with the question, whether the new technique outperforms the older or current state of the art. Due to time constraints, data limitations or lack of historical available forecasts or measurements, this is often a difficult question to answer.

Table 15.4 List of possible performance monitoring types for evaluation of operational forecasts, incentive scheme benchmarks, tests and trials. The types are not meant to be stand-alone and may also be combined.

Performance Measure	Comment/Recommendation
Improvement over persistence	Comparison against persistence is the same as comparing "not having a forecast" to having one. Useful measure for short-term forecasts as a mean of evaluating the improvement of applying forecast information to measurements. Note: be aware of data quality issues when evaluating, especially in the case of constant values that benefit persistence, while the forecast provides a realistic view.
Improvement over past evaluation period / forecast	If improvement is important, the comparison to a past evaluation can be useful, especially in long-term contracts. In this way, the forecaster is forced to continue to improve and the target is moved with the improvements. The payment structure however needs to incorporate the fact that improvements reduce over time and have an upper limit.
Comparison against set targets	If the required performance of a forecasting system can be defined, clear targets should be set and the payment directed according to a percentage from 0–100% of the achieved target.
Categorized error evaluation	An effective evaluation format is categorize errors (e.g. large, medium and small errors) instead of setting a single error target. If large errors pose a critical issue, then improvement on these may be incentivized higher and vice versa. The end-user can in that way steer the development and focus of improvements.

The following example demonstrates such a typical situation and presents the overall considerations that need to be taken, followed by the choice of metrics and test on significance of the results.

Exemplary Initial Considerations

Let's think of a number of forecasting models that can accept various inputs, such as online measurements in an auto-regressive manner, weather forecasts and other predictive features but use using different methodologies to generate power forecasts, which estimate the future electricity production.

In order to decide which model is most suitable, it is necessary to evaluate its quality by comparing the forecast against power measurements.

Typically, the errors of a separate test data are compared against each other in order to decide in favor of one of the models. The selection of the error metric should be individually adjusted to the corresponding application.

The evaluation should be performed strictly on test data that were not used to calibrate the respective model. Otherwise, it can easily happen that models are favored, which have adapted too much to the training data without being able to generalize for future unknown situations. If several models are compared, they should also have been jointly trained on data that does not originate from the test set.

In the case of wind or solar power forecasts, it is furthermore essential to select the test data from a continuous period. The data cannot be considered temporally independent. If one were to randomly assign individual samples to a training and a test set, one would assign both sets of random samples that share a large part of the information. As a result, preference would also be given to models that are over-adapted to the training data.

In addition to the error metric, other factors can also play a role. For example, one is faced with the question whether an established model should be replaced. For several reasons it may seem attractive not to replace it even though another one shows a smaller error. For instance, because confidence in the model functionality has been built up, or because a change in the model requires additional effort. These issues make it necessary to examine the significance of the estimated error values. The critical question behind this is whether the extent of the test data considered is sufficient to form the basis for a decision.

Evaluation of Significance

One way to evaluate the significance of the forecast performance results is to evaluate the distribution of the error metrics of a forecast model across different locations. This can be illustrated using the results of the study in [85]. It compared different machine learning models to weather forecasting and real-time measurement based forecasting. The box plot shown in Fig. 15.4 shows the distribution of the error measures of 29 wind farms in northern Germany. The error metric in this case is the root mean square error (RMSE) which is applied to nominal power normalized time series. The individual boxes represent the error distribution of one of the six models used. The triangular markers indicate the confidence range of the median. If these ranges do not overlap for two models, the medians are different under normal distribution assumption to a 5% significance level. This corresponds to a visual representation of a t-test.

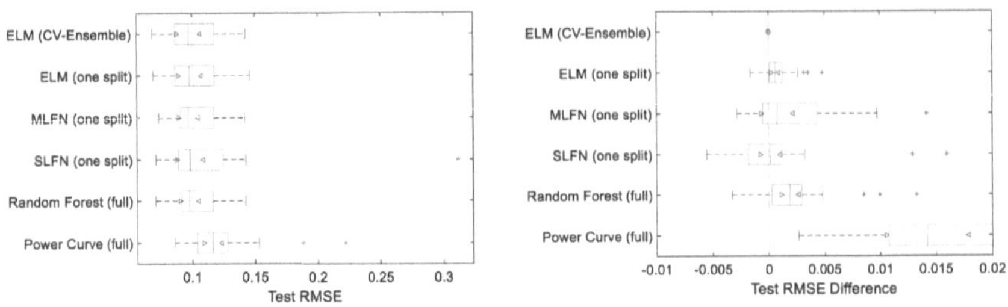

Figure 15.4 RMSE distribution of forecasts from six different prediction models for 29 wind farms in the north of Germany (left panel). Pairwise differences RMSE for each single model in comparison to the wind farm RMSE of the reference model ELM (CV-Ensemble) [85] (right panel).

Fig. 15.4 (left) shows, that only the power curve model has a significantly higher RMSE. All others cannot be clearly distinguished. The reason for this can be found in the broad distribution. This can be explained to a greater extent by the different local properties, such as the number of turbines per wind farm or the local orography. When considering the paired differences, local influences can be partially eliminated.

Fig. 15.4 (right) shows the distribution of the difference between a model and a reference model (ELM (CV-Ensemble)) across all 29 wind farms. If the distribution of a model is significantly in the positive range, it can be assumed that the reference model is significantly better. Thanks to these pairwise differences, it can now be established that two other models have a significantly worse result.

15.2.5 Incentivization

Operational forecasts may be tied to an incentive scheme by which monies are exchanged based on forecast performance. Examples of such arrangements exist in both commercial forecast services and regulation of monopoly businesses. As the terms of the incentive scheme typically include details of how forecasts are evaluated, this approach poses few risks. However, the evaluation methodology should be carefully considered when negotiating or subscribing to such incentive schemes.

Incentives may take the form of a linear relationship between reward/penalty and a forecast metric such as Mean Absolute Error, which may be normalized to installed capacity, and capped at some minimum/maximum reward/penalty. Similarly, incentives may be based on an event-based metric, such as an accuracy or hit-rate for specific events such as ramps or within-day minimum/maximum generation. The time period

over which such an incentive is calculated and settled will have a large impact on it's volatility as evaluation metrics may vary greatly on short time scales. Longer timescales are conducive to a stable incentive reflective of actual forecast performance rather than variations in weather conditions. The basic evaluation rules developed in section 12 and 14 are equally valid here and are recommended to be applied.
In summary, it is recommended that the formulation of incentive schemes should consider four factors:

- selection of relevant target parameters (see section 12.3)
- selection of relevant metrics (see sections 15.2, 15.1, 15.1.5, 15.2.3)
- selection of relevant verification horizons (see section 12.2)
- exclusion principles (see chapter 13, section 13.2, 13.4)

The selection process of relevant target parameters is highly dependent on the forecasting solution. The objective and proper setup of verification as well as evaluation metrics and frameworks can be found in 12, 14 and sections 15.1, 15.1.2, 15.3.1.

Recommendation: A set of relevant target parameters needs to be defined to provide a focus area for the forecaster. Comparison to a previous period, to a persistence forecast or a set target that is realistic can circumvent a number of constraints that are difficult to exclude in an evaluation. The most important consideration for any performance incentive scheme is that the scheme should put emphasis on the development and advancement of forecast methods for exactly those targets that are important for the end-user's applications. Table 15.4 provides a list of possible benchmark types for an incentive scheme.

15.3. Evaluation of benchmarks and trials

Key points

In order to maximize the probability of selecting an optimal forecast solution for an application the performance evaluation uncertainty process should be minimized and non-performance attributes of a forecast solution should be effectively considered.

Evaluation uncertainty can be minimized by a well-designed and implemented performance benchmark or trial protocol.

> A benchmark should have three well-designed phases: (1) preparation, (2) execution and (3) performance analysis that each address the key issues associated with the three primary attributes of an evaluation process.

As a general guideline, the evaluation of benchmarks and trials needs to follow the three principles of being:

1. **representative**
2. **significant and repeatable**
3. **relevant, fair and transparent**

The principles have been explained in detail in Chapter 12. This section addresses the consideration and application of these principles in benchmarks and trials.

15.3.1 Applying the principles of representativeness, significance, and relevance

The three key attributes of a forecast solution evaluation within a trial or benchmark (T/B) are (1) representativeness (2) significance and (3) relevance. If any one of these are not satisfactorily achieved the evaluation will not provide meaningful information to the forecast solution decision process and the resources employed in the trial or benchmark will effectively have been wasted. Unfortunately, it many not be obvious to the conductor of a T/B or the user of the information produced by the T/B, whether or not these three attributes have not been achieved in the evaluation. This section will present the issues associated with each attribute and provide guidance on how to maximize the likelihood that each will be achieved.

The conductors of a T/B should consider all the factors noted in the three key areas for a T/B. Part of these are described in detail in chapter 12 in sections 12.1, 12.2 and 12.3. The following is a reminder with specifics for the T/B case:

1. **Representativeness** (see section 12.1)
   Representativeness refers to the relationship between the results of a trial or benchmark evaluation and the performance that is ultimately obtained in the operational use of a forecast solution. It essentially addresses the question whether or not the results of the evaluation are likely to be a good predictor of the actual forecast performance that will be achieved for an operational application. There are many factors that influence the ability of the T/B evaluation results to be a good

predictor of future operational performance. Four of the most crucial factors here are:

   a. size and composition of the evaluation sample,
   b. quality of the data from the forecast target sites,
   c. the formulation and enforcement of rules governing the submission of T/B forecasts (sometimes referred to as "fairness"),
   d. availability of a complete and consistent set of T/B information to all T/B participants (sometimes referred to as "transparency")

2. **Significance** (see section 12.2) For benchmarks and trials it is important that a result obtained now, should also be obtainable when doing a second test. Or, if a test runs over 1 month, the same result should be obtainable over another randomly selected month.
   Often, especially in short intervals, this is not possible due to the different climatic and specific weather conditions that characterize specific periods of a year. In this case, it is necessary to establish mitigating measures in order to generate results that provide a correct basis for the respective decision making.
   Such a mitigating measure could be to consider potentially new forecasts in real-time and
   a. compare or blend them with a running system in order to test the value of such a new forecast
   b. evaluate the error structure of a potential new forecast to the error structure of your running system
   Both tests can be relatively easily incorporated and tested against the main forecast product, such as a day-ahead total portfolio forecast. It will not reflect the potential or performance and quality of a new forecast in it's entirety, but comparing error structures, for example, in the form of frequency distributions, ensures that a bias due to a lack of training or knowledge about operational specifics does not provide a misleading impression on quality. Chapter 14 details principles and section 15.1 provides details on suitable metrics.
3. **Relevance** (see section 12.3) Results obtained must reflect relevance in respect to the associated operational tasks. Forecasts for energy applications should follow physical principles and be evaluated accordingly. That means in fact that the b/t task must in some way reflect the future function of the forecasts. If this is not so, the results from a b/t should not be used to select a solution of vendor. Instead it may be used to evaluate other performance measures, such as service, support, delivery etc. Fairness in the evaluation, specific for benchmarks and trials

then means that the forecast providers are informed about this different objective. Forecasts also need to be evaluated on the same input and output. If assumptions are made, these assumptions must also be provided in a transparent way to all participants.

A useful approach is to create a evaluation plan matrix that lists all of the factors noted in the discussion in this section and how the user's evaluation plan addresses them.

15.3.2 Evaluation preparation in the execution phase

The evaluation of a T/B should start in the execution phase in order to prevent errors along the way from making results unusable.

Since there is usually a time constraint associated with T/B's there are a number of aspects that should be considered to ensure meaningful results.

Recommendations for the execution phase:

Data monitoring:

Measurement data and forecast delivery should be monitored and logged in order to prevent data losses and to ensure that all relevant data is available for the evaluation. It is recommended that the data monitoring should include:

- testing accuracy and delivery performance for fairness and transparency
- monitoring forecast reception to test reliability
- excluding from the evaluation all times for which any forecasts are missing to prevent manipulation on performance

Consistent Information

The fourth key factor is the availability of a complete and consistent set of T/B information to all participants in the T/B. Incomplete or inconsistent information distribution can occur in many ways. For example, one participant may ask a question and the reply is only provided to the participant who submitted the inquiry.

Develop and refine your own evaluation scripts:

Whether it is a user's first time b/t or a repeated exercise, the evaluation protocol should be carefully planned and prepared during the execution phase. It is recommended to verify metrics scripts or software tools and input/output structures as well as exclusion principles.

15.3.3 Performance analysis in the evaluation phase

The performance analysis has a number of key points that need consideration. These are:

1. Application-relevant accuracy measures of the forecasts
   The key point is that the metrics used in the verification must have relevance for the application. For example, if a ramp forecast is needed in the application, a mean average error only provides a overall performance measure and is not relevant for the target application. If a vendor knows that performance is measured with an average, the incentive would be to dampen forecasts to reduce the overall average error, which is the opposite of what is required for the needs of the application. Such an application should employ a scoring system for hits, misses and false alarms of pre-defined ramping events.
2. Performance in the timely delivery of forecasts
   The key pitfalls in an T/B are often associated with the failure to closely monitor the following items:
   a. Forecast delivery time
      If forecast delivery is not logged or checked, it is possible for a forecast provider to deliver forecasts at a later time (perhaps overwriting a forecast that was delivered at the required time) and use fresher information to add skill to their forecast or even wait until the outcome for the forecast period is known. Although one might think that such explicit cheating is not likely to occur in this type of technical evaluation, experience has indicated that it is not that uncommon if the situation enables its occurrence.
   b. Selective delivery of forecasts
      This is one way in which results might be manipulated without explicit cheating by taking advantage of loopholes in the rules. In this case the issue is that the B/T protocol does not specify any penalty for missing a forecast delivery and the evaluation metrics are simply computed on whatever forecasts are submitted by each provider. As a forecast provider it is easy to estimate the "difficulty" of each forecast period and to simply not deliver any forecasts during periods that are likely to be difficult and therefore prone to large errors.

      This is an excellent way to improve forecast performance scores. Of course, it makes the results unrepresentative of what is actually needed by the user. Often it is good performance during the difficult forecast periods that are most valuable to a user.
3. Ease of working with the forecast provider
   A T/B is also an opportunity to assess the support provided by the forecast vendor in understanding forecast results and error patterns. Effec-

tive communication with the forecast provider is important especially if forecaster support is a selection criterion. This factor is particularly important to explicitly address if it is an unfunded B/T (i.e. the forecaster is not compensated), where resources are used differently than in contractual relationships.

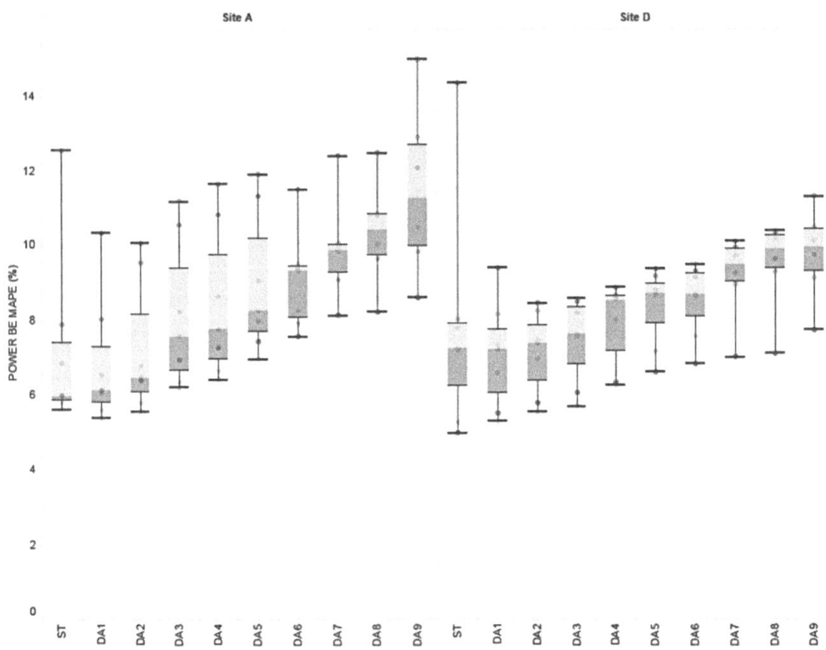

Figure 15.5 Example of a box-and-whisker-plot verification at two different sites (left and right panel) for different look ahead times (x-axis; DAx is x^{th} hour of day-ahead forecast) and mean absolute percentage error (MAPE; y-axis). Image from [87] with permission from Energynautics GmbH.

15.3.4 Evaluation examples from a benchmark

Fig. 15.5 shows an example of a forecast evaluation using a box-and-whiskers-plot to visualize the spread in MAPE (mean absolute error as percentage of nominal power) of 5 forecasts of different day-ahead time periods (each column) at two different sites. The distribution within each time period is shown for the 5 forecasts errors. In that way, the spread of forecast performance in each hour of the day-ahead horizon can be visualized. It also shows how some forecasts in some hours show very low errors

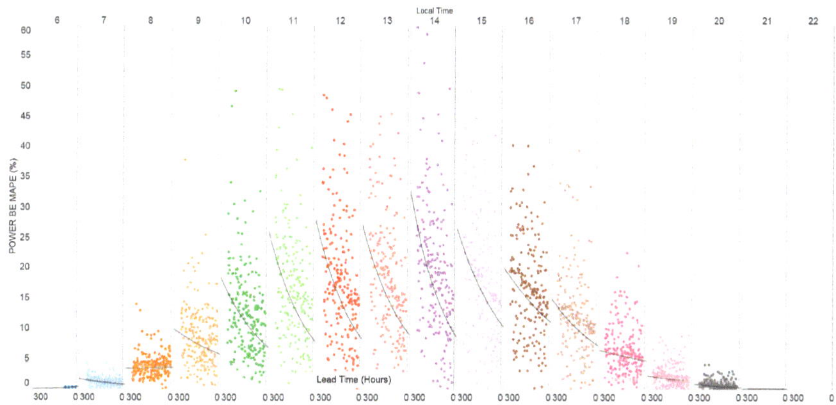

Figure 15.6 Example of a forecast error scatter plot by time of the day (top x-axis) for 3-hours lead times and forecast error (y-axis). (Image from [88] with permission from Energynautics GmbH).

compared to the average error in that hour, as well as occasionally very high errors.

Fig. 15.6 shows an example of an evaluation of errors by time of day for a fixed lead time of 3 hours. It illustrates a very large spread in errors during certain times of the day, as would be expected.

Nevertheless, if such evaluations are compared between different forecast providers an evaluation of the "most costly errors" may reveal a very different result than, if only an average metric per forecaster is used.

15.4. Use cases

Key points

The section presents a number of use cases that illustrate how an evaluation of forecast solutions in a specific part of the power and energy sector should ideally be designed and executed. In the **Energy Trading and Balancing, ramping forecast in general and for reserve allocation**, forecasts are a crucial part of the processes for balance-responsible parties as well as system operators. And yet, many mistakes are made in the evaluation and incentivization of forecasts that effectively often lead to results that are unsatisfactory and create mistrust in the ability of forecast service providers to provide useful forecasts.

Example code for evaluation, verification and validation can be found in Appendix G.

15.4.1 Energy trading and balancing

In energy trading, forecasts of multiple variables are used in order to provide situational awareness and support quantitative decision-making. Costs accrue on the basis of power production forecasts and energy prices at multiple look-ahead times. An example is forecasts used at the day-ahead stage and then again at an intra-day look-ahead time frame for the same trading period, and the relative price of buying and selling energy at different times.

Furthermore, prices, particularly imbalance prices, may be influenced by the cumulative forecasts and forecast errors of all market participants creating a significant correlation between renewable power forecast errors and the price at which resulting imbalances are settled. In addition, unrelated events may cause large price movements that result in an otherwise unremarkable forecast error having a large financial impact. Therefore, care must be taken when designing an evaluation scheme that is reflective of forecast performance and not externalities.

15.4.1.1 Forecast error cost functions

If trading decisions are based on a deterministic power production forecast, it is tempting to try to evaluate the 'cost' of forecast errors based on energy prices.

For example, this evaluation is sometimes performed by taking the cost of "under forecasting" to be equal to the difference between the day-ahead price and the system sell price (the opportunity cost of having to sell at the system sell price rather than day-ahead price), and taking the cost of "over forecasting" to be equal to the difference between the system buy price and the day-ahead price (the cost of having to buy back the energy not produced at a higher price than it was sold for).

This approach has several problems:

1. price asymmetry:
   Traders are aware of the asymmetry in imbalance prices and have a view of whether the market is likely to be long or short, as such they do not naively trade the forecast production and will hedge against penalizing prices. It is therefore not representative to assume the day-ahead forecast is contracted.
2. adjustment opportunities:

The intra-day market and flexibility within the traders portfolio provide opportunities for adjustment between the day-ahead market and imbalance settlement which may influence both the value and volume of traded energy, and potentially the imbalance price.

3. forecast error correlation:
Renewable power forecast errors are often highly correlated across the entire market and therefore to the market length and total imbalance. As a result, evaluating forecast errors based on imbalance cost will not discriminate between forecast performance and correlation with imbalance prices and one may incorrectly interpret reduced 'cost' as improved forecast skill.

For these reasons it is recommended that (normalized) mean absolute error be used as part of an evaluation matrix that also contains other relevant metrics when evaluating deterministic renewable power forecast performance for trading applications (see 14, 15.1). Additionally, a real example of a market analysis and evaluation of how different trading strategies influence the costs in comparison to the revenue is available at [17], and [18].

If trading decisions are based on probabilistic power production forecasts those forecasts should be evaluated as described in section 14.2. If probabilistic forecasts of both power production and prices are used, it is important that the dependency structure between power and price forecast errors is correct. Various metrics exists to measure this, such as the multivariate energy score [48] and p-variogram score [54,78]. Details are beyond the scope of this document.

15.4.2 General ramping forecasts

Power production ramps can have significant impact on power system and electricity market operation and are of interest to decision-makers in both domains. However, as ramps comprise a sequence of two or more forecasts, metrics that only compare predictions and observations at single time points are not suitable for evaluating ramp forecasts. Event-based evaluation in the form of contingency tables and associated metrics provide a tool-set for evaluating these forecasts.

Once an event is defined, such as ramp defined as a particular change in wind energy production over a particular time period, occurrences in forecasts and observations can be labeled and a table of true-positive, false-positive, true-negative and false-negative forecasts can be produced. From this, the skill of the forecast at predicting such events can be evaluated.

The definition of a ramp will influence the forecast tuning and evaluation results. It is recommended that the definition reflects the decision(s) being influenced by the forecast. For example, this could be related to a commercial ramp product definition, or the ramp rates of thermal power plant used in balancing. Furthermore, if an economic cost can be assigned to each outcome, then the forecasting system can be tuned to minimize costs, and the relative value of different forecasting systems can be compared.

In general terms, the following methods and metrics are recommended as basis for the evaluation of ramp forecasts:

- Contingency tables and statistics derived from the tables provide an evaluation framework
- Ramp definitions should reflect operational decision-making
- The cost implications of different types of errors should be considered when comparing different forecasting systems

In the next sections, a number of examples are described to demonstrate how evaluation should be planned and that illustrates the pitfalls in the metric selection process.

15.4.2.1 Amplitude versus phase

Ramping events cause shortage or overproduction and risk for congestion in the power system for relatively short time frames. For this reason, many system operators have different levels of reserve time frames and also forecasting time frames that provide the possibility to allocate different types of reserve to counteract ramps that have been forecasted insufficiently strong (amplitude) and/or are wrong in phase. On system operator level it is often described that the amplitude is more important than the exact timing (phase).

In this case, it is necessary that the evaluation method does not punish the forecaster stronger for a phase error than an amplitude error. This means for example that using a root mean square error to evaluate ramps is incentivizing a forecaster to dampen amplitudes and optimize on phase. Sometimes it is referred to the **"forecaster's dilemma"** when the end-user defines a metric for evaluation such that the target is opposite of what the end-user asks for and needs. The forecast provider then either tunes forecasts to the metric or to what the end-user likes to see and risks to be punished (e.g. loose a contract), when evaluated. See also [80].

Recommendation: When a forecaster should be incentivized for amplitude in a ramp forecast, the evaluation metric cannot be an average error measure such as mean absolute error or root mean square error. If these average error metrics are used, the data to be evaluated has to be prepared to:

- reflect only cases that contain ramps of a certain strength
- widen ramp events with a forward/backward window of 1 – 2 hours to allow for phase errors

Additionally, either a contingency test with hit rate, misses and false alarms have to be used in the evaluation of the forecasts to reflect the focus on amplitude.

15.4.2.2 Costs of false alarms

Ramps can have different costs in a power system. In some systems, too fast up-ramping causes congestion or in some way over-production that needs to be dealt with (case 1). The opposite case, the down-ramping can cause that there is power missing on the grid that is not available and the fast primary reserve causes high costs (case 2). In case 1, the system operator has to be able to reduce ramping capacity of the wind farms or have other highly flexible resources on the grid to level out the overproduction. In case 2, lacking energy can cause high costs for fast ramping resources on primary reserve level or outages, which are unwanted.

The consequence is that the cost profile for up-ramping and down-ramping is usually different. Also, the cost of not forecasting a ramp that occurs (false-negative) can be significantly higher than the cost of preparing for a ramp, which does not occur (false-positive). The only way to verify, whether a forecast is sufficiently good in predicting a specific type of ramping event is to use contingency tables, where the forecast skill can be computed and visualized.

15.4.3 Evaluation of probabilistic ramp forecasts for reserve allocation

The primary scope of reserve predictions is to reduce balancing costs via dynamic allocation of reserve and if possible with the help of non-fossil fuel capacity.

If a system operator (SO) or balance responsible party (BRP) can more dynamically schedule reserve, the costs for imbalances become lower and the energy system more efficient.

This was the scope of a study that will be presented as an example of the evaluation of a real-time environment application that needed a practical solution in order to reduce costs for reserve allocation for the end-user [79]. The evaluation strategy and results of the study can be considered a kind of guideline on how to best manage renewable energy imbalances in a market system.

In this sample control area there are approximately 40 wind farms. The permanent allocation of reserves for the control area amounted at the outset to +/-10% and up to +/−30% of installed capacity of wind, dependent on the time of the year, i.e. there are large seasonal reserve allocation differences. In our example area the wind generation is correlated and strong ramps occur. However, it is seldom to observe that the wind generation ramps down in a dramatic speed. Ramp-ups are faster than down-ramps and it is very unlikely that an instant total wind ramp down to zero can occur in the control area.

15.4.3.1 Definition of error conditions for the forecast

Fundamental for forecasting is that criteria for success and error can be defined. Given the fact that certain swings in the data are unrealistic or possibly so extreme that the operational cost of self-balancing would be too high, there was a need to work with probabilities. One way of doing this is to define that, if a forecast value lies within a band, the result is a success and if it lies outside the band, it is a false alarm. A constant very wide reserve band would imply 100% success, but would not be affordable.

The gain lies in finding a balanced criterion considering the following questions:

- How many failures can be tolerated?
- What is the allowed maximum error?
- Which frequency of reserve under-prediction is allowed?
- What is the cost of spilled reserve?

These questions are related or determined by the SO's operational experience and standards to which the SO must be conforming. Fig. 15.7 illustrates the challenges of deciding how many outliers can be accepted to reduce costly spill, a dilemma every balance responsible party has to deal with. The static allocation of reserves is very expensive, especially if all extremes should be covered. Even, if extremes are not covered always, there is a lot of spills (black areas in Fig. 15.7) in comparison to a dynamic allocation of reserves.

The difficulty for such a situation is to find objective criteria suitable for evaluation of a model result, which relates to operation and presents incentives for the forecaster to reduce the spill by maximizing coverage of extremes. Standard statistical metrics do not provide answers to this optimization task, because (1) it is not the error of 1 forecast any more and (2)

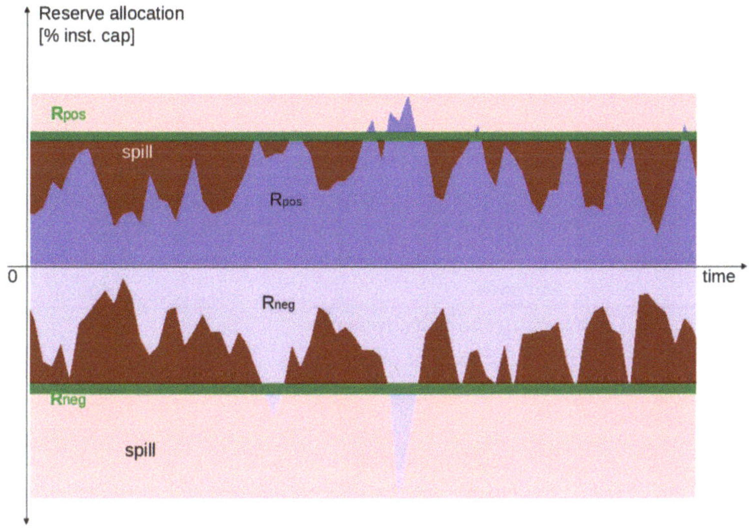

Figure 15.7 Illustration of the "reserve allocation dilemma" of costly spill versus covering all possible ramping events. Here, R_{pos} is the dynamic positive reserve, R_{neg} is the dynamic negative Reserve, the upper linear borders R_{pos} and R_{neg} are the static reserve allocation, the black area and the outer light grey areas are the spill for the dynamic and static allocation of reserves, respectively. Reproduced and modified image from [4] under the Creative Commons CC-BY license.

the target is whether the allocation was sufficient and cheaper than allocating with a constant "security band".

With contingency statistics it is possible to ask the right questions:

- Hits and Misses Analysis show the percentage of time the band was too small
- Positive and negative reserve allocation can be split up to reflect use of tertiary reserve allocation (cheaper) instead of primary reserve (high expenses)

The following analysis was carried out to reflect these objectives:

1. A BIAS, MAE and RMSE provide an overview of the plain statistical capabilities of the various forecasts
2. Contingency tables for hit rate, misses, spill and reserve coverage have been computed to provide metrics for further optimization of the task

Table 15.5 shows the evaluation matrix of metrics and their purpose in the verification and further optimization. The study [79] concluded that the real reserve deployment will not be able to cover the shortage or overcapacity for about two hours per day in average. Their 5760 hours of evaluation was not considered very robust to draw final conclusions and to set long-term strategies, it was found that the results provided the information necessary to enhance the optimization task and follow its progress closely over some time.

Table 15.5 Applied metrics in the evaluation matrix for the reserve allocation example in [79]. The input forecasts are split up in 9 percentile bands from P10..P90 and a minimum and maximum.

Metrics		Purpose	Input forecasts
BIAS		average to gain overview	MIN
MAE		average to gain overview	P10
RMSE		average to gain overview	P20
Inside Band		consistency forecast-deployment	P30
$R_{coverage}$		forecasted reserve deployment	P40
Hit rate	Total	achievable percent of activated reserve	P50
	R_{pos}	as above for pos reserve	P60
	R_{neg}	as above for neg. reserve	P70
Misses	Total	avg under-predicted reserve	P80
	R_{pos}	as above for pos reserve	P90
	R_{neg}	as above for neg. reserve	MAX
Spill	Total	avg over-predicted reserve	
	R_{pos}	as above for pos reserve	
	R_{neg}	as above for neg reserve	

In [64] statistical post-processing of ensemble forecasts are discussed and provide useful information and guidelines on how to carry out post-processing in support of renewable energy applications, and post-processing of long-range forecasts from months to decades. Finally, one chapter [53] provides guidelines and software code in the R programming language in order to assist developers, researchers and end-users to implement post-processing.

PART FOUR

Meteorological and power data requirements for real-time forecasting applications

Editors (1) and Authors (2):
Dr. Corinna Möhrlen, WEPROG, DK, DE[1,2]
Dr. John W. Zack, MESO Inc., USA[1,2]
Dr. Gregor Giebel, Technical University of Denmark, DK[1]

Contributing Authors:
Dr. Jethro Browell, University of Glasgow, UK
Dr. Stefan Wilbert, German Aerospace Center, DLR, ES
Dr.-Ing. Ines Würth, TGU enviConnect, TTI GmbH, DE
Dr. Martin Felder, ZSW Baden-Württemberg, DE

Contributions:

Dr. Jie Yan, North China Electric Power University, CN
Rui Pestana, REN, PT
Anton Kaifel, ZSW Baden-Württemberg, DE
Jan Remund, Meteotest AG, CH

CHAPTER SIXTEEN

Meteorological and power data requirements for real-time forecasting applications

16.1. Before you start reading

This is the **fourth part** of the IEA Wind recommended practice for the implementation of renewable energy forecasting solutions.

In this **fourth part**, guidance for the selection, deployment and maintenance of meteorological sensors, power measurements and associated data quality control relevant to real-time forecasting is provided. In the **first part**, *Forecast solution selection process*, the design of a customized process to select an optimal forecast solution for a user's specific situation and application is addressed. The focus of the **second part**, *Design and execution of benchmarks and trials*, is the design, execution and analysis of customized forecasting benchmarks and trials. In the **third part**, *Forecast solution evaluation* methods and guidelines for the meaningful evaluation of alternative forecasts, operational and non-operational forecasts and entire forecast solutions are presented.

If your main interest is in (1) selecting a forecasting solution, (2) testing or evaluating different forecasting solutions against each other, or (3) verifying the quality of your forecast solution, please go to parts 1, 2 or 3 of this recommended practice guideline to obtain recommendations on these specific topics.

It is recommended using the table of contents actively to find the relevant topics.

16.2. Background and introduction

Meteorological measurements from sensors within or in close proximity to renewable generation facilities provide data about the wind and solar resource and weather situation at a given time that is independent of the power generation data. This information is, not only an obligation that stems from the technical requirements of many system operators, but is also typically used to optimize the operation of renewable power plants and

IEA Wind Recommended Practice for the Implementation of Renewable Energy Forecasting Solutions
https://doi.org/10.1016/B978-0-44-318681-3.00029-5

electricity grids. For both the system operator and the power plant operator, these measurements provide an independent signal that can warn about critical weather and provide an indication of whether the generation facilities are operating at their expected performance level. For the transmission system operator (TSO), such measurements can also be used for situational awareness of the weather in the control area that may affect the transmission lines. This information also provides a second means of verifying whether the power signal from a specific power plant is malfunctioning in situations that may be critical for grid operation.

The assimilation of meteorological data from renewable generation facilities into forecast models has been tested by meteorological centres (e.g. [89]). One of the most important findings in these investigations is that the quality of data provided by the facilities is the most essential issue to be solved in order to gain higher quality forecasts with such measurements. In other words, if there is no specific effort put into standardization of requirements in the power industry, the benefits can not be achieved.

This part of the recommended practice (RP) series aims to provide background information on meteorological instrumentation, their recommended setup, maintenance, quality control and use in the real-time environment of wind and solar power generation plants. Information on the use of real-time power and other operational data in forecasting systems is also included. The document provides practical guidelines for quality control and recommended standards to be applied in the setup and calibration of instrumentation when entering the operational phase of wind and solar projects and for applications relevant to plant operators, system operators, power traders or balance-responsible parties.

16.3. Structure and recommended use

The structure of this part follows the order of a typical decision-making process that is used to select, deploy, operate and maintain meteorological sensors, to collect and quality control data from those sensors and power data from SCADA systems of generating units for real-time forecasting applications. The user of this document is encouraged to actively use the table of contents to find the desired information, either in the summary of recommendations (Chapter 22) or in the chapters, sections and subsections, whose content is briefly described below.

- **Chapter 18:** ***Meteorological instrumentation***
  In order to forecast wind or solar power, meteorological conditions such as wind speed or solar radiation need to be known. There are several measurement devices in use, which come with different attributes and requirements. The chapter provides an overview of those instruments.
- **Chapter 19:** ***Power measurements***
  Power measurements are a key input to minutes to hours-ahead forecasts and are also used to check the operational capacity and actual produced power to validate forecasts. This chapter provides an overview of relevant data types and their usage in forecasting applications.
- **Chapter 20:** ***Setup and calibration***
  When working with measurement data, it is crucial to follow best practices for the measurement setup and calibration to ensure the highest standard of data quality. The chapter provides an overview of different measurement setups and calibration procedures.
- **Chapter 21:** ***Instrumentation performance***
  There is a saying "he who measures, measures garbage", meaning that measurements are prone to errors and therefore ongoing checking of the performance of measurement signals is crucial to ensure high quality of forecasts. The chapter provides an overview of measures for quality control of measurements.
- **Chapter 22:** ***Best practices summary***
  This is the short-cut to the recommendations. Here, we collect and summarize all recommendations in the use of measurements in real-time forecasting applications without explanations or justification and link them to the respective background information.

CHAPTER SEVENTEEN

Use and application of real-time meteorological measurements

17.1. Application-specific requirements

This section defines and discusses the use of meteorological measurements for real-time applications and especially makes the distinction to the use of data in non-real-time applications such as resource assessment.

17.1.1 Application-specific requirements for meteorological data

Meteorological measurements made at the sites of current or future wind or solar generation facilities can be used for several different types of applications. Although there are many common requirements, there are significant differences in the required attributes of the meteorological data gathering among these applications. The primary applications for on-facility meteorological data are:

1. **Short-term Forecasting**
   Short-term (minutes to days ahead) forecasting utilizes on-facility meteorological data for the training of the statistical components of forecast systems as well as input into the production of forecasts. It is the "input to forecast production" application that creates the most demanding requirements since in order to have maximum value the data must be quickly quality controlled and available to the forecast production process with minimal time lags. This application is the primary focus of this document.
2. **Resource Assessment**
   The resource assessment application employs meteorological data to assess the general generation resource over a region (resource mapping) as guidance for the planning of future development or at a specific location (generation yield estimation) for the purpose of estimating the future production of a proposed project in order to assess its the economic viability. This does not require near-real-time access to the meteorological data.

IEA Wind Recommended Practice for the Implementation of Renewable Energy Forecasting Solutions
https://doi.org/10.1016/B978-0-44-318681-3.00030-1

3. **Generation Asset Performance Assessment**
   The performance assessment application uses meteorological data to estimate the expected generation from a wind or solar facility in order to assess the performance of the generation hardware at a specific facility relative to the manufacturer's performance specifications. This does not generally require near-real-time access to the meteorological data.
4. **Turbine Control**
   The turbine control application is specific to wind generation facilities and uses meteorological data to optimally orient the turbine for maximum generation efficiency. Typically only wind speed and direction data is required in real-time so that timely adjustments to the turbine position can be made.
5. **Plant Monitoring and Situational Awareness**
   The plant monitoring and situational awareness application employs meteorological data to facilitate the awareness of plant operators and possibly also grid system operators to the operating status of the generation facility and the likelihood of very-short-term changes in production. Meteorological data is employed as an independent check on the generation and availability status of the facility and also to identify very short-term trends in the resource that may not be evident from the generation data (such as in the case of wind generation facilities that are operating at rated power but may be near thresholds such as those for high-speed shutdown). The near real-time availability of data is important for this application.

A summary of the differences in required measurement attributes among these applications is provided in Table 17.1. It should be noted that the short-term forecasting application has specific requirements that are different from those of other applications. A meteorological measurement system designed primarily for use in a different type of application may not be ideal or even adequate for real-time short-term forecasting.

17.1.2 Applications in system operation, balancing and trading

The key applications in system operation and the balancing and trading of wind and solar power, where real-time meteorological measurements are required, are:

- **Situational awareness in critical weather events**
  Critical weather events can cause severe security risks in grid operation. Forecasting and measurements assist to a large extent to make such

events predictable and provide the necessary information to be able to act in advance. Such situational awareness is an important planning tool in grid operation, where penetration levels are above ca. 30% of energy consumption. Especially for wind generating power extreme winds can only be predicted by meteorological signals, due to the flattening of wind power curves in wind ranges > 12 m/s. In this range, the power signal provides no local information to the system operator or the wind farm operator or balancing authority.

- **High-Speed Shutdown events**
  During storm events, the critical parameter for the grid operation is the proportion of wind farms that are expected to enter into high-speed shutdown (HSSD) in any high penetration area. The risk and increased uncertainty for HSSD during storm events can result in the System Operator having to limit the wind generation in advance so that sufficient reserve is available.
- **Grid related down-regulation or curtailments**
  Grid related down-regulations or curtailments can be due to extreme weather events or technical problems with the electrical lines or controllers. Wind speed or solar radiation measurements can provide an independent signal to the system operator on the available active power potential, where this is not broadcasted and also provide the possibility to compute the lost power production due to the down/regulation.
- **Short-term Forecasting with updates from measurements**
  Short-term forecasting with time horizons of minutes up to a few hours need to rely on measurements as additional information to weather data from NWP models, due to the 6-hourly schedule of most operational NWP model deliveries. Improvements can however only be expected, if the real-time measurements to update the forecasts have a sufficient quality. If too much of the data needs to be blacklisted, or the filters have difficulties to capture erroneous measurement values, such data can actually make the forecast worse than without the additional data. Quality of these data is therefore imperative.
- **Intra-day power plant balancing**
  Intra-day power plant balancing is equally dependent on a high quality measurement data quality as the short-term forecasting, and usually relies on short-term forecasts.

Table 17.1 Summary of the required attributes of meteorological measurements among the major renewable energy applications.

Attribute	Forecasting	Resource Assessment	Performance Assessment	Turbine Control	Plant Monitoring
		General			
Availability in near real-time	essential	not necessary	not necessary	essential	essential
Availability in extreme weather conditions	essential	not critical	not critical	essential	essential
Measurement bias	not critical if trends are accurate	near zero bias critical	low bias important	not critical	not critical
Additional met variables (other than resource variables)	useful especially in specific weather scenarios	minimal value	not needed	not needed	useful in some weather scenarios
Plant outages / curtailment	essential	not relevant	not relevant	not relevant	useful
		Wind Power specific			
Deployment location considers wakes	important	not relevant	not an issue	not an issue	not critical
		Solar Power specific			
Obstacle Shading	must be representative of facility	must be representative of site	must be representative of facility	not applicable	documentation required

17.1.3 Applications in wind turbine and wind farm operation

The key applications for wind plant operation, where real-time meteorological measurements are required, are:

- **Wind turbine control**

Due to wake effects on nacelle anemometers, independent site data from a met mast or LIDAR can help the turbine controller to operate more safely and efficiently. Preview information of the turbine inflow from a nacelle-based lidar system can be used to induce blade pitch action and thus reduce loads and improve turbine power performance.

- **Wind farm control**
  Wake measurements of scanning lidars or nacelle-based lidars that measure the wake of turbines, can assist to redirect those wakes and thus reduce loads on downstream turbines and increase their power production.
- **Condition Monitoring**
  Knowledge about the wind conditions that affect a wind turbine or wind farm help to estimate the load budget that the turbines have experienced during their lifetime. This information can be used for lifetime extension measures thus increasing the energy yield of a wind farm and its profit.

17.1.4 Solar/PV plant operation

The key applications for solar plant operation, where real-time meteorological measurements are required are:

- Yield forecasting for the next minutes, hours and days
  - ramp rate control in PV power plants
  - dispatch optimization of power plans with storage
  - optimization of power plant operation for thermal plants (e.g. start up decisions)
- Power Plant Control
  - optimization of tracking of tracked PV or concentrating collectors
    - timing of transition into/out of stow position for high wind speeds/gusts
    - optimal tracking angle for non concentrating tracked PV according to sky radiance distribution and shading
    - de-focusing of concentrating collectors at high DNIs
  - mass flow control in thermal collectors
  - aim point control for solar tower plants

Most of the real-time meteorological measurements are only required for large scale power plants. For tracking collectors of any size wind speed and direction measurements are required to allow for securing the collectors in the stow positions at high wind speeds. Meteorological measurements may also be required for smaller systems depending on the solar thermal technology that is employed.

In the handbook [90] and [91], it is noted that measurements of irradiance are complex and more expensive as general meteorological instruments, especially for measuring direct normal irradiance (DNI). The applications named in [90] and [91] that utilize irradiance data are:

- Site resource analysis
- System design
- Plant operation
- Developing, improving and testing models that use remote satellite sensing techniques or available surface meteorological observations
- Developing, improving and testing solar resource forecasting techniques.

17.2. Available and applicable standards for real-time meteorological and power measurements

There are to date no standards available that specifically address real-time meteorological and power measurements for real-time wind and solar forecasting applications. Nevertheless, there are a number of standards available from the three areas of meteorological monitoring, wind and solar power resource assessment and monitoring that provide useful guidelines for measurement collection, monitoring, setup and calibration of instrumentation, verification and validation of measured data etc. This section introduces existing guidelines and standards from these three areas and analyzes them for their applicability in real-time wind and solar forecasting environments.

17.2.1 Standards and guidelines for wind measurements

For resource or site assessment in the planning phase of a wind farm an IEC standard exists IEC [92] with an updated version 2 (IEC 61400-12-2:2013), that specifies which tests and what kind of criteria the instrumentation has to fulfill when used for the required tests to be carried out. The IEC 61400-12-2:2013 rules contain the following items:

- Extreme winds
- Shear of vertical wind profile
- Flow inclination
- Background turbulence

- Wake turbulence
- Wind-speed distribution

The results of these tests have to be within a pre-defined range to be acceptable. In Appendix F of the 61400-12-1:2005 "Cup anemometer calibration procedure" the calibration of the instruments for measuring wind are specified.

The use of remote sensing for wind measurement was introduced in a new version 61400-12-1:2017. In Annex L guidelines for the classifications of remote sensing devices, for the verification of the performance and for the evaluation of uncertainties of the measurements are given.

MEASNET (MEASuring NETwork), the "international network for harmonized and recognized measurements in wind energy" has defined so called "Round Robin rules" for calibration of cup anemometers for wind energy [93], which are widely used. MEASNET has also under the EU project ACCUWIND published a number of guidelines regarding instrument calibration and measurement campaigns for the wind industry [94–96]. Lee [97] found a way of calibrating wind direction sensors with an optical camera.

In 2016 MEASNET published Version 2.0 of a "Procedure for the evaluation of site-specific wind conditions" [98]. This document gives guidance on measuring wind characteristics, and comprises an annex on wind measurement using remote sensing devices. It also includes guidance on how to set up measurement campaigns depending on the data required.

IEA Wind Task 32 and Task 11 published recommended practices RP-15 for ground-based remote sensing for wind resource assessment in 2013 [99]. It covers different aspects of using lidars and sodars. An updated review version of 2020 [100] identifies recommendations from the relevant normative documents (RP-15, MEASNET 2016, IEC 61400-12-1:2017 Annex L) concerning characterization, installation, operation, data analysis and verification of wind lidar.

The Annex D in IEC 61400-12-1:2005 standard states that the "implicit assumption of the method of this standard is that the 10 min mean power yield from a wind turbine is fully explained by the simultaneous 10 min mean wind speed measured at hub height, and the air density" [IEC, 2005, Annex D, Table D.1 [92]] and describes the associated measurement uncertainty evaluation principles.

In this respect, the standard refers to the "ISO Guide to the expression of Uncertainty in Measurements" [101,102], and its 2 supplements [103, 104] from the Joint Committee for Guides in Meteorology (JCGM), where there are two types of measurement uncertainty that are to be accounted for in any standardized measurement taking:

1. systematic errors, often associated with offsets/bias of the measured quantity
2. random errors, which are associated with the fact that 2 measurements of the same quantity are seldom the same

In section 3.1.2 of the guide, [103,104] it is stated that "the result of a measurement. is only an approximation or estimate.. of the value of the measurand and thus is complete only when accompanied by a statement of the uncertainty... of that estimate". Considering this definition, all measurements should ideally have an uncertainty term associated with it. This is impractical in real-time operations, where the value of the measurements lies in the availability of the data at a given time. Therefore, it is unrealistic to request uncertainty measures. However, it could be a standing data value that is determined at the setup of the instrument and provided as part of the standing data. In that way, the instrument-specific uncertainty could be accounted for in the handling of measurements (for other mitigation methods see 21.3.2).

In the introduction to the Guide [102], it is stated that "..the principles of this Guide are intended to be applicable to a broad spectrum of measurements", including those required for:

- maintaining quality control and quality assurance in production
- complying with and enforcing laws and regulations
- calibrating standards and instruments and performing tests throughout a national
- measurement system in order to achieve tractability to national standards developing, maintaining, and comparing international and national physical reference standards, including reference materials

To summarize, the handling and integration of wind power into the electric grid is an equally important step to harness the full potential of the energy resource in an efficient and environmentally friendly way. This requires that measurements are trustworthy and maintained to a quality that allows for their use in forecasting tools in order to produce high quality forecasts and thereby reduce the need of reserves. These guides in combination with the IEC 61400-1 standard would provide a good foundation for any grid code technical requirement specifications.

17.2.2 Standards and guidelines for solar measurements

A general guideline for meteorological measurements for solar energy is available in the IEA PVPS handbook [91]. The handbook summarizes important information for all steps of a solar energy project – reaching from required measurements and the design of measurement stations to forecasting the potential solar radiation. Measurement instruments and their application, as well as other sources for solar measurement data are presented. The handbook links to relevant further standards and guidelines. The standards and guidelines that are relevant for real-time applications are briefly summarized in the following paragraphs. For resource assessment purposes, we refer the reader to the IEA PVPS handbooks original version [105], version 1 [90] and 2 [91].

One of the frequently cited guidelines for measuring radiation is chapter 7 of the WMO CIMO guide [106]. There, guidelines are presented for meteorological measurements in general which mostly also apply for solar energy related measurements. However, some guidelines are different for solar energy as the conditions relevant for the power systems must be measured. For example, these conditions are often affected by nearby objects such as the solar collectors themselves, trees or buildings which should be avoided for other meteorological measurements.

In the ISO 9060 standard radiometers are classified according to their measurement errors caused by different effects, such as sensor temperature, or calibration stability. Classes are defined for both pyranometers (used to measure global radiation of the hemisphere above the sensor) and pyrheliometers (used to measure the direct normal irradiance). There are several ISO and ASTM standards for the radiometer calibration (ISO, 9059, ISO 9847, ISO 9846, ASTM G207, ASTM 824, ASTM 167). Guidelines for the application of pyranometers can be found in ISO 9901 and guidelines for the application of pyranometers and pyrheliometers are found in ASTM 183.

IEC 61724 on PV system performance monitoring describes how radiometers and other meteorological instruments should be integrated and used in PV plants. Accuracy classes of the resulting monitoring systems are defined. Also the recommended number of sensors to be deployed based on the peak power of the PV system is given. Additionally, the standard defines cleaning and calibration intervals for pyranometers.

17.3. Standards and guidelines for general meteorological measurements

As mentioned in section 17.2.1 and 17.2.2, the *Guide to Instruments and Methods of Observation* from the WMO (World Meteorological Organisation) [106] provides instrumentation standards for surface winds in chapter 5 and for radiation in chapter 7. Other meteorological parameters covered in the WMO Guide are measurement of:

- Surface and upper air temperature ([106] in chapter 2 and 10)
- Atmospheric and upper air pressure ([106] in chapter 3 and 10)
- Surface and upper-air Humidity ([106] in chapter 4 and 10)
- Surface and upper air wind ([106] in chapter 5 and 13)
- Sunshine Duration ([106] in chapter 6)
- Radiation ([106] in chapter 7)
- Visibility ([106] in chapter 8)
- Evaporation ([106] in chapter 9)
- Clouds ([106] in chapter 15)
- Atmospheric Compositions ([106] in chapter 16).

The United States Environmental Protection Agency (EPA) provides "Meteorological Monitoring Guidance for Regulatory modeling Applications" [107], which is a guideline on the collection of meteorological data for use in regulatory modeling applications such as air quality. It provides recommendations for instruments, measurements and reporting for all main meteorological variables used in meteorological modeling. In Section 4 of the guideline, the EPA provides recommended system accuracies and resolutions for wind speed, wind direction, ambient and dew point temperatures, humidity, pressure and precipitation, which are useful for wind and solar applications as well and will be discussed in the measurement setup and calibration chapter 20.

These guidelines and recommendations have been assessed for the purpose of wind and/or solar projects and are the basis for a number of the best practice recommendations in chapter 22.

17.4. Data communication

An important component of the gathering of on-facility meteorological data for short-term forecasting is the timely retrieval of the data from the sensors and dissemination to the forecast production process. This requires efficient and standardized data communication protocols and well-documented descriptions and formats of the data elements so that the data can be correctly and efficiently interfaced with the forecast production process. Part of this process will be dictated by the type of sensor hardware and software used to make the measurements and retrieve the data from the sensor site.

However, there will typically also be a component of that process that provides an interface between the process that gathers data from the sensors and the process that disseminates data to the forecast providers. Proposed standards and options for the data descriptions, format and exchange protocols for the latter process are presented in chapter 4 of part 1 "Forecast solution selection process".

CHAPTER EIGHTEEN

Meteorological instrumentation for real-time operation

Key points

This section describes and analyzes instrumentation that is currently in routine operational use as well as sensor types that are under development in the context of real-time forecasting applications for both wind and solar projects.

For wind projects, this chapter provides guidelines for establishing requirements for alternatives to meteorological masts, where this is part of the solution (e.g. diversity), cost savings, or ease of setup and implementation (e.g. if hub height winds are required at > 100 m).

For solar projects currently used standard meteorological instrumentation is described and compared to more advanced solar radiation instruments and measurement methods.

The focus of the measurement and methodology analyzes is to provide a knowledge base of the benefits and associated resources and requirements necessary to make fair and transparent evaluations and comparisons of the instrumentation, e.g. for a qualifying process.

The purpose of meteorological measurements as a supplement to the power measurements at wind and solar plants is to provide a measure of the resource and weather situation at the specific location and any given time. This information should not only be considered as an obligation of wind and solar plant operators due to technical requirements of system operation, but also as a tool to optimize the operation of wind turbines and solar plants by the operators.

For both the system operator and the plant operator, these measurements are an independent signal at the plant location that can warn about critical weather and provide an indication on whether the wind turbines and solar panels are performing at their expected level. For the transmission system operator, such measurements can additionally be used for situational awareness of the weather in the control area that may affect the transmission lines. They also provide a second means of verification, whether the power output at a given wind or solar plant is according to expectations or malfunctioning. This can be important for the economics of the plant, but also valuable for operators in critical situations. Meteorological centres have also shown an interest in these data for input into the initialization process (i.e.

IEA Wind Recommended Practice for the Implementation of Renewable Energy Forecasting Solutions
https://doi.org/10.1016/B978-0-44-318681-3.00031-3

the data assimilation process) of operational numerical weather prediction models (e.g. [89,108]) that typically lack input data at hub height levels.

One of the most important findings so far has been that the quality of data provided is the most essential parameter and an issue to be solved in order to gain higher quality forecasts through the use of such measurements. In fact, it has been identified that if there is no specific effort put into standardization of meteorological data requirements in the power industry, the benefits cannot harvested.

The following is a list of typical instrumentation used for wind and solar projects. These will be the focal point of this recommended practice guideline and recommendations will be made in how to setup these instruments and the implications that the use of the various instruments have on data quality and usability in the operational real-time context in the energy industry.

18.1. Instrumentation for wind projects

From a wind power forecasting perspective, there is potential value in the measurement of a comprehensive set of meteorological variables on or in the vicinity of operating wind projects. Of course, the most critical variable to measure is the wind speed and direction at heights that correspond to the levels swept by the turbine rotors with the hub height level generally considered to be the most important measurement level, if measurements can be made at only one height. The measurement of wind speed and direction at heights in the vicinity of the turbine hub can be achieved in two primary ways: (1) deploy one or more in-situ wind measurement devices at near hub-height and (2) deploy a ground-based remote wind sensing device. However, recent sensor technology advances have also made it feasible to consider the deployment of remote wind sensing devices at hub height.

The in-situ wind sensors consist of various types of anemometers and possibly wind vanes. Historically, the most commonly deployed in-situ wind measurement devices have been cup anemometers and wind vanes. However, the current trend is to deploy sonic-type anemometers rather than cup anemometers and wind vanes. In either case the sensor must be physically deployed at the desired measurement level. There are two primary options to achieve that goal:

(1) deploy the sensor on a meteorological mast of appropriate height that is sited in a representative location

(2) deploy the sensor on the nacelle of the turbines.

The measurement issues associated with each type of in-situ sensor and their deployment locations are discussed in the following subsections.

The other major wind measurement option is to deploy a ground-based remote sensing device. There are two primary types of devices in operational use for wind power applications:

(1) SODAR (Sound Detection and Ranging)

(2) LIDAR (Light Detection and Ranging)

Recent advances in LIDAR technology have made it feasible to deploy LIDAR units on the turbine nacelle. The key characteristics of these remote sensing devices and the issues associated with the data from these sensors are presented in following subsections.

In addition to wind speed and direction measurements, there is often value in measuring other meteorological parameters. Additional sensors that are often deployed are:

- Temperature sensors
- Hygrometers
- Air pressure sensors or microbarographs
- Precipitation sensors and/or Rain Gauges

Temperature and air pressure measurements enable the calculations of air density which is a factor in a turbine power curve. The temperature measurements can also be valuable for the monitoring of conditions that could result in low or high temperature turbine shutdown. The combination of temperature, humidity and precipitation sensors can be useful in identifying conditions favorable for turbine icing (or ice shedding) and possibly estimating the amount of ice accumulation.

In addition to these fairly standard sensors, other types of sensors have also been infrequently deployed at wind projects. These include:

- Microwave Radiometers (measures energy emitted at sub-millimeter-to-centimeter wavelengths at frequencies of 1–1000 GHz), which can be used to derive vertical profiles of temperature and moisture above the sensor site
- Ceilometer (light source to determine the height of a cloud base. Ceilometers can also be used to measure the aerosol concentration)
- Icing Sensor (measures the amount of ice accumulation on the sensor)

These sensors are more commonly used in research measurement campaigns and in meteorological projects. Literature on these types such as microwave radiometers are described by e.g. [109,110], for ceilometers by [111], or microbarographs by [112].

In addition to the deployment of the sensors, additional infrastructure must be installed to provide power to the sensors and infrastructure systems, temporarily store the data until it is transmitted and communicate the data for use in the applications. These include data loggers, communication systems and power supply components.

18.1.1 Cup anemometers

Cup anemometers with wind vanes for direction measurements are the most common sensor used for wind speed and direction measurements. There are the IEC 61400-12-1, the 61400-12-2 and the ISO/IEC 17025 standards that describe how these instruments must be calibrated and mounted as well as describing the process and the integrity of the measurement processes and the design of the mast, instruments and measuring procedures.

Fig. 18.1 shows the top of a Robinson cup anemometer, the first cup anemometer developed in 1899 [113], a mast mounted cup anemometer of today's standard and a propeller anemometer.

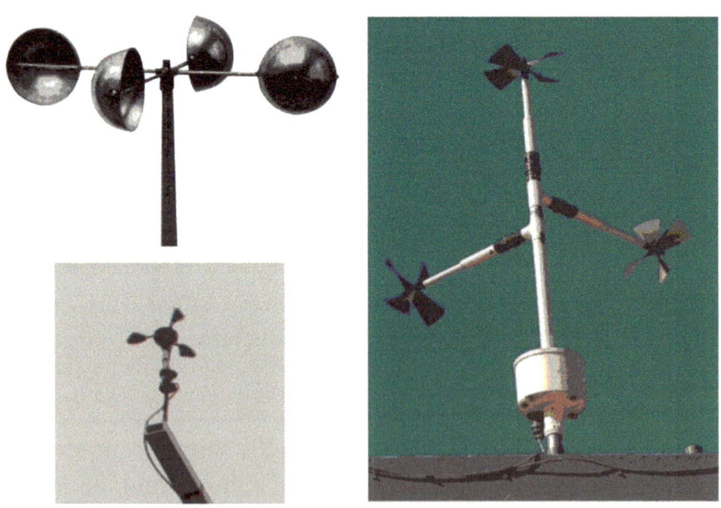

Figure 18.1 Example of an Robinson cup anemometer [113] (left upper), a cup anomometer at a field campain at Ambros Light (left lower image by Jeffrey F. Freedman with kind permission) and a propeller anemometer (right image by Jeffrey F. Freedman with kind permission).

18.1.2 Sonic and ultra-sonic anemometers

The sonic and ultra-sonic 3D anemometers have a long tradition in atmospheric science and meteorology to gather data for boundary layer studies of turbulence intensity and phenomena like low level jets.

These instruments are well tested and can be used for real-time operations, but have been considered too expensive for traditional wind measurements (e.g. [114–117]).

However, recent technological advances have lowered the cost of sonic anemometers and they now often provide an economically feasible high quality measurement alternative. Fig. 18.2 shows examples of a 2D sonic anemometer, a 3D sonic anemometer and an acoustic resonance anemometer.

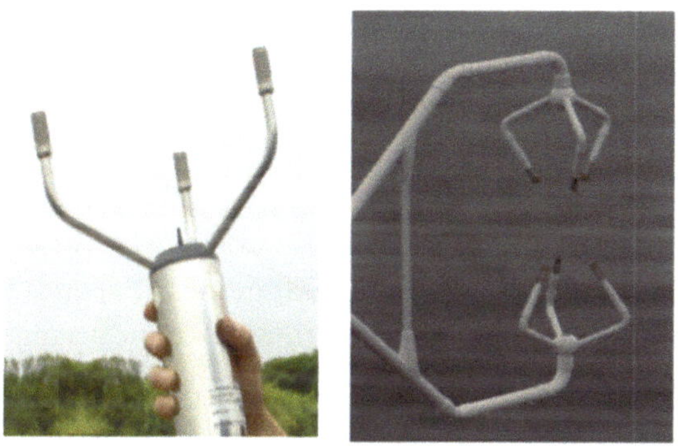

Figure 18.2 Example of a 2D sonic anemometer (left image by Jeffrey F. Freedman with kind permission), a 3D ultrasonic anemomenter (middle image by Jeffrey F. Freedman with kind permission) and an acoustic resonance anemometer (right), a technology that uses resonating acoustic (ultrasonic) waves within a small purpose-built cavity instead of the time of flight measurement of conventional sonic anemometers [118].

18.1.3 Remote sensing devices

Remote sensing has a long tradition in geology, atmospheric science, hydrology and oceanography and other earth sciences. The earliest remote sensing "devices" were aerial photographs that were analyzed with the heights and the geographical space in which the pictures were taken.

Today, remote sensing devices are used in wind energy applications to measure wind speed and direction [119]. They are based on the emission of radiation or sound that interacts with the atmosphere, e.g. with aerosols that move with the wind speed. The sensor measures the signal that is reflected or back-scattered from the particles and has experienced a frequency shift due to the Doppler effect. The frequency shift is proportional to the line-of-sight (LOS) wind speed along the direction of the emitted beam or sound. Horizontal wind speeds and directions are derived from the LOS data through the use of wind field reconstruction algorithms.

Examples of such devices are RADAR (RAdio Detection And Ranging sensor), SODAR (SOund/SOnic Detection And Ranging sensor) and LIDAR (LIght Detection And Ranging sensor). These sensors have been deployed on the ground, elevated platforms, aircraft or even satellites. For wind energy applications such as site assessment or real-time applications, mostly ground-based devices are used to measure the LOS wind speed vertically and then the horizontal wind speed and wind direction is derived. The quality of remote sensing data is dependent on its spatial, temporal, spectral, and radiometric resolutions. Technology developments and/or the instrument's signal processing therefore may have to vary depending on where and for which purpose the instrument will be deployed.

SODAR and LIDAR are the most commonly used technologies in wind power applications. The SODAR devices are typically a phased array or a three-antenna type. SODARs typically provide a vertical profile of wind speed and direction. The range of measurement depends on the power of the unit and the atmospheric conditions. A typical range for a lower cost device is about 200 m but high power SODARs can be measured to 600 m or higher about the level of the unit.

LIDARS can be operated in either a vertical profiling mode or horizontal scanning mode. In the vertical profiling mode, the LIDAR provides a vertical profile of the wind direction and speed. The range depends on the unit's power and the atmospheric conditions. A typical vertical range for a lower cost unit is about 2 km but high power units can have a substantially longer range under favorable atmospheric conditions. In a horizontal scanning mode the LIDAR emits the beam horizontally (i.e. at a very low elevation angle such 0.5 or 1 degree above the ground) and thus is able to measure the LOS wind speed at various horizontal distances in the scanned directions. These can be converted to estimate the horizontal wind speed an direction and thus can provide an indication of the wind perturbations approaching a location in the next seconds or even minutes. In addition to ground-based deployment, LIDARS have also been horizontally mounted on the nacelle of turbines to "look" upstream and provide information about the wind perturbations approaching the turbine location (see section 18.1.5).

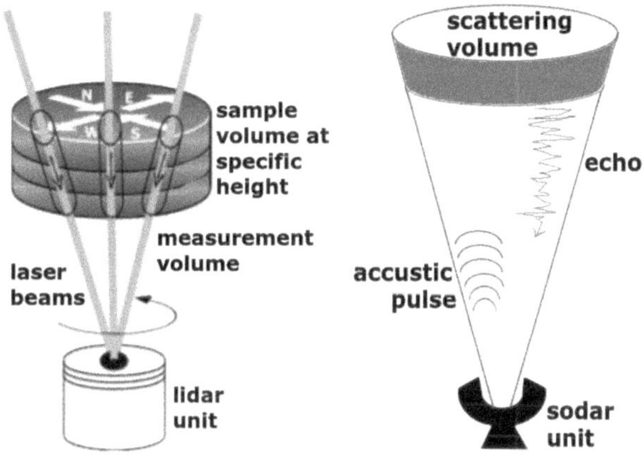

Figure 18.3 Principle of the remote sensing devices' scanning with light (left) and sound (right).

Ground-based remote sensing in wind energy has for a long time been driven mostly by a desire to find alternatives to the expensive or at times difficult installation of met masts. Especially with increasing hub heights, met mast heights have grown to a size, where the erection of the mast requires planning permission and cranes of significant size. Hence, it has become so expensive that previously not considered alternatives from the remote sensing area have become interesting. Developments of SODARs for the wind industry, where larger parabolic dishes are used, but reduced in size to capture data up to 200 m rather than up to 1000 m have also reduced the cost and increased the availability of the signals significantly in recent years. Fig. 18.3 shows the principle of these two devices.

The main driver of ongoing developments has been the competitiveness in price, the ease of installation and the increasing heights of wind turbines and size of the projects, where it is often no longer sufficient to measure at only one location per wind farm. Fig. 18.4 shows examples of where SODARs and LIDARS have proven to be valuable alternatives to traditional met masts.

Measuring turbulence and wind profiles also have found their way into real-time wind farm control applications [4]. Nevertheless, the disadvantage of not directly measuring the target parameter is still present [120]. With increasing experience and technical advances in computational science and technology, the remote sensing devices have however become a realistic alternative, not only for resource assessment, but also for real-time forecasting applications. This has also been reflected in the IEC 61400-12:2005 standard, where remote sensing devices have been incorporated as possible devices to carry out wind measurements for wind energy applications in the 2017 update (IEC 61400-12:2017).

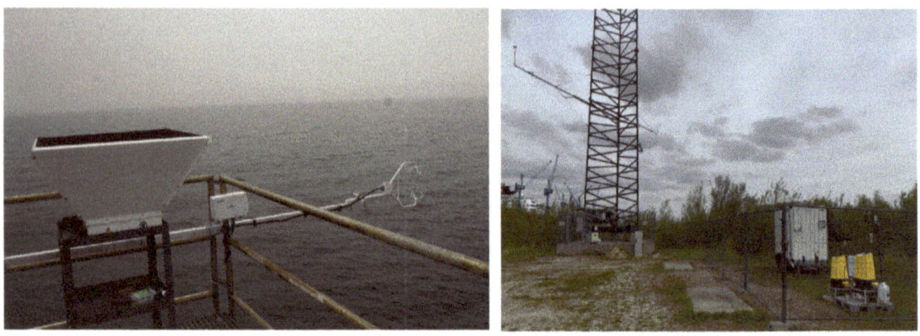

Figure 18.4 Examples of a SODAR and a 3D sonic at an offshore platform (left image by Jeffrey M. Freedman with kind permission) and two LIDARs besides a met mast of 80 m height, illustrating the dimensions and space requirements of these devices (right image by Julia Gottschall, Fraunhofer IWES, with kind permission).

Looking at the benefits outlined by manufacturers and users of remote sensing devices the following list of key advantages of using remote sensing devices in wind energy applications can be summarized:

- Minimal environmental impact
- Short installation time
- Highly portable
- Short lead times
- Wind profiling over the whole rotor area up to 300 m
- Flexible measurement heights

The main technical advantage to be considered is the ability to measure over an area or volume rather than at pre-defined fixed heights above the ground. This is also how forecasting models work. NWP models compute variables across grid cells as volume averages and area or volume verification of variables is widely applied for model verification in meteorology.

The drawbacks of remote sensing devices so far have been for both SODAR and LIDAR inaccuracies of signals in complex terrain. According to the white paper of the Deutsche Windguard and DTU [121] and also Bradley [122], especially "in complex terrain sites, influence of the relatively large scanning volume of LIDARs and SODARs must be carefully considered in terms of its influence on the measurement accuracy." This has been a general observation and a large research topic (see e.g. [122–126]). Issues and preliminary recommendations of using LIDAR in complex terrain are summarized by a group from IEA Wind Task 32 in [127]. The task also formed a working group which is carrying out a group study on several different transfer methods for the use of LIDAR in complex terrain. It is recommended to follow this group[1] for recommended use and up to date advances when considering LIDARs in real-time environments.

When used in real-time applications, remote sensing devices require special treatment. Due to the physics of the measurement principle, the measurement availability is dependent on environmental conditions [128]. If there are too many (e.g. fog) or too few aerosols in the atmosphere (e.g. after a rain shower), a LIDAR does not provide a useful signal. Or, if there are very stable or neurally stratified conditions without turbulence, SODAR signals disappear. Filter algorithms need to detect these data gaps and the real-time forecast algorithms need to be able to handle them. The common findings of all the experimental measuring campaigns as well as real-time testing are that the instruments need to be well serviced and are maintained similar to any other real-time instrument operating under changing conditions throughout the yearly cycles. If this is not done, echoes, interfering noise sources, laser beam disturbances deteriorate the instruments and make the further processing of the data impossible. It is also commonly understood that it requires skilled personnel to install and maintain such instrumentation, if it is expected to run continuously and reliably. For a real-time application it is additionally crucial that the measurement signals can be used as is and need no further processing.

18.1.4 Met mast sensor deployment

Meteorological masts are still the most commonly used way to deploy meteorological sensors for the planning and operation of wind farms. The most common types of masts are telescoping or tubular masts and lattice masts. Lattice masts are typically used to deploy sensors at higher levels such as 80 m. Sensors are frequently deployed at multiple levels on a mast in order to get information about the vertical profile of the wind and estimate important properties of the profile such as the vertical wind shear. An example of a met mast is shown in Fig. 18.5.

[1] IEA Wind Task 32 LIDAR (2016–2021) and Task 52 LIDAR (2022–2026) can be found on IEA Winds homepage https://iea-wind.org under "Research Tasks".

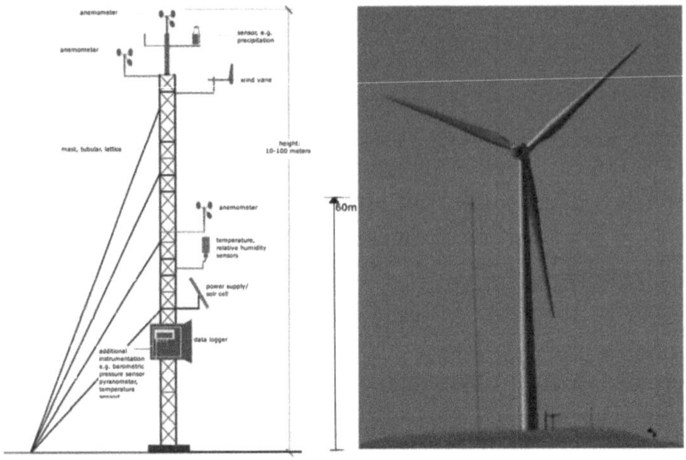

Figure 18.5 Example of a typical met mast with various instrumentation, data logger, power supply and wiring. Typical instrumentation are cup anemometers or sonic anemometers, wind vanes, temperature, humidity pressure, air density and precipitation sensors and pyranometers (left) and example of a 60 m met mast at a wind farm (right image by Jeffrey M. Freedman with kind permission).

18.1.5 Nacelle sensor deployment

There are three types of nacelle measurement devices that are commonly used:

- cup and sonic anemometers
- ultra sonic 3D spinner anemometer
- horizontally mounted LIDAR

Cup- and Sonic Anemometer

The cup anemometers at the nacelle have one distinctive advantage over any other instruments: they are installed at the turbine and connected to the SCADA system that is delivering data to the system operator. However, this advantage comes with a downside:

the measurements taken at the nacelle are affected by two major disturbances:

(1) the rotating turbine blades, which extract energy from the wind speed and increase turbulence

(2) wake effects from other upstream wind turbines.

To counteract (1) the cup anemometers are usually calibrated with a nacelle transfer function which transfers the signal measured behind the rotor into a free stream measurement. However, in the worst collection hours both phenomena disturb the signal of the nacelle instrument and the signals can cause deterioration of the forecast, if they are used in the data assimilation process of forecast models.

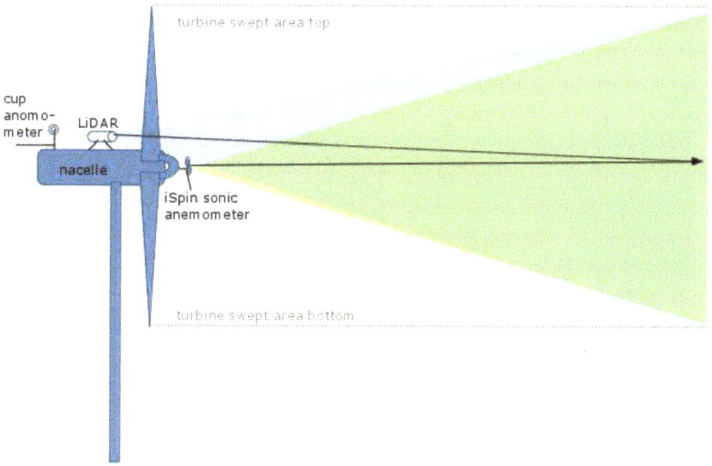

Figure 18.6 Schematic of the nacelle-mounted instruments cup anemometer, LIDAR and iSpin ultra-sonic anemometer. The latter two instruments look forward into the wind eye and cover the rotor swept area.

Fig. 18.6 shows a schematic of the instruments and how and where they are mounted at the turbine's nacelle. The cup or (less often) sonic anemometers are typically mounted at the back of the nacelle. The horizontally mounted LIDAR is mounted approximately in the middle of the nacelle with a slight displaced angle in order to cover the total swept area of the rotor upwind of the turbine. The iSpin ultra-sonic anemometers are mounted at the front of the spinner, measuring wind characteristics directly in front of the rotor.

Ultra-sonic 3D spinner anemometer

A newer type of sonic anemometer is the ultra-sonic 3D spinner anemometer, which is typically shortened to "iSpin". These have recently found their way into wind energy applications.

With the update of the IEC standard 61400-12-2, the iSpin technology has become part of the measurement types used to define the absolute power curve. The iSpin instrument strictly speaking is a sonic anemometer that is mounted at the tip of the spinner of the rotor, in front of the turbine blades, looking forward in wind direction and rotating with the blades. This means that the velocity of the rotating blades is taken into the computation of the signals and wake effects and yaw misalignment are measured instead of the signal being disturbed by the rotating blades.

There are a number of studies that have been carried out since 2011, when the instruments were first launched. Reviews made by DNV GL [129] and ECN [130] provide a comprehensive overview of the technology and it's development phase.

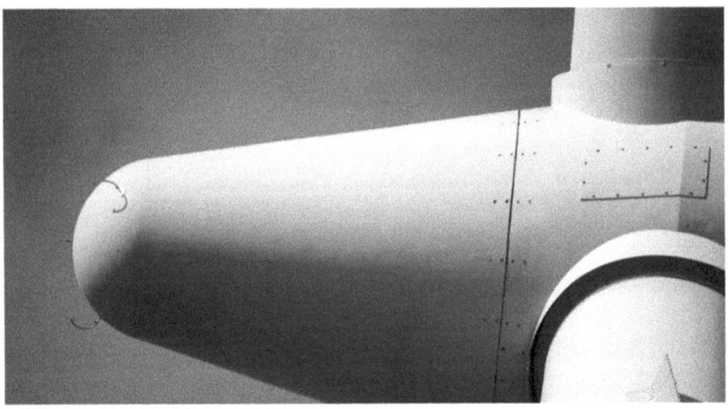

Figure 18.7 Ultra-sonic anemometer spinner technology "iSpin" example mounted at a turbine nacelle top. Image provided by Troels Friis Pedersen with kind permission.

DTU Wind (Ris/o Laboratory) has published a number of technical reports describing the technology characteristics and basic principles [131–133]. The "iSpin" instrument was installed for the first time on a fleet of wind turbines in Denmark in 2016, and delivered, implemented and maintained by ROMO WIND A/S [134,135]. There is a research and demonstration project "Performance Transparency Project" (PTP) associated in the first phase after the launch that provides developed Spinner Transfer Functions (STF) technology for different turbine models and conducted test of the iSpin technology to be used in wind turbine performance evaluations in various terrain settings. The project is a systematic demonstration project for wind measurement systems with around 90 iSpin systems on wind turbines in 9 different wind farms, 3 different turbine types, each of them installed at wind farms in 3 different terrain classes: flat, semi-complex, and complex or offshore [136]. See Fig. 18.7.

Nacelle-mounted LIDAR

Another type of nacelle-mounted wind measurement device is a LIDAR that is horizontally mounted on the turbine nacelle. However, the space and requirements for a LIDAR on top of the wind turbine are very different than for a ground-based deployment.

There are several commercially available instruments on the market at present (Fig. 18.8). All are compact in form and are able to measure the wind speed upstream of the turbine over several distances in front of the turbine. The devices are typically mounted at the back of the nacelle similar to the classical cup anemometer. Because nacelle LIDARs measure the wind speed at several points and in several distances upstream of the rotor, they are able to estimate wind characteristics such as shear over the whole rotor plane. They are also able to measure the wind before it actually impacts the turbine operation, thus gathering preview information of the wind characteristics. This makes the instrument an interesting device not only for performance measurements, but also for very short-term forecasting.

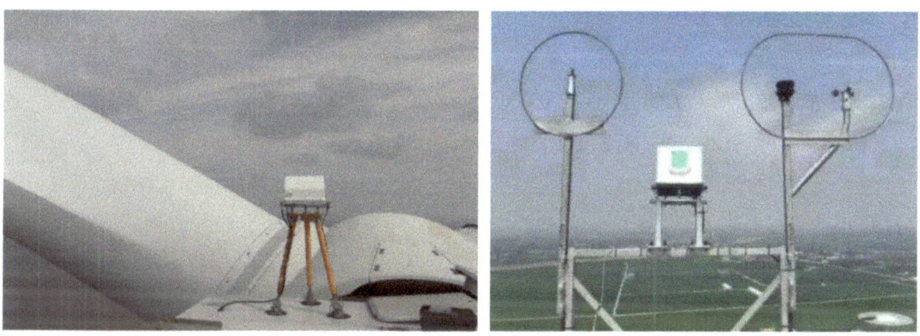

Figure 18.8 Example of nacelle mounted instruments. A LIDAR (left) and cup anemometer and wind vane in the backgound (Images by Jie Yan, NCEPU, with kind permission).

The advantages of nacelle LIDARs are:

- compact and small devices
- measurement of turbine inflow at several distances in front of the rotor over the whole rotor plane
- measurement of wind characteristics such as shear and turbulence intensity
- detection of yaw misalignment
- information about the upcoming inflow wind characteristics for the turbine

It should be noted however, that the turbulence intensity measured by a LIDAR is not the same as the one provided by a cup or sonic anemometer. Due to the measurement volume of the LIDAR, which acts as a low pass filter for the measured wind speed fluctuations, the measured turbulence is smaller. However, a recent study shows that "the LIDAR-based along-wind unfiltered variances with those from a cup anemometer installed on a meteorological mast close to the turbine shows a bias of just 2%" [137].

18.2. Instrumentation for solar projects

The "Best Practices Handbook for the Collection and Use of Solar Resource Data for Solar Energy Applications" (referred to also as "PVPS solar resource handbook") [91] presents detailed descriptions of the relevant meteorological measurements and specific references to even more detailed publications. Here, the focus is on those instruments relevant to real-time forecasting purposes as defined in section 17.1.4.

Different applications may require different and specific measurements in order to get relevant irradiation information from a solar site. The two primary components of sun's radiation at the earth's surface are:

- Direct normal irradiation (DNI)
- Diffuse horizontal irradiation (DHI)

These are linked through the equation for global horizontal irradiation (GHI):

$$GHI = DHI + DNI \times cos(\theta) \tag{18.1}$$

where θ is the solar zenith angle, GHI is the global horizontal irrandiance, which is the total amount of solar radiation per unit area on a horizontal (i.e. perpendicular to gravity) surface.

There are various components that can and others that are recommended to be measured at a solar plant for solar energy forecasting applications. The most common measurements that are relevant for solar energy forecasting are GHI and DNI, as DHI can be easily computed from the other two components, but not so easily measured.

1. **System components for Radiation Measurements:**
   - **a.** Data logger
   - **b.** Steel cabinet with solar power supply and communication system
   - **c.** Pyranometer
   - **d.** Pyrheliometer
   - **e.** Optional:
     - 2 solar reference cells (horizontal and tilted)
     - Pyranometer tilted at the same angle as the solar module to measure GTI

   - Rotating Shadowband Irradiometer to measure GHI, DHI (DNI calculated)
   - Delta-T SPN1 Pyranometer to measure GHI, DHI (DNI calculated)
  f. Meteorological components relevant for forecasting:
   - solar irradiance (various components)
   - Wind Speed anemometers
   - Ambient Temperature and Relative Humidity sensors
   - Atmospheric Pressure sensor
   - Precipitation sensor or gauge
   - Aerosols and Water Vapor

2. **Associated measurement parameters**
  a. Radiation Measurements:
   - Spectral Irradiance
   - Ultraviolet Irradiance
   - Soiling
   - All sky imagers
   - Circumsolar Radiation
   - Beam Attenuation between Heliostats and Receiver
   - Surface Albedo measurement/calculation
  b. Met Stations:
   - Ambient temperature
   - Wind speed and wind direction
   - Air humidity
   - Air pressure
   - Precipitation amount and frequency
   - Soiling

For the purpose of short-term solar forecasting, the optimal use of different instruments and data can be viewed as a cascade, as indicated in Fig. 18.9. When targeting a particular range of forecast horizons for a given application, this should be taken into account before excessive instrumentation is deployed. The corresponding instruments are described in more detail in the following sections.

18.2.1 Point measurements

Most instruments used for solar energy provide point measurements, e.g. a pyranometer measures the solar irradiance in units W/m^2 incoming from the hemisphere above the sensor plane using a roughly 1 cm^2 sensor element. Compared to the size of the solar power plants or pixels of satellite-derived irradiance data this can be described as a point in space.

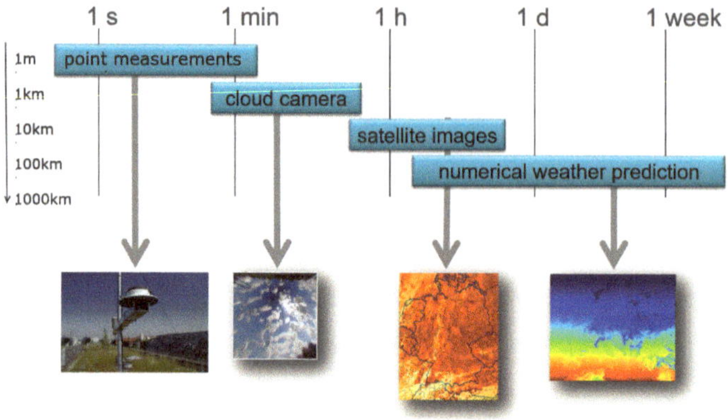

Figure 18.9 Application of different data sources in the frame of short-term PV forecasting. Persistence in this case encompasses time series based statistical methods in general; cloud camera is an alternative name for all-sky imager.

Pyranometers

Pyranometers can be used to measure GHI (global horizontal irradiance), if they are installed horizontally facing the sky or GTI (global tilted irradiance), if installed tilted. GTI is also called POA (plane of array irradiance), if it refers to the plane of the solar collectors. Pyranometers can also be used to measure the DHI (diffuse horizontal irradiance), if they are shaded by a specific shading structure. Such a shading structure can be a shading ball or shading disk that tracks the solar position through the use of a solar tracker. Also shading rings are used at times, but the accuracy of such systems is lower as they cover not only the sun, but the whole daily solar path as seen from the pyranometer which also excludes part of the diffuse radiation from the measurement. In order to measure the albedo, the GHI can be compared to the RHI (reflected horizontal irradiance) which is measured by a horizontally mounted ground facing pyranometer.

Reference cells

Reference cells can be used to measure the GTI. Actually the measurement signal of the reference cells is only an approximation of the GTI, but it is helpful as it is closer to the power generated by a PV module than the GTI itself. This is because the spectral and incidence angle behavior of reference cells are quite similar to PV modules of the same PV technology. DNI (direct normal irradiance) can be measured by a pyrheliometer mounted on a sun tracker. Solar trackers are expensive, and they require a significant maintenance effort. Other instruments, for example RSIs (Rotating Shadowband Irradiometers), exist that also allow the determination of DNI and consist of a horizontally leveled pyranometer and a shadowband, that rotates around the pyranometer frequently, e.g. each minute. While the shadowband is beneath the sensor plane the pyranometer measures GHI. During the rotation the shadowband shades the pyranometer at some point and then DHI is measured. The DNI can then be derived using the DHI, GHI and the solar elevation angle. Also, systems of several pyranometers under a specific shading mask can be used to measure DHI and GHI (SPN1). Other approaches to avoid solar trackers e.g. by using sunshine duration sensors also exist.

Soiling

Soiling measurements can be done by measuring the short circuit current of a pair of reference cells if one of the cells is cleaned and the other not. The approach can also be used with a pair of PV modules. Specific soiling sensors with active light sources or camera systems are other valuable instruments.

Circumsolar Radiation

For concentrating systems the measurement of circumsolar radiation can be beneficial. This can be done with rotating shadowband irradiometers, pyrheliometers with different acceptance angles or special camera systems. For solar tower plants further measurements are of interest to provide information on the beam attenuation between the mirrors and the receiver.

Point measurements related to met masts

Point measurements related to met masts with anemometers, temperature sensors, pressure sensors, hygrometer sensors and precipitation sensors have been described in section 18.1.4.

18.2.2 All sky imagers

All Sky Imagers (ASI) are cameras that take photos of the hemisphere above the ground. ASIs are used to provide now-casts of the solar irradiance for the next 10 to 30 min. Most ASIs use fish eye lenses to obtain such photos, but systems using curved mirrors are also used at times. The sky images can be common RGB photos, or infrared images. Clouds can be detected and even classified by image processing and/or machine learning techniques.

A physical approach may use two consecutive images e.g. every 30 seconds to derive the cloud motion vectors of individual clouds or groups of clouds. Assuming that the clouds will not change their form and velocity, their position can be predicted. Some ASI forecasting systems also include an estimation of the cloud's form and size. As only a limited area is covered by an ASI the forecast horizon is limited, and it depends on the cloud speed and cloud height.

If more than one ASI is used the cloud height can also be determined using e.g. stereo-photography. With such a cloud height measurement, alternative measurements or estimations of the cloud heights, spatially resolved maps of the solar irradiance can be derived from the ASI data. Such maps can then be projected forward in time by forecast methods.

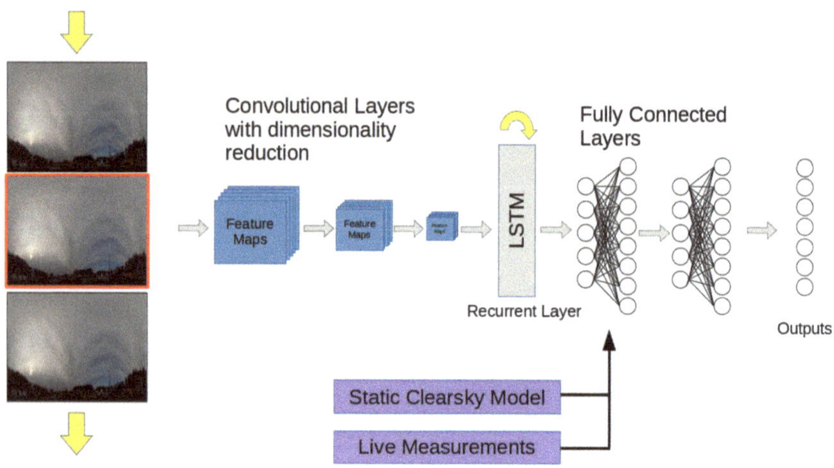

Figure 18.10 Example of a machine learning model for now-casting solar irradiance based on ASI images [138]. A series of cylindrically transformed ASI images is first compressed via a series of convolutional neural network layers. The resulting features are processed by a recurrent LSTM [139] layer, which remembers the evolution of the cloud field. Some fully connected layers can be used to incorporate other, low dimensional input data and assemble an irradiance or power forecast over the next few minutes.

If only a single ASI is available at a forecast target site, an alternative approach is to use machine learning (ML) for discerning patterns in the cloud field. As a data driven approach, this typically requires several weeks or months of ASI images plus corresponding irradiance and/or PV power measurements. Using image processing (convolutional) neural networks and related techniques, the motion and transformation of the cloud field and its impact on the target quantity can be learned, to a certain degree. Fig. 18.10 shows an example of such an ML model.

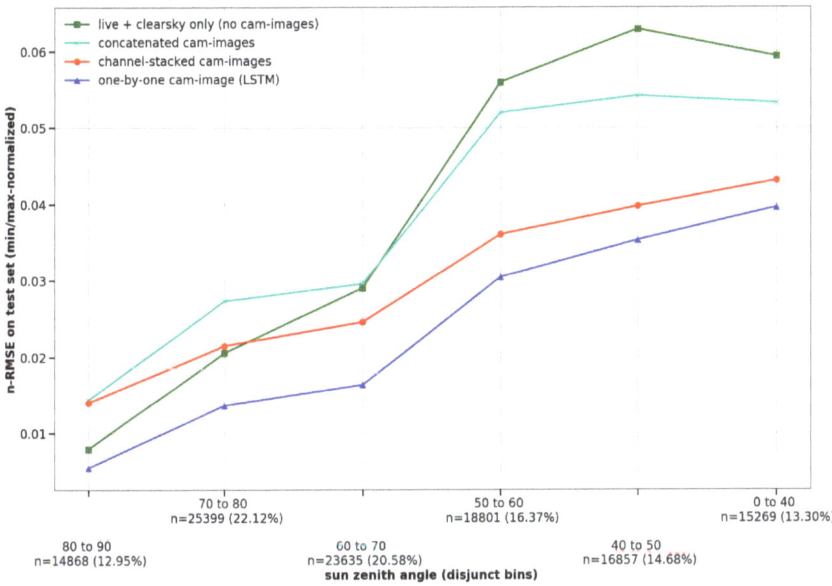

Figure 18.11 Evaluation of the ASI-based 5-minute forecast model from Fig. 18.10 (labeled *one-by-one cam-image*) and three other models, which vary image treatment and the internal neural network structure. At high sun elevation, the errors due to moving clouds are most pronounced, as is the improvement gained by the ASI forecast.

Note that there are many different ways of setting up such models, and a single best practice can not yet be identified. In Fig. 18.11, part of the evaluation of the described example now-cast model is shown.

To summarize, the data from ASIs can help to optimize the operation of solar power plants and the management of solar power variability on electricity grids. For example large amplitude PV power ramps that might cause technical issues in the grid can be avoided. Further reading on ASIs and their application can be found in the "PVPS solar resource handbook" [91] including several references on the topic.

18.2.3 Satellite data

Due to the global coverage of the earth with geostationary weather satellites (except at very high latitudes), one can obtain satellite-based solar irradiance data for any PV project. Both GHI and DNI, plus sometimes other components of the radiation field are available. Surface irradiances are typically produced from multi-spectral satellite images using one of the many variants of the HELIOSAT method [e.g. 140]. The basic principle is that clouds, as seen from the satellite, are always brighter than the surface. Thus, the amount of cloudiness at a fixed location (i.e. pixel) can be estimated from the difference between the albedo observed by the satellite, and the lowest albedo observed for this location during the course of (typically) a month. Surface irradiance is calculated from a clear-sky model and then reduced by factoring in the satellite derived cloudiness. More recent HELIOSAT methods also take changes in atmospheric composition, surface snow and ice, slanted viewing geometries and other factors into account (see [91]).

While using satellite data for PV power resource assessment is standard practice, its application to real-time forecasting is not quite as common. The standard image update rate for most of the globe is 15 min; in some areas new images are only updated once per hour. However, the next generation of satellites will have significantly shorter update intervals and higher spatial image resolutions. For example, visible images produced by the GOES-16 and GOES-17 satellites over North America are updated every 5 minutes and have a nominal spatial resolution of 500 m. Similarly to processing ASIs, cloud motion vectors can be calculated from sequential images, and used to provide short-term forecasts of cloudiness and hence, surface irradiance. Part or all of these calculations can be aided with machine learning techniques, if sufficient training data are available.

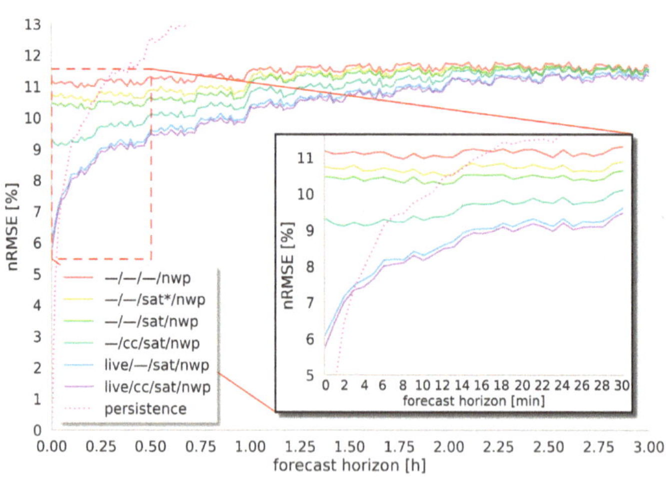

Figure 18.12 Forecast error for different input data combinations in an ML-based irradiance forecast model. *sat* and *sat**: different satellite data setups, *cc*: cloud camera, *live*: live data from the pyranometer.

In contrast to ASIs, data from meteorological satellites are constantly being assimilated into weather forecast models. Hence, the advantage of using real-time satellite data diminishes within the first few forecasted hours, if NWP forecasts are also utilized. To illustrate this point, Fig. 18.12 shows the contributions of different types of sensor and model data in a short-range forecast experiment. Note that this model was not tuned towards very short-term accuracy and uses a simplified ASI processing method. However, the contribution of the inputs towards error reduction of the forecasts including live data (blue and purple) in comparison to persistence (red dotted line) is obvious, as well as the typical relaxation towards the pure NWP-based forecast (red and green lines) at longer forecast lead times.

CHAPTER NINETEEN

Power measurements for real-time operation

Key points

- Live power production data are a valuable input to very short-term forecasting systems, especially those with frequent updates and high temporal granularity.
- Additional operational data such as plant set-points, operational capacity, and power available signals are critical for robust forecasting and forecast evaluation.
- Real-time data should be collected at the same or higher temporal resolution and frequency than that of the desired forecasts.

Real-time forecasting systems rely on input data that are highly correlated with future values of the quantity to be predicted. In the case of wind and solar power, recent measurements of power production are highly correlated with future measurements on very short time scales, those from seconds to minutes and hours ahead. Furthermore, as these are measurements of the target variable itself, they are not subject to errors from data processing, such as mathematical models of the weather-to-power conversion process, which may be applied to recent weather observations for example. Therefore, real-time measurement of power production can be extremely valuable inputs for forecasting systems. Furthermore, as wind and solar plants are subject to partial or complete outages due to maintenance or instructions from network operators or traders, data describing the operational capacity of a plant are also critical for successful forecasting.

19.1. Live power and related measurements

Real-time measurements of power production from wind and solar farms are a valuable input to very short-term forecasting systems, those with lead-times of minutes to hours ahead. This and related data can also assist monitoring of plant availability, which is important for operational forecasting. Real-time power data has the potential to significantly increase the accuracy of very short-term forecasts compared to those based on Numerical Weather Prediction and/or those which incorporate real-time meteorological data. Power measurements have the advantage of being the

IEA Wind Recommended Practice for the Implementation of Renewable Energy Forecasting Solutions
https://doi.org/10.1016/B978-0-44-318681-3.00032-5

quantity that is being forecast, and therefore not subject to errors when converting measured meteorological variables to power estimates. However, power production is affected by non-weather effects, such as control actions from system operators, which should be accounted for by forecasters.

Power production may be measured at multiple points between individual generators (individual wind turbines or solar panels) and the point of connection to the electricity network. In the majority of cases, the energy metered at the connection point and used in settlement of the electricity market is the quantity to be forecast. Accuracy standards for settlement meters are generally high, and live data are typically available to at least the plant and relevant electricity system operator. Power from individual generators or other points in a wind or solar park's internal network will be subject to losses so will not match the settlement meter. This data may however be utilized to improve forecasts.

Temporal resolution is an important factor when considering the use of live data in forecasting systems. Different users may be concerned with power/energy production on different time scales. The primary concern of Market participants is energy in a given settlement period, which differ in length between countries/regions, and between financial products for energy and other services, such as reserve products. Settlement periods with 5, 15, 30, 60, 240 minute duration are common. System operators, on the other hand, may be more concerned with shorter periods (one minute or less), or even instantaneous power, for balancing purposes. In practice, instantaneous is difficult to define and measure, and may therefore be approximated by averaging over a short time period or filtering/smoothing. Real-time data should be collected at the same or higher resolution than the user requires for their forecasts. If the user requires forecast for each 15 minute period, data should be gathered at 15 minute resolution or higher. Higher resolution data also enables more frequent updates to forecasts as new data becomes available more frequently.

A list of common measurements and their potential uses in forecasting systems is provided in Table 19.1, and are discussed in more detail in the following section. In general, they are collected by the plant's Supervisory Control and Data Acquisition (SCADA) system, or by dedicated metering/monitoring devices that communicate with the electricity system and/or market operator.

Table 19.1 List of power-related quantities measured at wind (W) and solar (S) plants that have a role in forecasting and examples of how they may be used.

Quantity	Type	Location	Use
Active Power	Wind/ Solar	SCADA or Connection Point	Input/feature in short-term forecasting models, indicator of plant availability, if combined with met measurements
Plant Effective Capacity (live and future)	Wind/ Solar	SCADA, operator systems	Forecast input and quality control for system operation
Controller Set-point	Wind/ Solar	SCADA	Flagging curtailment and other control actions
Capacity in operation	Wind/ Solar	SCADA	Scaling forecast based on available capacity
Voltage	Wind/ Solar	SCADA or Connection Point	Flagging plant unavailability
Status of breakers	Wind/ Solar	Energy Mangement System (EMS)	Flagging plant unavailability
Temperature	Wind/ Solar	Plant	Forecast input: PV efficiency, snow, icing
Wind Speed	Wind	Turbine SCADA or met instrument	Forecast input and quality control
Wind Direction	Wind	Turbine SCADA or met instrument	Forecast input and quality control
Wind Turbine Yaw Angle	Wind	Turbine SCADA	To check alignment of wind vane(s) and other data quality control
High Speed Shutdown Flag	Wind	Turbine/Plant SCADA	Forecast model training and evaluation
Icing Shutdown Flag	Wind	Turbine/Plant SCADA	Forecast model training and evaluation
Global Horizontal Irradiance (GHI)	Solar	Plant	Forecast input and quality control
Panel Tilt	Solar	Plant	Forecast input and quality control
Sky images	Solar	Plant	Forecast input

19.2. Measurement systems

19.2.1 Connection-point meters

The interface between a power plant and the electricity system, the so-called connection-point, is typically metered to a high degree of precision as the data is used in electricity market settlement and as a live feed to plant and system operators. The minimum precision of such measurements is usually dictated by network codes and/or market rules in a given region. For example, international standard IEC 62053-21 and IEC 62053-23 describe classes of active and reactive power meters, respectively. These standards are references in the Great Britain Balancing and Settlement Code, where active power meter errors are required to be less than 1.5% under normal conditions, or 2.5% if the power factor is beyond 0.5 lag or 0.8 lead, or active power is below 20% or rated import/export. It should be noted that these measurements may not match those recorded by plant SCADA systems (the topic of the next section) due to differences in equipment or location of measurement devices relative to other balance of plant equipment.

Live power data is often streamed to plant and system operators and made available to control room engineers and their support systems. It is often visualized along side forecasts to track deviations from the forecasts continuously. Live data is also a key input to very short-term forecasting systems with high temporal granularity, which is discussed in Section 19.4.2.

Energy is typically metered according to the duration of market settlement periods, which typically range from 5 to 60 minutes. Since it represents the volume of energy used in market settlement, predicting the volume of energy measured by these meters is the objective of the majority of forecasting systems, especially those used by market participants.

19.2.2 Wind power SCADA systems

Wind turbines routinely measure operational variables for their control and operation. Several of these are valuable in forecasting, particularly on the very short-term horizons if provided in (close to) real-time to forecasting systems. These are listed in Table 19.1 and include variables for measuring both power production and plant availability. It is important to note the particular characteristics of these, in particular of the nacelle mounted anemometer and wind vane, which are impacted by the up-wind rotor, see Section 18.1.5 for more details. The sampling frequency is also significant. Typically 10-minute mean values are stored and communicated to control centres, but higher resolution may be of value, particularly if maximizing forecast accuracy on lead-times of 10-minutes or less is a high priority. Live feed of instantaneous active power can be valuable in very short-term forecasting, though it is important to treat both instantaneous power and power averaged over different time periods as distinct variables.

Plant availability is an important factor in forecast production and evaluation. This includes unavailability due to fault or maintenance outage, either of wind turbines or balance of plant equipment, as well as control actions that reduce availability, notably high speed shut down and icing. Live availability alone is useful in forecasting but future changes in availability are also important. Signals indicating future availability are therefore valuable and should be made available to forecast systems.

Finally, data quality is very important. These variables can be a source of error in forecast production if they are not of high enough quality or availability.

(i) **Live active power measurements** are a key input to very short-term forecasting systems and status variables (e.g. availability, activity, potential power, available active power) provide important information regarding plant availability.

(ii) **Active power set-point** is the maximum power the wind farm controller will allow to be produced, e.g. if instructed to limit output by the system operator.

(iii) **Current outages and 'effective capacity'** are not necessarily a predictor of continued outage/effective capacity, but it is an important input on very short-time scales and when diagnosing errors in longer-term forecasts. These are:
- Turbine reduced capacity
- Turbine outage
- Strings of turbines out of service
- Voltage and breaker status at connection point

(iv) **Nacelle wind speed and direction measurement** can indicate the operating regime of the turbine, and be used to verify whether it is operating a full or reduced capacity.

(v) **Power available signals** accurately estimate the amount of power that could be produced in the absence of control actions, such as reduced set-points.

(vi) **Turbine yaw angle** indicates the direction that the turbine is facing, and can be used to verify normal operation, e.g. by comparing to the necelle measured wind direction.

19.2.3 Solar power SCADA systems

Solar power plants routinely measure operational variables for their control and operation. Several of these are valuable in forecasting, particularly on the very short-term horizons if provided in (close to) real-time to forecasting systems. These are listed in Table 19.1 and include variables for measuring both power production and plant availability. The sampling frequency is also significant. Typically, 10-minute mean values are stored and communicated to control centres, but higher resolution may be of value, particularly if maximizing forecast accuracy on lead-times of 10-minutes or less is a high priority. Live feed of instantaneous active power can be valuable in very short-term forecasting, though it is important to treat both instantaneous power and power averaged over different time periods as distinct.

(i) **Live active power measurements** are a key input to very short-term forecasting systems and status variables provide important information regarding plant availability.

(ii) **Current outages** are not necessarily a predictor of continued outage, but it is an important input on very short-time scales and when diagnosing errors in longer-term forecasts. These may be recorded using SCADA flags as outages of:
- Inverters
- String(s) of panels
- Specific outages at lower levels
- Voltage and breaker status at connection point

(iii) **Irradiance measurements** allow the efficiency of the plant to be determined by comparing to output and can be used in forecast model tuning.

(iv) **Back panel temperature** effect panel efficiency and can be used in forecasting systems directly, and in combination with other variables to determine plant efficiency.

(v) **Panel tilt** if measured, can also be useful since trackers may be miscalibrated or faulty, and this data can be used to aid in cleaning of training data and identifying issues with live forecasts

Meteorological stations measuring temperature and wind speed, which has been described in detail in section 18, especially in section 18.2 can be combined with irradiance measurements to provide other meteorological data.

Finally, data quality is very important. These variables can be a source of error in forecast production, if they are not of high enough quality or availability.

19.3. Power available signals

Power Available (PA), sometimes also referred to as Available Active Power (AAP), signals provide an estimate of the potential power that could be produced by a wind or solar plant, if not constrained in any way. Constraints are typically enacted by controller set-points issued by the plant or electricity system operator. PA is equal to active power under normal operation, or the power that could be produced, if any constraints were lifted. Modern wind and solar plants typically produce PA signals internally for control purposes and can be made available as SCADA data feeds. In some jurisdictions, these are shared with electricity system operators and are subject to accuracy requirements.

Wind and solar power forecasts are typically configured to forecast the power that would be produced in the absence of constraints, which therefore corresponds to PA signals when such actions are in place. Furthermore, forecasts that use live power as an input should switch to taking PA as an input during constraints, or at least flag power data accordingly.

19.3.1 Embedded wind and solar "behind the meter"

Embedded wind and solar, which is connected 'behind the meter' is in many electricity systems handled as negative demand. This poses a challenge as both the installed capacity, location, and power output of these generators may be unknown.

Various actors require forecasts of net-load with gross load and embedded generation disaggregated. In this case, a combination of net-load metering, meteorological observations, and wind and solar production data all add value to forecasting systems. Key variables that should be made available to forecasting systems are:

(i) **Installed capacity** of embedded wind and solar generation are crucial information for forecasting. National and commercial databases are often available, but levels of accuracy and detail vary; establishing a high accuracy is recommended.

(ii) **Metered production** of embedded wind and solar generation, most likely a sub-set of total installations that is deemed to be representative of the total generation in a given region.

(iii) **Geographically distributed meteorological observations** measuring wind speed and direction, solar irradiance, and temperature, as a minimum.

19.4. Live power data in forecasting

Live measurements of the quantity that is being forecast are the most important inputs to any forecasting system on very short lead-times. Their recency and locality cannot be matched by modeling due to latency and epistemic uncertainty introduced by modeling, except in the case, where live measurements are corrupted or information abour the location and installed capacity is unknown. In general, methods based on live data outperform NWP-based forecasts for lead-times shorter than 2 to 8 hours, depending on the specific target variable and the reference NWP system. State-of-the-art forecasting systems combine both approaches for optimal performance at all lead-times, and may also include live data from multiple neighboring measurement locations for added benefit.

In addition to live measurements of the forecast variable, operational data such as plant availability (e.g. proportion of turbines/panels in service) and control actions (e.g. curtailments) are also required as they change the nature of the power measurement. State-of-the-art forecasting systems will adapt to changing operational regimes and must be calibrated to predict the variable of interest to the user: what the actual power production is expected to be in the future, or, the power production would be expected to be in the future if no control actions were in effect. Forecasting systems must also be robust to missing data and able to either adapt to the loss of a live feed, or impute missing values.

19.4.1 Specifics for producers of forecasts

It is best practice for those who produce forecasts for internal use or to supply to external users to incorporate live data into their forecasting system for both continuous forecast verification (see chapter 11) and production of very short-term forecasts. As discussed above, live data is a valuable input to very short-term forecasting systems, and depending on the nature of forecast produce/service, may be necessary for post-processing to account for plant availability. Live data may also be included in forecast visualization so that users may see recent history in the same figure as a forecast.

19.4.2 Specifics for consumers/users of forecasts

Consumers/users of forecasts should be aware of whether their forecast provider is using live data when producing forecasts, especially for very short-term lead-times. Some benefit of including live data may be realized by rudimentary methods, such as blending live data with forecasts or simply visualizing recent observations alongside forecasts. However, to maximize forecast performance, it is recommended to employ a forecasting system/provider that leverages live data.

19.5. Summary of best practices

In summary, the following are recommended practices for use of power measurements in real-time operation and forecasting of wind and solar power:

1. Live/real-time power measurements should be used in very short-term wind and solar power forecasting, i.e. for lead-times from minutes to hours ahead.
2. Power data should be recorded at the same or higher temporal resolution and frequency than that for the forecasting system.
   - For electricity system operation temporal resolution may be one minute or less, for trading operations this should match the duration of the shortest traded product or settlement period.
   - Forecast update frequency should match the highest frequency with which new information becomes available, within the constraints of IT infrastructure.
3. The power measurement should be taken from the metering point that is most relevant to the forecast user, this will usually be the metering system at the connection point to the electricity network.
4. Live data on plant operating conditions (e.g. control actions that effect maximum output) and availability (e.g. maintenance outages) should be used in forecast production and evaluation. Where direct data is not available, indirect measurements should be inferred.
5. Data on future plant availability (e.g. maintenance actions) should be used in forecast production. Typically, power forecasts do not include the effect of control actions issued by electricity system operators.
6. Live power available signals should be used in forecast production in place of live power production data during periods when output is curtailed due to control actions.

CHAPTER TWENTY

Measurement setup and calibration

Key points

- Instrumentation Selection
  1. Evaluation of the required data accuracy or uncertainty levels
  2. Cost-benefit analysis of instrumentation regarding quality and maintenance requirements
  3. Specification on redundancy levels.
- Representativeness of Measurements.
- Verification of Correctness of Installation and Calibration.
- Setup and Calibration Logging.
- Maintenance Schedules of Instrumentation.

20.1. Selection of instrumentation

This section describes the best practice for the selection of instrumentation for forecasting applications for wind and solar projects. The focus is not on instruments, but rather on the requirements and necessary considerations for the selection of instrument classes that are appropriate for pre-defined requirements.

The first step in the selection procedure is the specification of requirements for the forecasting application at hand. The following priority regarding the selection process of instrumentation is recommended for both wind and solar forecasting applications [91]:

1. **Accuracy requirements**:
   Accuracy requirements need to be defined for the application/project and aligned with the associated levels of effort necessary to operate and maintain the measurement system under these constraints. An overall cost-performance determination should be carried out to adapt the budget to the accuracy requirements and vice versa.
2. **Reliability requirements**:
   Reliability can be achieved with redundant instrumentation and/or high quality instrumentation. Redundancy enhances and ensures confidence in data quality. Selection of multiple instruments needs to be aligned with the accuracy needs.

IEA Wind Recommended Practice for the Implementation of Renewable Energy Forecasting Solutions
https://doi.org/10.1016/B978-0-44-318681-3.00033-7

Table 20.1 Forecast applications and respective recommended requirements for appropriate instrumentation.

Forecast Application	Requirements for Wind according to IEC 61400 Part 12-1 [142]	Requirements for Solar according to ISO9060: 2018, IEC61724-1:2021 and WMO Guide No. 8 [106,143,144]
System Operation Forecasting	Class A	Class A or B
Utility Scale Forecasting	Class A	Class A or B
Wind/Solar Park control	Class A	Class A
Park / Turbine Monitoring	Class S	Class B or C
Electricity Market Trading	Class B	Class B

Table 20.1 additionally provides typical forecasting applications and respective appropriate requirement classes or standards.

The above classification in Table 20.1 is only a categorization of a best practice, and is at best a rough guideline of requirements for forecasting applications to ensure high quality measurements to establish the potential for improved forecasting. For those applications in which there are 2 specified classes, the second (lower) class should be understood as minimum requirement and the higher class as a requirement if high quality is required and the associated cost is justifiable.

The classes for wind projects are defined in detail in the IEC 61400 Part 12-1 [142] and explained in Annex D of the standard. The classes for solar or PV systems are defined in the ISO 9060:2018 [143], the WMO Guideline No.8 [106] and the IEC 61724-1:2021 [144], where differences, consistency and overlapping areas are explained in detail by the IEA Task 16 PVPS in their "Best Practices Handbook for the Collection and Use of Solar Resource Data for Solar Energy Applications" (PVPS-Handbook) [91] and a few more detailed differences for specific forecasting project types in section 20.1.2.

20.1.1 Selection of instrumentation for wind projects

The selection of instrumentation of meteorological measurements for forecasting applications of operational wind farms should ensure (1) an independent source of measurement to the power generation and (2) a strong relationship to the power generation of the wind farm.

In other words, there is a need for measurement equipment that satisfactorily addresses the following factors:

1. **Accuracy**
   - appropriate quality of instrumentation
   - uncertainty evaluation of instrumentation
2. **Reliability**
   - correct installation of instrumentation
   - correct calibration of instrumentation
   - if needed, redundant setup of instrumentation and logging
3. **Availability**
   - if needed, redundant instruments
   - loggers and instruments being fail safe
4. **Weather resistance and safety**
   - meet local requirements of climate
   - meet local requirements of landscape
   - meet safety requirements (e.g. flight safe in case of met masts at hub height)

This list provides general guidance for the five most important aspects that need consideration in the selection process of instrumentation for real-time forecasting applications.

It is important for any authority (e.g. TSO, DSO, utility or balance responsible party), assessment party or advisor to go through these aspects, when setting requirements for the instrumentation. Dependent on these aspects, there are standards available that guide the power plant operators to the instrumentation that is appropriate for the requirements.

In this recommended practice guideline, the focus is on the procedure and instrument classes rather than the individual instrumentation, as these are handled by available standards (see section 17.3 for a description of the applicable standards).

For wind measurements, the IEC 61400 [145] standard distinguishes between three classes of instruments (class A, B and S) dependent on the requirements for accuracy and reliability and also associated differences in cost levels (see Table 20.2). It is therefore recommended to first define the requirements, before identifying a specific instrumentation quality standard that is appropriate for the application.

The "Guide to Instruments and Methods of Observation – volume I" [106] defines important requirements for meteorological instruments to:

1. Simplicity of design which is consistent with requirements
2. Durability
3. Convenience of operation, calibration and maintenance
4. Acceptable cost of instrument, consumables and spare parts
5. Safe for staff and the environment

It is recommended that authorities refer to the classification of instruments in their requirements or provide accuracy limits.

The IEC 61400 standard [145], for example, provides information on anemometers according to class A, class B or class S types, where the classes of instrumentation are dependent on the terrain structure defined in Annex B of the standard. In areas with complex terrain, the class B standard requires e.g. specific setup of instrumentation to accommodate the influence of turbulence from varying terrain etc.

Table 20.2 Wind instrument classes for various environments.

Environment type	Environment description	Instrument class
Standard terrain	Flat terrain with few obstacles	class A
Complex terrain	varying heights and many obstacles	class B
Offshore	wave/current driven turbulence, salty air	class S

The class S is associated with specific requirements, "where the influence parameter ranges are restricted to allow for the specified accuracy of the anemometer" [145]. Manufacturers of wind instrumentation that sell instruments for wind projects provide information about the class of instrumentation to make it easy for wind farm owners to purchase the appropriate instruments.

Table 20.2 describes the main and applicable types of instrument classes in their respective environments.

20.1.2 Selection of instrumentation for solar power plants

In the IEA PVPS handbook for the collection and use of solar resource data [91] the authors present recommendations for the selection of instruments. These recommendations also apply for the real-time applications. Depending on the solar technology used, different radiation components must be measured. The requirements for fixed monofacial PV or thermal collectors, bifacial PV, concentrating systems and tracked non-concentrating PV are different. Besides, radiometers also further meteorological parameters should be measured as stated above.

A useful guideline for the selection of instrumentation may be the following:

1. **Accuracy requirements**:
   Accuracy requirements need to be defined for the application/project and aligned with the associated levels of effort necessary to operate and maintain the measurement system under these constraints. An overall cost-performance determination should be carried out to adapt the budget to the accuracy requirements and vice versa.
2. **Reliability requirements**:
   Reliability can be achieved with redundant instrumentation and/or high quality instrumentation. Redundancy enhances and ensures confidence in data quality. Selection of multiple instruments needs to be aligned with the accuracy needs.

For selecting the instrumentation, the user must also evaluate the required data accuracy and consider the effort necessary to operate and maintain the measurement system. Specifically, the most accurate instrumentation should not be purchased, if the project resources cannot support the maintenance required to ensure measurement quality consistent with the radiometer design specifications and manufacturer recommendations.

In other words, the accuracy of instruments needs to be considered under the aspect of its purpose of measuring and the expectation on the accuracy of the measured quantity. For example, if the accuracy of an instrument is ∓ 0.3 and the target is an accuracy of 0.1, neither the instrument nor the measured quantity can provide a representative picture.

Various radiometers of the same type should be considered for big power plants and are also helpful to ensure a higher data quality. The number of required instruments for PV parks of different peak power is given in IEC 61724-1 along to further requirements on instrument accuracy, maintenance and data logging. Multiple radiometers within a project location and/or providing for the measurement of all three solar irradiance components (GHI, DHI, and DNI) can greatly enhance opportunities for post-measurement data quality assessment.

To summarize, the following considerations should be taken in the selection process:

1. Evaluation of required parameters, data accuracy, uncertainty levels
2. Cost-benefit analysis of instrumentation regarding quality and maintenance requirements
3. Specification of number of instruments

For the selection of pyranometers, the ISO 9060 standard "Solar energy – Specification and classification of instruments for measuring hemispherical solar and direct solar radiation" [143] separates since 2018 between 3 main classes of pyranometers A, B and C and four classes of pyrheliometers (AA, A, B, C).

Furthermore, the characteristics "spectrally flat" and "fast response" were defined and made up the largest change from the 1990 version of the standard to the newer 2018 version, aligning it to the WMO Guide No.8 on *Instruments and Methods of Observation* [106] and from IEC 61724-1 [144]; here, the performance verification for temperature dependence and directional response must now be included with every individual instrument of the highest accuracy class A. In general they were added to the class to further specify the instrument's characteristics. It should also be noted that the IEC 61724-1 PV system performance monitoring standard requires compliance with the latest ISO 9060:2018 version [143], so that requirements for the highest accuracy, Class A PV monitoring systems, also changed.

The purpose of the WMO Guide No. 8 and IEC 61724-1 standard, specifying "Spectrally Flat" instruments is to ensure "...continuity of performance" [106,144]. In that sense, the newer ISO 9060:2018 specifies since 2018 the spectral error by using a clear sky spectrum and horizontally installed instruments, where the "Spectrally Flat" category is defined for instruments installed non-horizontal, potentially measuring a different spectrum, using the more stricter WMO Guide, IEC and ISO definition of the so-called "spectral selectivity".

These standards state the use of "Spectrally Flat" instruments for:

1. reflected solar radiation
2. albedo
3. plane of Array (including reflected) irradiance
4. diffuse irradiance (diffusometers)

Details and more practical explanations on the interception and interplay for the selection of instrumentation according to the three standards WMO Guide No. 8 [106], IEC 61724-1:2021 [144] and ISO 9060:2018 [143] can be found in the NREL Handbook for PV [91] or with instrument manufacturer and service providers (e.g. [146,147]). The following Table 20.3 provides a summary of the applications using pyranometer signals for forecasting and maps these applications to possible instrument classes, where there exist standards, for which the quality and accuracy is considered relevant and appropriate when using in the respective solar energy forecasting applications.

Table 20.3 Pyranometer classes for various applications. Note that where there are multiple classes recommended, the classes should always be compared with the requirements and desired outcome (quality of data) at stake. If a sufficient quality can be achieved with a lower instrument class, the "quality of data" criteria should prevail and the lower class chosen.

Application	Instrument class	Instrument description
Meteorological or Energy forecasting/ modeling for utility scale PV systems	Class B or A Spectrally Flat (ISO9060: 2018) Class A or B (IEC 61724-1:2021) Class 1 or 2 (WMO Guide No. 8)	Scientific quality, highest accuracy High quality
Measurements for high level monitoring of large commercial scale PV systems	Class B (ISO9060:2018) Class B (IEC 61724-1:2021) Class 2–3 (WMO Guide No.8)	Good quality
Economic solutions for routine measurements and small PV systems	Class C (ISO9060: 2018) Class C (IEC 61724-1:2021) Class 4–5 (WMO Guide No. 8)	Medium quality Moderate quality

Note that these are recommendations that are based on experience from existing campaigns at end-users and the respective analysis of challenges associated with the choice of instrumentation in the absence of a standard for forecasting applications. The third column, the instrument description, provides an indication of the quality criteria that the recommended instrument classes reflect.

When choosing requirements for instrumentation, it should be emphasized, that the recommended classes should always be compared with the instrument description and desired outcome (quality of data) at stake. If a sufficient quality can be achieved with lower instrument classes, the quality of data criteria should prevail and the lower instrument class chosen.

For anyone changing requirements from the 1990-standard with the classes Secondary Standard (now Class A), First Class (class B) and Second Class (class C), the most sensible way is to let stakeholders contact the manufacturers or service providers to find out about the costs for upgrading instruments to the new standard. Especially for pyranometers, the newer 2018 ISO 9060 standard defines for each class the required instrument heating, azimuth and tilt angle accuracy. It also defines cleaning and calibration intervals for pyranometers and requirements for measurement of module- and air temperature, wind speed and direction, soiling ratio, and (AC and DC) current and voltage [146].

For the selection of requirements for real-time forecasting purposes, it is crucial to identify the needs regarding the quality of the instrumentation, as costs for the instrumentation, but also for operation and maintenance are significantly different.

For example, compliance with IEC61724-1 Class A pyranometers with directional response and temperature response test results is equivalent to ISO 9060 Spectrally Flat Class A instruments. In some cases, older instruments from the ISO 9060:1990 standard's [148] highest quality "Secondary standard" (now Class A), may be updated, if a pyranometer lacks the required test reports for the performance verification on temperature dependence and directional response (e.g. [146]).

20.1.3 Measurement characteristics of different technologies

20.1.3.1 Measurement characteristics of LIDARs

An advantage of the remote sensing device's ability to measure the wind profile is its ability to "detect" low-level jets [149] that can have significant influence for the power production forecasting. The low-level jets are a meteorological phenomenon that is a well-known and extensively researched topic in meteorology since the 1950s (e.g. [150,151]) and has been a topic in wind energy research since forecasting started.

Recent progress with the help of wind profilers (SODAR, LIDAR) as well as comparisons with a 120 m mast has been made in the Lamar Low-Level Jet Program, reported by Kelly et al. [149] over a 1-year period.

20.1.3.2 Lightning effects on instrumentation

It is a know phenomena (e.g. [149]) that lightning can cause high frequency noise contamination to instruments. This is applicable for:

- Remote Sensing instruments (LIDAR, SODAR, RADAR)
- Sonic Anemometers

In the case of LIDAR or SODAR lightning contaminates the signal processing with echoes. Such echo reflections can make it impossible for the signal software to process the signal correctly and hence the data cannot be used. In resource assessment of research projects, such noise can be corrected and the data re-processed to provide valuable data. In real-time this is not possible.

In the case of sonic anemometers, high-frequency noise contamination disturbes the sonic signals of wind velocity and temperature and usually makes the data unusable.

Maintenance and mitigation methods

These examples show that the maintenance and upgrades of software to make use of fixes in the signal processing algorithms of the devices are a key technical requirement for real-time use of the devices, or alternatively that the raw data needs to be sent and the processing takes place where the data is used.

Therefore, we can conclude that the reliability of any measurement device in real-time operation requires a maintenance schedule to be a technical requirement in order for it not to deteriorate. If this is done, the remote sensing instruments as well as sonic anemometers have proven to provide reliable time series of wind speeds and gusts.

20.1.3.3 Measurement characteristics of SODARs

There are a number of SODAR manufacturers using a variety of product designs. Some are designed for general meteorology information, and a few are validated for use within the wind industry according to the IEC 61400-12-1: 2017 standard (e.g. AQ510, PA-0, PCS.2000).

SODARS are generally more cost effective than other instrument solutions but some items need to be considered when selecting a specific SODAR instrument.

There is basically two types of Sodar technologies, parabolic dish and phased array, where the phased array solution is more compact and less expensive but the parabolic dish Sodar may have better data availability and quality.

Data availability and quality are important aspects and this may vary between different designs and is determined by:

- Effective sound power directed to the atmosphere
- Level of internal electrical noise in the instrument
- Maturity of algorithm to filter out incorrect data
- Attenuation material / components surrounding the instrument
- Sensitivity to pick up available atmospheric backscatter
- Fixed echo sensitivity

Specification:

- Measurement height span
- Number of measurement heights

Reliability:
- Performance during various environmental conditions (classification)
- Power solutions available and related performance

Market acceptance and maturity of the product:
- availability of independent verification of the performance
- Valid comparisons to approve references
- Successful usage in wind energy projects

20.2. Location of measurements

The WMO Report Nr. 55 [152] describes the site and instrumentation selection as a 6-tier problem:

1. selection of a suitable site
2. correct exposure of instruments
3. determination of the area of representativeness of measurements
4. description of the site and its facilities
5. homogeneity of the meteorological/climatological data
6. access to information*

The last two tiers require international collaboration to ensure measured data can be compared and the precision and accuracy of the measured data follows a common understanding for the use in models and methods to improve or interpret model results. We will not deal with these aspects in this document, but want to highlight these topics to anyone dealing with measurements and that the meteorological community has solved these critical problems by establishing international data networks to provide modelers, researchers, instrument developers and end-users the possibility to progress by exchanging high-quality information.

The fifth tier deals with the lack of international homogeneity on measuring standards that has been a problem in meteorology and can also be observed in the definition of measurement requirements for real-time purposes of wind and solar projects on an international scale (e.g. [153]). If data measuring standards are not international, it is difficult to obtain homogeneity in data and therefore also in forecast models and methods, where such data are used.

The WMO Guide for Meteorological Measurements [106] ("WMO Guide 8") contains in its *ANNEX 1.D. SITING CLASSIFICATIONS FOR SURFACE OBSERVING STATIONS ON LAND* information about siting of instrumentation to ensure representativeness. The guide covers all meteorological instrumentation that are relevant for wind and solar projects and operation. The WMO Guide 8 states that "...the environmental conditions of a site may influence measurement results. These conditions must be carefully analyzed, in addition to assessing characteristics of the instrument itself, so as to avoid distorting the measurement results and affecting their representativeness..." and recognizes that "...there are sites that do not respect the recommended exposure rules".

Out of these conditions, the WMO has developed a classification system with 5 classes to "help determine the given site's representativeness on a small scale (impact of the surrounding environment)" and help to better take their exposure rules into consideration. The classes are however not clearly defined, but are deviations from a standard class with minimum impact of the surrounding environment. For wind projects, the IEC 61400-12-1 [142] standard classifies 2 classes, (1) simple terrain and (2) complex terrain (see next section 20.2.1), and recommends to adjust any instrumentation requirements for sites that fall outside these well-defined classes.

In the following two sections, we will define and discuss specific requirements for wind and solar projects, respectively. The most relevant and useful rules to consider and to apply for the definition of requirements for both wind and solar projects can be summarized with the following **5 rules**:

1. The classification is based on the place of the instrument, not the site as a whole
2. The classification of each site should be reviewed periodically as environmental circumstances can change over a period of time
3. An update of the site classes should be done at least every five years
4. An uncertainty factor due to siting has to be added in the uncertainty budget of the measurement
5. The primary objective of a classification should be to document the presence of obstacles close to the measurement site

20.2.1 Location of representative measurements for wind projects

The representativeness of instrumentation for a specific purpose is defined and explained in the MEASNET guideline [98] "Evaluation of site-specific wind conditions" in section 6.4 and are valid for "conditions which will influence the installation, operation and maintenance (O&M), loading, durability, performance and energy yield of wind turbines installed at a site". This guideline thereby provides "...a traceable basis concerning the conformity of the design parameters with site-specific conditions according to IEC 61400-1 standard [142,145]" and can hence also be applied for operational real-time measurement campaigns for wind power projects.

For operational purposes, the minimum requirements for representative measurements of a wind project are defined in the guide through 2 factors:

1. height of the primary wind speed measurement level
2. representativeness radius of a measurement

The MEASNET guideline [98] recommends that these two most important factors for the representativeness of measurements are defined by a "site-specific expert analysis", but also provides minimum requirements for the (1) height of measurement levels in order to reduce the "uncertainty of the vertical extrapolation of the wind conditions"; and (2) the radius around a mast or other instrument at which "the wind conditions measured at the position can be extrapolated with tolerable uncertainty" and where "all wind turbines shall be located in the representativeness radius of at least one measurement". The guideline differentiates between two terrain classes [98]. The United States Environmental Protection Agency (EPA) provides a "Meteorological Monitoring Guidance for Regulatory modelling applications" [107] add to these two terrain types a type that represents a coastal or offshore location:

- **simple terrain class**
  flat terrain with no noticeable terrain elevation variations, where the wind conditions are mainly influenced by homogeneous roughness conditions.
- **complex terrain class**
  complex terrain with considerable orographic variation (relief), significant slopes and non-homogeneous roughness conditions.
- **Coastal and Offshore Locations**
  the unique meteorological conditions associated with offshore and local scale land-sea breeze circulations necessitate special considerations; the latter especially, if the land side is characterized by complex terrain

This ensures the representativeness of measurements to capture the wind conditions reaching the entire wind farm.

Table 20.4 provide these minimum requirements that can be assumed also valid for the operational part of a wind farm, where the purpose is to measure the wind conditions reaching the wind turbines.

Table 20.4 Definition of measurement campaign requirements for different terrain classes according to MEASNET "Evaluation of site-specific wind conditions" [98].

Terrain type	Minimum measurement height	Representativeness radius of a measurement (max. distance of any wind turbine to the next mast)
Simple terrain	2/3 hub height	10 km
Complex terrain	2/3 hub height	2 km

20.2.2 Location of representative measurements for solar projects

For solar power plants, the location of the instruments is of importance for the representativeness of the measurements as the irradiance can vary within the solar park due to clouds or shading. Soiling, albedo, wind speed and temperature can also vary strongly. For PV plants, a recommendation for the number and position of the instruments can be found in IEC 61724-1 [144].

The most important rules can be summarized to:

- **Distribution of sensors:**
  Sensors should be distributed over the whole area of the power plant and of course not concentrated at a single site
- **Location of the instruments:**
  The location should be selected as representative for the area surrounding the power plant
- **Radiometers**:
  - Avoid shading for radiometers mounted on the front side of the PV modules
  - For rear side instruments and albedo measurements, the number of required radiometers depends also on the variability of the ground
  - For rear side sensors multiple sensors are recommended at different positions on the module, as the illumination profile is not uniform
  - Specific information on the installation of radiometric stations can be found in the PVPS handbook [91].

20.3. Maintenance and inspection schedules

Data quality is usually dependent on the care taken for routine and preventive maintenance. While this can be a requirement in a real-time environment, it is difficult to control. The alternative to setting maintenance reports on the requirement list, is to routinely quality check the delivered data and set time limits for repair of instrumentation into the requirement list with a recommendation to follow the manufacturer's maintenance schedules. In chapter 14 "Assessment of Instrumentation Performance", the assessment of the data for the monitoring of the data quality provides recommendations that may make it unnecessary to require reports on maintenance schedules. It can in many cases be more straight forward to have a data quality measure in place. Nevertheless, if such a maintenance and inspection schedule is part of the requirement list, the "Meteorological Monitoring Guidance for Regulatory Modelling Applications" [107] provides useful recommendation for all common meteorological parameters and their respective routine and preventive maintenance schedules. For most modeling applications, a 6 monthly schedule or a schedule according to the manufacturer's recommendation, whichever is the shorter time period, is recommended. The following list provides the most important components that such a protocols and reports should contain. A station checklist may be developed, which should include the following components according to the monitoring guidance [107]:

- A list of safety and emergency equipment
- A list of items to be inspected following severe weather
- A check to ensure there is adequate disk space for on-site storage of the raw data
- A check to indicate that backup of data has been completed
- A check to indicate that clocks have been checked and adjusted as necessary
- A check for the cables and guy wires securing the equipment
- All routine and preventive maintenance activities should be recorded in the station log and/or on the appropriate checklist
- The station log and checklist provide the necessary paper trail to support claims of accuracy

In the following section maintenance requirements for specific instrumentation is being described and discussed in case the data quality monitoring requirements should contain maintenance schedule reporting.

20.3.1 Maintenance of radiometers

The maintenance of the radiometers is often challenging. IEC 61724-1 [144], ASTM G183 and ISO TR9901 recommend maintenance and inspection tasks including

- cleaning
- leveling/tracking

- ventilation
- desiccant
- general instrument status incl. cables
- quality control of the acquired data sets.

Also the intervals for the different tasks are given. With modern radiometers, and professional installation of the instruments, the task that has to be performed most frequently at the station itself is the cleaning of the sensors. The recommendations for cleaning are between daily (ISO), daily inspection and at least weekly cleaning (ASTM) and weekly cleaning (IEC). In fact the required maintenance frequency depends on the site, the instruments and the accuracy requirement as discussed in [91]. The quality control of the data must also be performed frequently as discussed above. Further information of the maintenance and inspection of solar measurement stations can be found in [91].

CHAPTER TWENTY-ONE

Assessment of instrumentation performance

Key points

- High measurement data quality requires continuous maintenance.
- In real-time environments, it is not possible to compensate for insufficient data quality.
- Uncertainty in measurements is attributable to:
  1. the calibration (and possibly installation) as part of standing data
  2. known issues in the operation of instrumentation in data delivery for real-time operation.
- Quality assurance (QA) and quality control (QC) require a quality assurance project plan (QAPP), which is the management and documentation of QC and QA procedures and should include:
  1. Project description and organization
  2. QA procedures and monitoring
  3. Design of QC procedures.

The quality of measured data intended to be used in real-time applications is of immense importance. Modern technologies to assimilate measured data into forecasting models and processes usually have automatic algorithms that blacklist data that is out of range or in other ways suspicious, because bad data is often worse for the forecast models than no data.

While low-quality data can be compensated with longer collection periods or in general longer time-series for non-real-time applications such as plant assessment and configuration, resource assessment, etc; this is not possible in real-time environments, where the data has to be quality checked at the time of retrieval and processed or dismissed. Quality control and clear assessment criteria are therefore important tools for the success of an application that uses real-time measurements. This chapter describes the challenges and mitigation strategies for processing and quality control of measurement data.

21.1. Measurement data processing

Measurement data processing is a non-trivial task due to the expectation that measurements are to show the real conditions of the measurand.

IEA Wind Recommended Practice for the Implementation of Renewable Energy Forecasting Solutions
https://doi.org/10.1016/B978-0-44-318681-3.00034-9

This may be so in laboratory experiments, but is seldom the case in atmospheric monitoring. The uncertainty in the correctness of measurements is due to two primary factors:

1. instrument uncertainty:
    - incorrect calibration
    - failures/errors in signal processing (e.g. inexact values of constants and other parameters obtained from external sources*)
    - finite instrument resolution or discrimination threshold*
    - inexact values of measurement standards and reference materials*
    - approximations and assumptions incorporated in the measurement method and procedure*
    - variations in repeated observations of the measurand under apparently identical conditions
    - incorrect mounting
    - yaw misalignment
    - limitation of line-of-sight
2. environmental uncertainty:
    - obstacles
    - interfering signals
    - wake effects in wind projects
    - shading in solar projects

Items marked with a "*" are items also mentioned in [102].

There are many more uncertainties in measurements of atmospheric monitoring (see e.g. 3.3 Uncertainty in [102]). Nevertheless, the above list is sufficient evidence to point out how important quality assurance and control as well as the knowledge of the specific instrumentation uncertainty is for real-time forecasting purposes. The following sections will describe a number of *known issues* in relation to wind and solar forecasting that are relevant considerations for the end-users to understand possible quality issues in the received data, and for stakeholders to acknowledge the importance of not underestimating the resources that are required for high-quality data collection and processing for forecast models.

In the next two sections, some of the important aspects of uncertainty expression in measurements, and *known issues* for measurements associated with real-time forecasting for wind and solar projects will be discussed.

21.2. Uncertainty expression in measurements

The "Guide to the expression of uncertainty in measurement" describes the *result of a measurement only as an approximation or estimate of the value of the measurand and thus is complete only when accompanied by a statement of the uncertainty of that estimate* [102].

In section 20.1 and 20.3 it was noted that obtaining uncertainty measures from instrumentation in real-time is complex. Although often too limited, the first step to integrate a solution, is to provide a standing uncertainty value as a percentage that is determined at the setup/calibration of the instrument and provided as part of the standing data. In that way, at least the instrument specific uncertainty can be considered in the handling of measurements.

1. **Formal requirement for uncertainty expression in measurements**:

   For a standardized technical requirement on uncertainty expression in measurements, the JCGM guides [101–104,154] offer a valuable general source that is also applied in meteorology and oceanography. In that way, a harmonization of "best practices" with these directly related real-time disciplines can be achieved. In fact, the guides do not only consider the measurand as a physical quantity, but also provide guidance to the conceptual design and the theoretical analysis of measurements and methods.

   One way to carry out an uncertainty estimation is with the Monte-Carlo method described in [104] (pp. 23–33).

2. **Informal practical solution for uncertainty expression in measurements**:

   For wind measurements, a practical solution for the expression of uncertainty is to add a mean uncertainty value to raw measurements, such as applied by Pinson and Hagedorn [155] in an experiment over Ireland and Denmark with wind measurements from standard met masts.

   For solar projects it is well known that maintenance and ambient conditions of the measurement heavily influence the uncertainty (see section 7.2 Measurement Uncertainty in the PVPS Handbook [91] for more details). These influences should be included in the uncertainty estimates. Influences such as the solar position or ambient temperature can be considered automatically. Other influences such as, e.g. the leveling or soiling of instruments are more difficult to include in the uncertainty estimates, but may be added to the standing data as described above or in [102].

Whether the formal or informal way is chosen for the quantification of uncertainty in measurements, it is recommended to account for the uncertainty of the instrumentation for a real-time forecasting application in the following way:

1. **Standing data**: uncertainty from the calibration (and possibly installation) should be part of the standing data of the instrumentation. This enables forecasters to take this uncertainty into account in there quality control and data screening.
2. **Data Provision Flag**: uncertainty from known issues in the operation of instrumentation should be flagged as part of the data provision in real-time operation, if the instruments provide such a flag. Most atmospheric instruments complying to e.g. class A and B (IEC 61400 [145], PVPS Handbook [91]) provide such flags and only require the IT solution to allow for an additional value.

21.3. Known issues of uncertainty in specific instrumentation

This section provides a few *known issues* associated with the specific use of instrumentation at the nacelle of wind turbines and in radiation measurements.

21.3.1 Effects of uncertainty in nacelle wind speed measurements and mitigation methods

Today, there are different types of nacelle wind measurements available and used in real-time applications such as forecasting and monitoring (see section 18.1.5). Some instruments are mounted at the wind turbine (e.g. LIDAR, ultra-sonic spinner anemometer), always aligned with the wind turbine's yaw to provide important information on the wind conditions reaching the wind turbine or wind farm, other stationary sensors, especially cup anemometers, measure the wind at the back of the turbine's gondola. All of these measurement types show different pattern of uncertainty. For the use in real-time applications, it is necessary to consider the uncertainties for all types of instrumentation and compare how well such uncertainties can be quantified and mitigated.

The three most significant impacts of uncertainty are:

1. wind speed reduction in induction zone (overall in rotor plane)
2. wake effects from rotating blades
3. yaw misalignment of wind turbine

In order to make use of nacelle mounted instrumentation, corrections or the quantification of the associated uncertainty are necessary. The challenges and possible correction methodologies related to these known issues are described in the following subsections.

21.3.1.1 Wind speed reduction in the induction zone

The wind speed measured by an anemometer on the nacelle of an operating turbine is lower than the undisturbed wind speed due to the energy extraction by the turbine. The area in front of the wind turbine with reduced wind speed is usually referred to as "induction zone", is wind speed dependent and usually considered to be negligible for distances more than 2.5 rotor diameters. Therefore, the wind speed measured by a nacelle anemometer is usually corrected by a so-called "nacelle transfer function" obtained from comparing anemometers on the nacelle and a met mast outside the induction zone from the turbine prototype.

LIDAR systems can measure outside the induction zone, but wind field characteristics such as horizontal wind speed and wind direction from line-of-sight wind speed measurements have to be reconstructed using a wind flow model rather than being directly measured [156]. Several sources of errors and uncertainties exist, including the ability to detect only radial velocities, spatial averaging, and wind evolution [157].

In comparison to cup anemometers, the LIDAR can outperform the cups in many, but not all cases due to the fact that lateral de-correlation is usually stronger than longitudinal [158].

Further, LIDAR systems can use several measurements within the induction zone and an induction zone model to reconstruct the undisturbed wind speed [159]. This is helpful, if the wind turbine is operating in complex terrain or has a large rotor diameter.

To summarize, it is recommended to follow recent research regarding the reduction possibilities for these error sources by e.g. addressing the alignment of the turbines and precision versus accuracy and to take uncertainty estimation into consideration when using such measurements.

21.3.1.2 Wake effects from rotating blades

From a theoretical perspective, wake effects from the rotating blades that affect the mean wind flows are strongest at high and low speeds, but not so much in the "normal" operating range. When plotting nacelle anemometer measured data in a scatter plot, where the linear relationship is strong in the range 3–12 m/s and along the monotonically increasing part of the power curve, this becomes most apparent. Below cut-in and above the wind speed where the power curve gets flat, the linear relationship does not hold. It has also been shown with frequency distributions that met mast anemometers produce an approximate Weibull distribution, where nacelle mounted instruments often produce strong biases at the lower wind speeds affected by wake effects.

Drechsel et al. [160] found out that the wake effects on nacelle-measured wind speeds are highest up until the cut-in wind speed and above approximately 10 m/s, where the power curve starts getting flat. Allik et al. [161] found out in a study with nacelle-mounted cup anemometers, nacelle mounted sonic anemometers and a reference met mast that the mean of the three measurements did not coincide very well. The nacelle wind speed measurements, due to the wake effects of the blades, have a much lower mean. The correlations however were strong between cup anemometer and met mast anemometer and even stronger between sonic anemometer and met mast readings within the range of 3–12 m/s.

Jing et al. [162] also found that blade wakes affect the measurement of nacelle anemometer and result in the inconsistency between nacelle wind speed (NWS) and free stream wind speed, which seriously affects the power forecasting and performance evaluation of wind turbines. They propose a practical way of overcoming such wake effects by developing a site calibration model with a NWP model or CFD model and an independent measurement from a met mast or scanning LIDAR to have a model calibrated for free wind-stream. This model can then be used to correct for the wake effects. In their data-driven calibration method, reported in [162], a "Relevance Vector Machine" was used to establish a site calibration model between a LIDAR wind speed (LWS) and a numerical weather forecasted wind speed. Once the model is calibrated, the calibrated LWS can be used to replace the free stream wind speed and wake effects on nacelle anemometers.

21.3.1.3 Yaw misalignment of wind turbine for scanning LIDARs

A LIDAR system needs to estimate the horizontal wind speed from the measured line-of-sight (LOS) wind speeds using a wind flow model and applying wind field reconstruction (WFR) methods. This is the reason, why the uncertainty in LIDAR measurements is often assumed to be higher than the one from cup anemometers, which is justified when focusing on a point measurement [158]. However, in real-world applications such as forecasting or power performance monitoring, it is the wind conditions around the wind turbine or wind farm that are of interest.

There are two types of uncertainties having impact on the resulting wind speed estimates from scanning LIDARS: [156]:

1. uncertainty caused by measurement errors of the line-of-sight wind speeds
2. uncertainty caused by model errors assuming stationary instead of turbulent wind conditions

Held et al. [163] also reports that due to the limitation of line-of-sight measurements and the limited number of focus positions of a scanning LIDAR, assumptions are necessary to derive useful inflow characteristics at the turbine nacelle. The horizontally homogeneous inflow assumption is violated, if a wake impinges the field of view of one of the LIDAR beams. In such situations, the turbine yaw misalignment estimate shows large biases which require the detection and correction of these observations. In e.g. Schlipf et al. [156] an approach to model the uncertainties in wind field reconstruction has been shown. If such methods are applied, a flag can be used in the real-time applications to quantify the uncertainty and thereby assist the forecaster to detect measurements that may not provide a correct picture of the current wind conditions.

21.3.2 Application of nacelle wind speeds in real-time NWP data assimilation

The only recorded project to date that carried out dedicated real-time studies with nacelle wind speeds in a real-time forecasting environment is the US Department of Energy funded "Wind Forecasting Improvement Project" (WFIP). The project had a demonstration phase of 1-year and used 410 nacelle wind speeds for the data assimilation into NOAA's models [89,153].

One of the main findings in the experiment was that the nacelle wind speeds were contaminated too much by wake effects to be useful as individual measurements. Due to the constraints in the data assimilation techniques, it was important to find a strategy that made it possible to use the raw data from the cup anemometers. The research team of NOAA found that the best way to handle the contaminated data was to average the individual turbine data per wind farm and then blacklist those measurements that were outside the range of 2 standard deviations from the mean of the wind farm. This is a reasonable constraint to ensure that measurements contaminated by wake effects will not be passed into the assimilation process.

Additionally, the measurements were averaged over the nearest model grid point in the numerical weather prediction model. By doing this, it was possible to remove systematic biases and make use of the direct outcome of the model at the grid points.

To summarize, the strategy to use all 411 nacelle-measured wind speeds at 23 wind farms was:

- averaging wind speed measurements over each wind farm
- blacklisting measurements that were more than two times the STD from the mean
- averaging the farm-averaged nacelle wind speed data to the nearest grid point of the NWP model
- BIAS correcting at the model grid points

The advantage of this approach is that wake effects are smoothed out through the averaging within the wind farm and averaging at the NWP model grid points ensures that bias corrections are brought forward to the model result, i.e. the wind power forecast. In this way, it could be demonstrated that nacelle wind speeds can become useful signals seen from a general forecasting perspective.

Pinson and Hagedorn [155] used a different path to reduce uncertainty of the 633 meteorological stations with cup anemometers that they compared to model results. Their assumption was made according to the recorded uncertainty of unbiased state-of-the-art anemometer uncertainty, which is a standard deviation of around 0.5 m/s. It was shown that this was a reasonable and valid assumption. However, it is not known how much this assumption is dependent on the number of measurement units and their distribution. Therefore, such assumptions must be considered with care.

21.3.3 Known uncertainty in radiation measurements

In the PVPS handbook [91], the recommendation is to treat uncertainty according to the Guide to the Expression of Uncertainty in Measurements (GUM) [102].

Here, a detailed description of the "Estimation of Calibration and Field Measurement Uncertainty" and mitigation methods are described, specific for solar applications.

Section 7.2.1 of the PVPS handbook describes the details of the GUM procedure that is specific for solar applications in six steps [91]:

1. Define the measurement equation for the calibration and/or measurement system
This refers to the mathematical description of the relation between sensor voltage and any other independent variable and the desired output (calibration response or engineering units for measurements)
2. Determine the sources of uncertainty
   a. uncertainty from statistical calculations, specifications from manufacturers, and previously published reports on radiometric data uncertainty or professional experience
   b. uncertainty associated with SZA[1] response, spectral response, nonlinearity, temperature response, thermal loss, data logger accuracy, soiling, and calibration, including the drift of the calibration constant(s)
3. Calculate the standard uncertainty, U
Calculate an u value for each variable in the measurement equation by using:
   a. Type A: statistical method
   b. Type B: uncertainty component from manufacturer specifications, calibration results, and experimental or engineering experience
4. Compute the sensitivity coefficient, c
The coefficient weighs the various uncertainties of the variables in a measurement equation and provides appropriate contributions of uncertainty of each input factor for the irradiance value.
5. Calculate the combined standard uncertainty, U_c
This is the combined standard uncertainty using the propagation of errors formula and quadrature (square root sum of squares) method. It is applicable to both Type A and Type B sources of uncertainty.
6. Calculate the expanded uncertainty (U_{95})
The expanded uncertainty is calculated by multiplying the combined standard uncertainty by the coverage factor, typically by applying the Student's t-analysis to determine the appropriate value of k (typically 1.96 for 95% and 3 for 98% confidence, respectively, for large data sets assuming a Gaussian distribution).

These six steps are considered a cycle when quantifying the uncertainty of radiation measurements. Step 6 can be used as an input to calculations of the performance ratio of solar conversion systems: to calculate the ratio of system output/solar input, the expanded uncertainty in Step 6 is used as an

[1] Solar Zenith Angle.

input to evaluate the denominator (solar input), and the cycle continues to ultimately quantify the expanded uncertainty of the performance ratio.

Further, these steps are applicable to the quantification of the uncertainty in both calibration and field measurements (see section 7.2.1 [91]).

Fig. 21.1 provides typical calibration uncertainty for pyrheliometers and pyranometers and provides a guideline and recommendation on how uncertainty of pyranometer and pyrheliometer instruments may be provided in standing data or limited as an accuracy requirement.

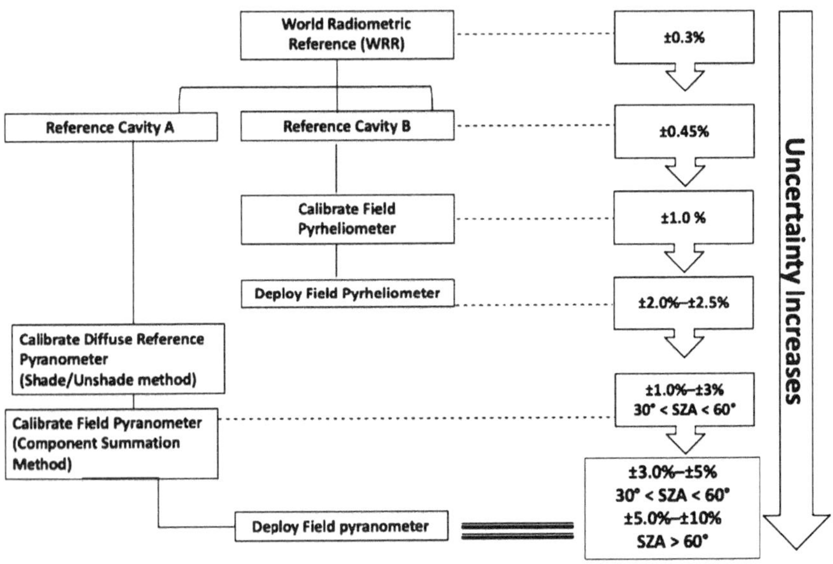

Figure 21.1 Calibration traceability and accumulation of measurement uncertainty for pyrheliometers and pyranometers (coverage factor $k = 2$). Image reprinted from Report No. NREL/TP-5D00-77635 (Online Access to original report: https://www.nrel.gov/docs/fy21osti/77635.pdf) with permission from the National Renewable Energy Laboratory, accessed July 6, 2022.

21.4. General data quality control and quality assurance (QCQA)

The following general data quality and assurance process recommendations are based on the *Meteorological Monitoring Guidance for Regulatory Modeling Applications* [107] of the Environmental Protection Agency's (EPA) definition of QC, QA and QCQAPP.

These guidelines have been translated for use in real-time wind and solar power forecasting with support from meteorological and power measurements.

The underlying principle, in line with EPA's Quality Assurance/Quality Control (QA/QC) procedures, is to ensure that the data collected meet standards of reliability and accuracy.

- **Quality Control (QC)** is defined as those operational procedures that will be routinely followed during the normal operation of the monitoring system to ensure that a measurement process is working properly. These procedures include periodic calibration of the instruments, site inspections, data screening, data validation, and preventive maintenance. The QC procedures should produce quantitative documentation to support claims of accuracy.
- **Quality Assurance (QA)** is defined as those procedures that will be performed on a more occasional basis to provide assurance that the measurement process is producing data that meets the data quality objectives (DQO). These procedures include routine evaluation of how the QC procedures are implemented (system audits) and assessments of instrument performance (performance audits).

  It is important that the person providing the QA be independent of the organization responsible for the collection of the data and the maintenance of the measurement systems. Ideally, there should not be any lines of intimidation possible on the QA provider, which might be used to influence the QA report and actions.
- **Quality Assurance Project Plan (QAPP)** is the management and documentation of QC and QA procedures and should include the following items (which are a subset of the EPS guideline [107]), relevant for real-time wind and solar projects:
  1. **Project Description and organization**
     - Description of Measurement Application and Usage in forecasting processes
     - Validity Support of Measurement Data by the end-user
     - QA objective and documentation for validity claims
     - Documentation of Calibration method (and frequency) requirements
     - Documentation of Data flow
       - from samples to archived valid values
       - from samples to archived valid

- Development of a Validation and reporting method for forecasting processes

2. **QA procedures and monitoring**
   - Performance monitoring by end-user
   - Data reporting validation and verification by independent agent
   - Procedures to implement QA objectives
   - Management support for corrective action and reports
3. **Design of QC procedures**
   - Analysis of time dependency of quality control
   - Analysis of required data quality for forecasting process
   - Analysis of sampling requirements
   - Selection of data screening methods
   - Selection of validation and verification methods

When followed, the QA task reduces to spot checks of performance and examination of records, thus providing the best data with the best documentation at the least cost. Once the QA and QAQPP are planned and setup, the quality control of measurements needs to be designed in order to ensure that the data quality is sufficient to be used in the forecasting processes. The following sections therefore provide recommendations separated for wind and solar forecasting purposes and on two different time horizons:

1. QC in real-time at the time of receipt: data "black- and white listing", possibly determination of uncertainty in measurements
2. QC in historic mode: quality control of specific time intervals such as day, month, year(s) for resource assessment, performance monitoring, model/forecast tuning etc.

21.5. Historic quality control (QC)

There are different ways of establishing a quality control procedure and management. Dependent on the level of quality that should be achieved, there are practical solutions that the forecasting party can take over, or an independent consultant or alternatively the end-users themselves. The decision on that is dependent on the purpose of the quality control, the requirements to the quality of the measurements and transparency requirements.

In the following, principles that are recommended QC processes in some standards or guidelines for site assessment auditing, resource assessment and meteorological monitoring, have been translated for real-time wind and solar power forecasting applications.

The recommendation section 22 will distinguish some of these principles with respect to the desire of conformity and relevance to the mentioned quality standards. Note that all selected principles assume that the end-user and forecast provider using the meteorological data in the forecasting process require high-quality data for their real-time applications.

21.5.1 QC for wind forecasting applications

In most cases the QC methodology should be designed for both long-term analysis of e.gà year and shorter periods such as weekly, monthly or quarterly examination of observational data signals. There are four targets for the validation and quality control:

1. To identify the amount of valid data submitted.
2. To produce a comprehensive analysis, which will provide the wind farm owner with a description of the root of the detected error(s) in the signals.
3. To limit the time from when an issue with data signals starts until it is diagnosed and solved.
4. To avoid cross correlations between measurement from different sources to fill data gaps.

The last item is suggested, because data quality when used to fill data gaps from irregular distances of the generating unit's locations is too challenging and usually only produces justifiable results, when done over long verification periods, which is often not possible in real-time applications.

The "ISO Guide to the Expression of Uncertainty in Measurements" [101,102,154] and its 2 supplements [103,104] from the Joint Committee for Guides in Meteorology (JCGM) distinguish between two types of measurement uncertainty that are to be addressed in any standardized measurement. These guidelines are relevant also for QC of measurements for the purpose of supporting real-time wind and solar power forecasting:

1. **systematic errors**, which are also known as measurement bias, often associated with offsets of the measured quantity
2. **random errors**, which are associated with the fact that 2 measurements of the same quantity are seldom the same

In section 3.1.2 of the guide, [101,104] it is stated that "the result of a measurement .. is only an approximation or estimate .. of the value of the measurand and thus is complete only when accompanied by a statement of the uncertainty ... of that estimate". Considering this definition, all measurements should ideally have an uncertainty term associated with it. This is impractical in real-time operations, where the value of the measurements lies in the availability of the data at a given time. Therefore, it is currently still unrealistic to request uncertainty measures. However, bringing awareness of the importance of this issue may pave the way for such signals to become part of the development strategy for a manufacturer. For now, it could be a standing data value that is determined at the setup of the instrument and provided as part of the standing data. In that way, the instrument-specific uncertainty could be considered in the handling of measurements.

The alternative is to carry out an uncertainty estimation with e.g. the Monte-Carlo method described in [104] pp. 23–33 or a mean uncertainty value must be added to raw measurements, as applied by Pinson and Hagedorn in an experiment over Ireland and Denmark with wind measurements from standard met masts ([155], p. 7). If a more standardized technical requirement is desirable, the JCGM guides offer a valuable general source, also applied in meteorology and oceanography. In that way, a harmonization of "best practices" with these directly related real-time disciplines can be achieved. In fact, the guides do not only consider the measurand as a physical quantity, but also provide guidance to the conceptual design and the theoretical analysis of measurements and methods.

In the introduction to the Guide [JCGM, 2009], it is stated that "..the principles of this Guide are intended to be applicable to a broad spectrum of measurements", including those required for:

- maintaining quality control and quality assurance in production
- complying with and enforcing laws and regulations
- calibrating standards and instruments and performing tests throughout a national measurement system in order to achieve tractability to national standards
- developing, maintaining, and comparing international and national physical reference standards, including reference materials.

In summary, the reliable and cost effective integration of wind and solar power into the electric grid requires that meteorological measurements from generation facilities are trustworthy and maintained to a quality that allows for their use in real-time forecasting tools in order to produce high-quality forecasts and thereby reduce the need for electric system reserves. These guides in combination with the IEC 61400-1 standard for wind and the PVPS handbook [91] for solar provide a good foundation for grid code technical requirement specifications.

21.5.1.1 Specific control procedures

In the following a few specific control procedures for the most common instrumentation are provided.

1. **Cup anemometer on a met mast:**

   The accuracy of a single value from a cup anemometer is not high without a 10 min time average. The purpose of the 10 min averaging process is to eliminate the impact of the turbulent motion, which is generated as a result of frictional forces from the terrain on the air as well as the imbalance in the diurnal cycle and the temperature difference between the air and the surface. From a 15-minute data delivery of a noise contaminated signal, it is almost impossible to prove the correctness or falsify the data signals, because some values are realistic and others are not.

   In contrast to the nacelle measurements, a single cup anemometer on a mast can be inspected at a much lower cost. Newer tools such as drones have made routine inspections economically feasible. Several anemometers can be mounted on the mast, and it is at least possible to submit the data directly without giving the wind farm software the possibility to delay, block or manipulate the data.

2. **Cup anemometer on a wind turbine nacelle**

   Previous studies [94,153,160,164,165] agree that the disturbances, whether it be flow induction or wake induced, are of significant size to have a significant impact on nacelle-mounted measurement. While there has been progress over the years in applying precautionary measures to reduce the risk of measurement errors and thereby reduce the uncertainty of the measurement signals, the physical aspects leading to the disturbances cannot be resolved for units that are placed behind the rotor. Unfortunately, all studies that looked at high wind speeds (> 15 m/s) up to cut-off wind speeds concluded that the relationship to the reference measurements from met masts were no longer linear and deteriorated strongly. This also means that nacelle mounted measurement units are unsuitable in the control room regarding ramping in high-speed wind events as well as pitch regulations due to curtailment or safety, because it is throughout these times, where the measurements are most unreliable. At the time of writing, there are limited peer-reviewed studies that would provide any hint of these instruments providing proven and consistent quality in a real-time operation.

3. **Remote sensing devices**
   Nacelle-mounted LIDAR system measurements are limited by the line-of-sight capability and the available number of focus positions of the instruments. The consequence of the limitations is a non-complete inflow measurement towards the wind turbines. The signal processing software typically produces a large BIAS if the assumption of homogeneous inflow over flat and homogeneous terrain is violated. This is the case at a wind site, if e.g. a wake impinges the field of view of one of the beams, and requires the detection and correction of these observations [163].
4. **Torque-inverted nacelle wind**
   A relatively new development is the nacelle wind speed computed with a method that inverts the power curve to compute wind speed from measured torque. This conversion is straight forward for the monotonically increasing part of the power curve and needs adjustment for the ranges up to the cut-in and from the flat full-load range (approx. 12 m/s) to cut-out.
   There are no publications on this method, as it is confidential manufacturer information. In some cases an evaluation of signals from blade pressure sensors may be applied to compute wind speeds for these wind ranges, where the turbine's blades are pitched. In one recent analysis in Ireland [166,167] the data signals from so-called "computed" nacelle wind show a significantly better fit of the met signals to the power production compared to the data signals from met masts. Among the nacelle sourced met signals, such signals often provide the most reliable sourced met data. The better fit of these data has been found due to the calibration of the signals to fit the wind turbine's and/or wind farm's power production.
   There are benefits and drawbacks with this method, which need to be examined before permission is given, and the signals also need to be quality controlled regularly: The alignment with the power production is probably the largest benefit, while costs are another.
   The drawback on the other hand is that the signal is not independent of the wind turbines and is prone to failures under cut-out or other outages of the turbine, where an independent measurement would still provide a representative picture of the weather situation at hand. Special care needs to be taken for these cases, i.e. when the blades are pitched and no longer provide a representative wind measurement.

The method is not a recommended alternative to a met mast for forecasting purposes with a time horizon of minutes or hours, unless there is a calibrated (against flow induction, wake effects and yaw misalignment) nacelle wind anemometer installed that provides or corrects the signals, when the turbine is in some sort of outage (wind induced or grid induced) and/or the turbine's blades are in some way pitched. If used, it is recommended to introduce a flag that indicates, which type of data is provided at any time.

Otherwise, these measurements, ideally in combination with a met mast at reduced height (lower than hub height), SODARs or LIDARs provide a cost-effective alternative to instruments mounted on hub height met masts when hub height wind measurements are necessary.

21.5.1.2 Practical methodology for quality control of measurement for wind applications

A practical methodology for the validation and quality control of meteorological measurements is a combination of different consistency checks:

- Missing values and time stamps
- Forecasted wind speed versus measured wind speed
- Forecasted temperature, wind direction against measured values
- Forecasted power versus active power checked with SCADA MW
- Computed active power from measured wind speed versus actual active power
- Comparison against previous years of the same wind farm
- Comparison to the average error level for wind farms in the same period.

21.5.1.3 Statistical tests and metrics for the QC process

One practical solution to test measurement signal quality is to use verification methods similar to the verification of forecast errors with the exception that a forecast or a forecast range of the respective variable is used as the reference, because it is the measurement that needs validation.

The forecast has a known accuracy level, which is used to find changes in quality in the measurement signals. By using e.g. ensemble forecasts, the uncertainty of the measurement signals can also be quantified (see e.g. [168]). By validating in different sub periods of the year, it can be shown whether the error pattern has been temporary or persists on a long-term basis.

The use of a set of different statistical tests as recommended in part 3, chapter 11 of this recommended practice, with datasets that are typically large enough allow the user to reliably interpret the measurement data's accuracy.

The following set of statistical metrics (formulas can be found in Appendix F) are recommended:

1. **BIAS:**
   The BIAS in itself should be low, but is no guarantee of correctness of the data, because a BIAS can be low for the incorrect reason.
2. **MAE:** MAE and BIAS together show, if the data has an offset.
3. **RMSE:** There are few extreme errors, if the ratio RMSE/MAE exceeds 1.3.
4. **CORRELATION:**
   The correlation allows for easy detection of constant measurements as well as sign errors.
5. **Frequency distribution:**
   The frequency distribution from e.g. a one year data set of 15-min mean values of a wind speed should be a smooth curve with decreasing probability of high wind speeds. A temporary instrument fault will be visible as a skewness of the curve. Comparing the frequency distributions of an ensemble mean forecast against measurements is recommended in this case, as a mean smooths outliers in the data set.

A graphical analysis of measurement signals with these metrics can then also be used to define acceptance limits for the meteorological variables that are to be delivered.

Figs. 21.2 and 21.3 show examples of results of a historic quality control procedure of data signals in form of CORRELATION, MAE and BIAS for the following 4 variables:

(a) wind speed
(b) wind direction
(c) air temperature
(d) air pressure.

Each metric is calculated for one wind farm. The ranking for the quality will always be variable dependent. For example temperature varies less than wind speed and therefore generally achieves a higher correlation. With such a graphical analysis it is possible to define acceptance limits for the quality of the data in terms of BIAS, MAE and CORRELATION.

This type of validation procedure has been found [166] to allow for the examination of met signal data in an anonymous form while also being

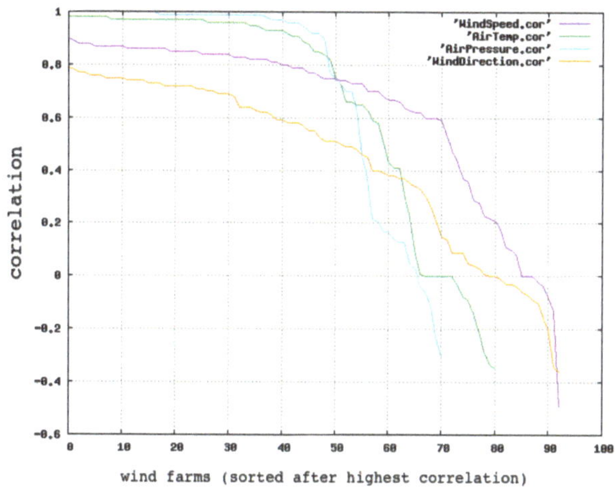

Figure 21.2 Example of a graphical analysis of met data signals for 4 variables to define acceptance limits. The x-axis shows the percent amount of wind farms ordered from lowest to highest error score (y-axis).

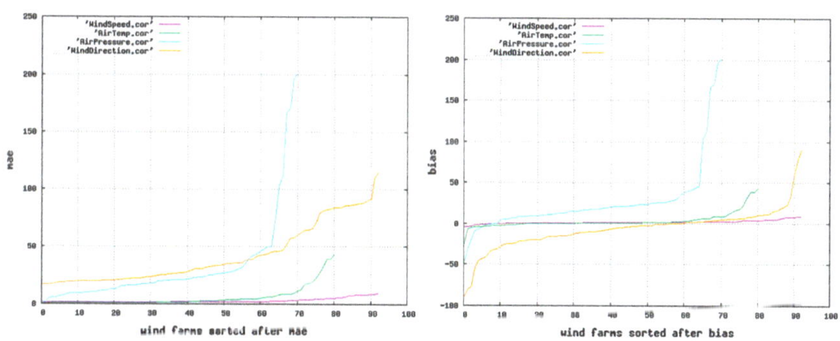

Figure 21.3 Example of a graphical analysis of met data signals for 4 variables to define acceptance limits for historic MAE QC (left) and hMAE QC (right). The x-axis shows the numeric order of wind farms with lowest to highest error score (y-axis).

suitable to produce a meaningful overview of the data quality. The graphs directly show the percentage of capacity that lacks quality. Usually, temporary outages show up as spikes in data time series. Although forecasting systems have to have an ad-hoc quality control and must contain a certain fault tolerance for blacklisting "spiky" data, some spikes are weather related and may in certain weather situations no longer be distinguishable from data that is realistic. Extreme errors often occur in individual months, after periods of higher reliability, and indicate a weather dependency [166].

21.5.2 QC for solar applications

There are several sets of limit-based QC tests for historic radiation data (BSRN, SERI QC, QCRad, MESOR, ENDORSE [169,170]). The tests in the literature use different limits for individual irradiance components (DHI, GHI, DNI) or parameters derived from these components together with solar position and at times clear sky irradiance. Types of limits are:

- physical possible limits
- rare limits
- extremely rare limits

The existing QC tests have been harmonized in the framework of IEA PVPS Task 16 for stations with measurements of all three irradiance components (GHI, DHI, DNI) or two (GHI and DHI or DNI) and are documented in the section 3.4.2 of the Data Inspection of the PVPS Handbook [91] in more detail.

The quality control consists of automatic tests and visual inspection by an expert. The QC results in one flag per time stamp and test. The flag's value is recommended to be:

- "data seems ok"
- "data point was detected as problematic"
- "test could not be performed".

The latter can occur for a missing time stamp/data, or if the test domain criteria was not satisfied and the test could not be applied.

The visual inspection of the data is of importance to detect bad data and manually assign the flag. This also includes the control of the metadata (logbook with comments, calibration information). Visual inspection can also help to determine, if the time stamps refer to the start or the end of the averaging interval (e.g. 1 min, 10 min or 1 h averaging). If test results are visualized, manual flagging may be used to improve the automatic test results in the real-time environment over time. Some tests may not be automated, but only used for visual inspections:

- Missing time stamps
- Missing values
- K-Tests[2]
- Baseline Surface Radiation Network (BSRN) QC

[2] The test compares three K values that are ratios of (1) the global irradiance to the extraterrestrial (i.e. top of atmosphere) irradiance, (2) the direct irradiance to the extraterrestrial irradiance and (3) the ratio of diffuse to global irradiance. The test verifies if these values are within specified intervals (see details in chapter 3 "Measuring Solar Radiation" of the PVPS handbook [91] and e.g. [171]).

- **(a)** Three-component test (if DNI, DHI and GHI are measured, one can calculate GHI from DHI and DNI and the solar elevation angle and compare it to the measured GHI)
- **(b)** Test of extremely rare limits
- **(c)** Test of physically possible limits (PPL)

- Tracker-off test verifying high GHI, low DHI at DNI close to zero
- Visual inspection

The PVPS handbook [91] provides some information about "gap filling" methods in section *3.4.2.1 Data Quality Control and Assurance* to fill in missing values or time stamps in time series. While this is relevant for the generation of bankable data in resource assessment or other monitoring tasks, it is more important in real-time applications to ensure that data gaps are not counted in the verification calculations, where they can lead to misleading results, if they are e.g. filled with zeros instead of a well-defined flag in the databases.

For the visual inspection, several plots are needed. Heat maps of the irradiance with axes hour of the day (y) and day of year (x) may be used. An example of such a heat map has been presented by El Alani et al. [171] and can be seen in Fig. 21.4.

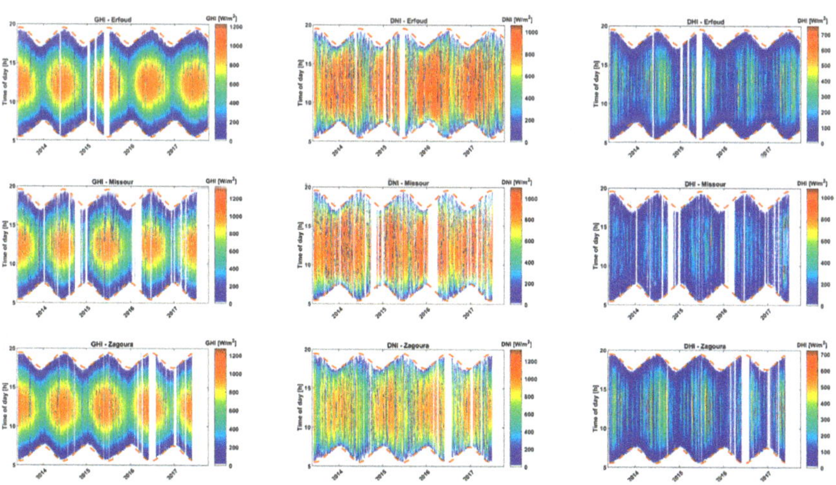

Figure 21.4 Two-dimensional representations of GHI, DNI and DHI measurements in Erfoud, Missour, and Zagoura. White color during daytime between sunrise and sunset times (represented in red dash lines) correspond to missing values, x-axis corresponds to days. (Image from El Alani et al. [171] under the Creative Commons Attribution 4.0 International licence [62]).

To check for shading, heat maps of the maximum irradiance in bins of the sun's elevation and the azimuth angle with axis elevation (y) and azimuth (x) are commonly used. Objects can be seen in this plot as patterns of low irradiance. The deviation of the DNI measurement from the DNI, when calculated from GHI and DHI, should also be inspected (e.g. in form of heat maps or a plot against time). The AM/PM symmetry of the GHI data should be visualized. Calibration changes can be made visible in a plot of the clear-sky index (measured GHI/extraterrestrial GHI) against time.

The decision to use a data point, should depend not only on the result of a single flag for a timestamp, but also all flags for that timestamp and surrounding timestamps.

For the validation of satellite and model derived radiation data, the following procedure is recommended: A data point is usable, if

- all individual QC flags are indicating that the data is ok
- the test could not be performed and all measured radiation components are available

Data should be excluded, if

- 30% or more of the timestamps (daytime, solar elevation > 0) from one day are flagged, exclude the entire day
- intervals between flagged data are shorter than 60 min.

For the determination of the length of the interval, only timestamps with elevation > 0 are considered. Less stringent exclusion rules could be applied for other purposes, such as the determination of yearly sums.

21.6. Real-time quality control (QC)

There are significant differences between real-time quality control and historic quality control (QC). The major difference is that real-time QC is restricted to the data values in real-time and hence the methods used need to relate to the historic validations, calibration results and pre-defined accuracy limits and levels, but not all can be conducted and validated in real-time.

For most general quality control of measurement data, there is no difference, whether the measurements are targeted to wind or solar forecasting applications. For this reason, the first part of this section describes the recommended quality control procedures that apply for both wind and solar forecasting applications.

A general description of errors in both wind and solar measurements can be summarized to (see e.g. [172,173]:

1. **data management errors:**
   - data transcription and collection
   - errors that occurred during data manipulation (e.g. duplication of data sequences)
   - standardization of practices (e.g. measurement units, reference times)
2. **measurement errors:**
   - temporal or spatial consistency in the data
   - errors produced at the moment of sampling as a result of:
     - instrumental malfunction
     - calibration
     - exposure problems.

The data management errors can be avoided or quickly solved in many cases, if there is a QCQA project plan (QCQAPP) as described for the historic QC in section 21.4 that contains the necessary documentation to identify the source of the errors.

21.6.1 Data screening in real-time wind and solar forecast applications

General rules for data screening in real-time forecasting applications apply to both, wind and solar. The most common data errors that a quality control system needs to catch are:

- repeated values
- values out of range limits (see Chapter 22)
- formatting of data file/decoding error
- chronological consistency of time stamps
- data sampling and time averaging definitions (see Section 21.6.2)
- site coordinates
- instrumentation identification.

21.6.2 Data sampling thresholds in real-time wind and solar forecast applications

Section *4.5 Sampling Rates* of the EPA guidance *on Meteorological Monitoring for Regulatory Modeling Applications* [107] deals with sampling of data signals and averaging of data. These recommendations are to a large extent relevant for the wind and solar real-time forecasting applications in the energy industry, as the recommendations are directed to the data quality required by numerical weather prediction models to add value. All state-of-the-art wind and solar forecasting processes above a few minutes forecast horizon are based on NWP models; hence, our recommendation to follow these guidelines.

The following recommendations are adjusted for wind and solar forecasting applications;

1. Estimates of means should be based on at least 60 samples (e.g., one sample per minute for an hourly mean)
2. Estimates of the variance (standard deviation to within 5 or 10%) should be based on at least 360 samples (e.g., six samples per minute for an hourly variance).
3. To compute the mean wind direction:
   - Single-pass processing wind direction sensor (wind vane): sampling once per second to ensure that consecutive values do not differ by more than 180 degrees
   - Multi point analogue recorders: sampling at least once per minute.

21.6.3 Real-time QC for wind and solar applications

21.6.3.1 Data screening

The recommended data screening criteria for wind and solar projects as a practical approach to data quality control and management follow the EPA guideline [107] and are suggested with some limits that are easy to control. Table 21.1 provides some useful and practical limits that can be recommended for the data screening task.

21.6.4 Solar forecasting specific real-time QC

For the real-time QC of solar radiation data, the QC methods for historic data can only be partly applied. QC methods requiring visual inspection cannot be applied in real-time systems that require automation.

The following tests can also be applied in a real-time environment (more details are provided in section 21.5.2):

- Missing time stamps
- Missing values
- K-Tests (see section 21.5.2 or the Glossary)
- Baseline Surface Radiation Network (BSRN) QC
  - (a) three component test
  - (b) extremely rare limits test
  - (c) physically possible limits (PPL) test

Table 21.1 Practical data screening criteria for quality control of wind/solar projects.

Variable	Screening Criteria: Flag data if the value
Wind Speed	– is less than zero or greater than 50 m/s – variation less than 0.1 m/s for 3 consecutive hours – variation less than 0.5 m/s for 12 consecutive hours
Wind Direction	– is less than zero or greater than 360 degrees – variation less than 1 deg. for 3 consecutive hours – variation less than 10 deg. for 18 consecutive hours
Temperature	– is greater than the local record high – is less than the local record low (limit could be applied on a monthly basis) – is greater than a 5°C change from the previous hour – variation less than 0.5° for 12 consecutive hours
Temperature Difference	– is greater than 0.1°C/m during the daytime – is less than −0.1°C/m during the night-time – is greater than 5.0°C or less than −3.0°C
Dew Point Temperature	– is greater than ambient temperature for given time period – is greater than a 5°C change from the previous hour – variation less than 0.5°C for 12 consecutive hours – equals the ambient temperature for 12 consecutive hours
Pressure	– is greater than 1060 mb (sea level) – is less than 940 mb (sea level) (values should be adjusted for elevations other than sea level) – changes by more than 6 mb in three hours
Radiation	– is greater than zero at night – is greater than max. possible for date and latitude

QC results indicating that the result is suspicious such as the above described tests for rare limits or some versions of the three component tests might lead to too many data gaps, depending on the real-time application. If this is the case, these strict QCs should be adapted with less strict limits or used only for further analysis of the data.

Limits should always be defined based on the required data quality for the target application and data availability, taking into consideration that limits differ for different measurement devices. The site-dependency of these limits should also be considered.

CHAPTER TWENTY-TWO

Best practice recommendations

Key points

Application Areas for the Recommendations

This summary chapter of recommended best practice contains the following application areas and associated applications:

1. System Operation, Balancing and Trading
    - Situational awareness in critical weather events
    - High-Speed Shutdown events
    - Grid related down-regulation or curtailments
    - Short-term forecasting with updates from measurements
    - Intra-day power plant balancing.
2. Wind Turbine, Wind Farm and Solar Plant Operation and Monitoring
    - Wind turbine and Power Plant Control
    - Condition Monitoring

Recommended Principles for the Selection of Instrumentation:

The recommendations for the selection of instrumentation in this section are based on the following set of principles:

1. Accuracy requirements:
   Accuracy requirements need to be defined for the application/project and aligned with the associated levels of effort necessary to operate and maintain the measurement system on under these constraints. An overall cost-performance determination should therefore always be carried out to adapt the budget to the accuracy requirements and vice versa.
2. Reliability requirements:
   Reliability can be achieved with redundant instrumentation and/or high quality instrumentation. Redundancy enhances and ensures confidence in data quality. Selection of multiple instruments need to be aligned with the accuracy needs.

Detailed information of short-cut Recommendations

The short-cut recommendations in this chapter are applicable for meteorological and power measurements used in real-time wind and solar forecasting applications. The detailed underlying information can be found in the following chapters:

- chapter 18: Description of meteorological instrumentation
- chapter 19: Description of power measurements
- chapter 20: Setup and calibration of instrumentation
- chapter 21: Quality Assurance and Quality Control

IEA Wind Recommended Practice for the Implementation of Renewable Energy Forecasting Solutions
https://doi.org/10.1016/B978-0-44-318681-3.00035-0

This chapter brings the principles developed in these four previous chapters to the application level. In other words, the somewhat theoretical considerations from the previous chapters are applied to real-world problems and expressed in a summary format with a focus on the recommendations. For ease of use, all underlying information, explanations and descriptions are linked to the associated chapters and sections of this document containing the detailed information.

22.1. Definitions

This recommended practice guideline is targeted to the use of meteorological measurements for real-time forecasting applications of wind and solar projects. We define real-time applications in the following way (see also section 17.1):

The aim of **real-time applications** is to have reliable information about the current weather situation; gaps (missing data) are more critical in this application type, because forecasts or plant control parameters can only be optimally generated or adapted with the help of measurements; raw forecasts and other control options with lower quality must otherwise be used; temporarily erroneous data is also more critical in real-time, as the forecasts or plant control might lead to energetic and economic inefficiencies, system security issues, economic loss, etc.

22.2. Instrumentation

This recommended practice guideline has investigated the usefulness and challenges associated with the use of the following instrumentation for real-time forecasting purposes:

1. **Instrumentation for Wind projects** (section 18.1)
   a. Remote Sensing for wind farms (sections 18.1.3, 22.4.1.2)
   b. Nacelle instrumentation (sections 18.1.5, 21.3.1, 21.3.2)
   c. Cup anemometers (section 18.1.1)
   d. Sonic and ultra-sonic anemometers (section 18.1.2)
   e. Horizontally mounted nacelle LiDAR (sections 18.1.5, 21.3.1.3)
2. **Instrumentation for Solar Projects** (section 18.2)
   a. Point Measurements (section 18.2.1)
   b. All sky imagers (section 18.2.2)
   c. Satellite Data (section 18.2.3)

3. **Power Measurements for real-time operation** (section 19)
   a. Live power and related measurements (section 19.4.1)
   b. Power available signals (section 19.3)
   c. Connection-point meters (section 19.2.1)
   d. SCADA Systems (sections 19.1, 19.2.3)

The purpose of describing these instrumentation types is to enable end-users to verify and specify requirements and selection criteria, such as (1) which resolution and/or accuracy ranges limit the use of certain instrumentation for pre-defined applications, or (2) which instrumentation can be applied for pre-defined criteria.

22.3. Recommendations for real-time measurements by application type

It is recommended that the choice of instruments be made according to a standardized classification, when the choice of requirements has led to the definition of specific quality criteria for the chosen application type.

Table 22.1 provides a guideline to a best practice categorization for the development of requirements in real-time forecasting applications to ensure high-quality measurement data. For those applications, where there are two classes provided, the second (lower) class should be understood as minimum requirement and the higher class as a requirement, if high quality is required and the respective budgets are justifiable.

The instrument classes for wind projects are in detail defined in the IEC 61400 Part 12-1 [142] and explained in Annex D of the standard. Further detail on the quality of the instrumentation can be obtained from this standard. Some more detailed explanation can be found in section 18.1.

The instrument classes for solar or PV systems are defined in the ISO 9060:2018 [143], the WMO Guideline No.8 [106] and the IEC 61724-1:2021 [144], where differences, consistency and overlapping areas are explained in detail by the IEA Task 16 PVPS in their "Best Practices Handbook for the Collection and Use of Solar Resource Data for Solar Energy Applications" (PVPS-Handbook) [91], the most important instrumentation for real-time forecasting has been described in detailed in section 18.2.

Resolution and accuracy for the respective applications and parameters are provided by the standard's categories for the instrumentation.

Table 22.1 Forecast applications and respective recommended requirements for appropriate instrumentation. Note that where there are multiple classes recommended, the classes should always be compared with the requirements and desired outcome (quality of data) at stake. If a sufficient quality can be achieved with a lower instrument class, the "quality of data" criteria should prevail and the lower instrument class chosen.

Forecast Application	Recommendations for Wind according to IEC 61400 Part-12-1-2021	Recommendations for Solar according to ISO9060: 2018, EC 61724-1:2021 and WMO Guide No. 8
System Operation Forecasting	Class A	Class A or B
Utility Scale Forecasting	Class A	Class A or B
Park Control	Class A	Class A
Park / Turbine Monitoring	Class S	Class B or C
Electricity Market Trading	Class B	Class B

Manufacturers of such instrumentation follow these classifications and provide a straight forward decision tool for requirements for wind and solar radiation measurements.

In the following sections 22.4, 22.5 and 22.6 recommendations for three different application areas are summerised.

22.4. Recommendations for real-time measurements for power grid and utility-scale operation

22.4.1 Recommendations on quality requirements

The choice of instrumentation should always take into account the need for appropriate measurement equipment in the sense of (see details in section 20.1):

1. Accuracy and Resolution
2. Reliability
3. Availability
4. Weather resistance and safety

Table 22.2 Instrument class recommendations for various environments.

Environment type	Environment description	Instrument class
Standard terrain	Flat terrain with few obstacles	Class A
Complex terrain	Varying heights and many obstacles	Class B
Offshore	Wave and current driven turbulence Salty air	Class S

22.4.1.1 *Requirements for wind forecasting applications according to environment*

Table 22.2 describes the main and applicable types of instrument classes in their respective environments (see section 18.1 for details).

The class S is associated with specific requirements, "where the influence parameter ranges are restricted to allow for the specified accuracy of the anemometer." [145]. Manufacturers of wind instrumentation that sell instruments for wind projects provide information about the class of instrumentation to make it easy for wind farm owners to purchase the appropriate instruments.

22.4.1.2 *Wind measurement alternatives to met masts*

There are various alternatives to met masts for the collection of meteorological measurements, such as ground-based LIDARs, SODARs, RADARs, nacelle-based cup or sonic anemometers, nacelle LIDARs, etc. (see more details in section 18.1). However, most of these have either a high measurement uncertainty (due to weather conditions, obstacles or other factors) that limit these instruments to the more non-critical, or non-real-time use. Also, some may simply not have been tested for the purpose yet.

The two alternatives to met masts, that are most common, tested and recommended at present for grid operation and utility-scale operation (see detailed information in sections 18.1.3, 18.1.5, 20.1.3.1, 21.3.1.3 and 21.5.1.1) are:

1. Remote Sensing Devices: LIDAR/SODARs

   LIDAR and SODARs can be an acceptable source of wind measurement in the real-time power system or utility scale operation, if the requirements for delivery rate and validity/uncertainty of the measured value can be kept within specific limits.

   The recommended technical requirements for LIDARs and SODARs is to ensure high-quality data in long-term real-time operation and as alternatives to met mast measurements are:

- raw measurements must also be stored or technical requirements must include maintenance and software updates at the manufacturers defined interval
- lightning protection and recovery strategy after lightning
- measurements should be taken at a height appropriate for the wind farm, either at one or preferable at both hub height and around 30 m above ground level
- instruments must be serviced and maintained, at the manufacturers defined intervals by skilled staff
- version control must be maintained for signal processing
- LIDARs/SODARs require special consideration in complex terrain

Details for these requirements can be found in section 18.1.3.

2. Torque-inverted nacelle wind speed:

This method can be recommended for the use of real-time measurements for forecasting purposes under the following conditions (see also sections 21.3.1 and 21.5.1.1):

- the portfolio of wind farms contains a minimum of 30% well distributed wind measurements from other independent sources such as instruments on met masts or from a LIDAR or SODAR
- a well calibrated transition from torque inverted computations to anemometer measurements at the nacelle in high-speed wind ranges, or down-regulation situations (pitched blades) (see sections 21.3.1 and 21.5.1.1)
- a combination of a met mast with instruments at lower levels, e.g. 10m, 20m and 30m together with the torque-inverted method to ensure coverage over the full wind speed range from 0–40 m/s

If these measures are taken into consideration, the torque-inverted wind observations provide a cost-effective alternative to instruments mounted on met masts or remote sensing devices, when hub height wind measurements are a requirement (See more details in section 21.5.1.1).

22.4.1.3 Recommendations for solar forecasting applications

For the formulation of requirements for real-time forecasting purposes, it is crucial to identify the needs regarding the quality of the instrumentation, as costs for the instrumentation and for operation and maintenance are significantly different.

Table 22.3 Pyranometer classes for power grid and utility-scale operation. Note that where there are multiple classes recommended, the classes should always be compared with the requirements and desired outcome (quality of data) at stake. If a sufficient quality can be achieved with a lower instrument class, the "quality of data" criteria should prevail and the lower class chosen.

Forecast Application	Instrument class	Instrument description
Meteorological or Energy forecasting/ modeling for utility scale PV systems	Class B or A Spectrally Flat (ISO9060: 2018) Class A or B (IEC 61724-1:2021) Class 1 or 2 (WMO Guide No. 8)	Scientific quality and highest accuracy high quality

The following considerations are recommended to take into account when selecting requirements for instruments to serve in real-time forecasting applications:

1. Evaluation of required parameters, data accuracy, uncertainty levels
2. Cost-benefit analysis of quality and maintenance requirements
3. Specification of the required number of instruments

Table 22.3 provides a very brief summary of the applicability of various instrument classes that are considered relevant for solar energy forecasting at power grid level or utility-scale operation. Details can be found in section 20.1.2.

When choosing requirements for instrumentation, it should therefore be emphasized that the recommended instrument classes should always be compared with the instrument description and desired outcome (quality of data). If a sufficient quality can be achieved with lower instrument classes, the quality of data criteria should prevail and the lower instrument class chosen.

For existing campaigns, there may be discrepancies on the compliance with e.g. the IEC61724-1 Class A pyranometers with directional response and temperature response test results. They are equivalent to ISO 9060 Spectrally Flat Class A instruments. And, in some cases, older instruments from the ISO 9060:1990 standard's [148] highest quality "Secondary standard" (now Class A), may be updated, if a pyranometer lacks the required test reports for the performance verification on temperature dependence and directional response (e.g. [146]). Details and decision support can be found in section 20.1.2.

22.4.1.4 Recommendations for power measurements for real-time wind and solar forecasting

In summary, the following are recommended practices for use of power measurements in real-time operation and forecasting of wind and solar power:

1. Live/real-time power measurements should be used in very short-term wind and solar power forecasting, i.e. for lead-times from minutes to hours ahead.
2. Power data should be recorded at the same or higher temporal resolution and frequency as necessary for the forecasting system.
   - For electricity system operation temporal resolution may be one minute or less; for trading operations, this should match the duration of the shortest traded product or settlement period.
   - Forecast update frequency should match the highest frequency with which new information becomes available, within the constraints of IT infrastructure.
3. Power measurements should be taken from the metering point that is most relevant to the forecast user, this will usually be the metering system at the connection point to the electricity network.
4. Live data on plant operating conditions (e.g. control actions, the effect of maximum output) and availability (e.g. maintenance outages) should be used in forecast production and evaluation.
   - Where direct data is not available, this should be inferred using indirect measurements.
5. Data on future plant availability (e.g. maintenance actions) should be used to forecast production. Typically, power forecasts do not include the effect of control actions issued by electricity system operators.
6. Live Power Availability signals should replace forecast production signals during periods of curtailment due to control actions

22.4.2 Accuracy and resolution recommendations

Table 22.4 and 22.5 show the accuracy and resolution recommendation for system operation tasks on grid or utility-scale in the energy area. The limits are partially adapted from EPA's *Guidance on Meteorological Monitoring for Regulatory Modeling Applications*, section 4.5 Sampling Rates and from the *Example Performance Specifications* of 8.1 Instrumentation Procurement [107], the WMO Guide No.8 "Guide to Instruments and Methods of Observation" [106] and the heights from IEC 61400-12-1 [142] and system operators (see examples in appendix H) that have gained experience with these and other relevant guidelines and standards adopted from meteorological monitoring for real-time applications.

It is also recommended to consider the uncertainty of the instrumentation. Section 21.2 provides a number of useful measures, how to define and request instrumentation to comply or to provide such uncertainty quantification from the calibration of instruments as part of the standing data.

Table 22.5 shows the accuracy recommendation for system operation tasks in the energy area. The limits are partially adapted from EPA's *Guidance on Meteorological Monitoring for Regulatory Modeling Applications*, section 4.5 Sampling Rates [107] and system operators that have gained experience with these tasks (see examples in appendix H) and other relevant recommendations from the WMO Guide No. 8 [106].

22.4.3 Validation and verification recommendations

The quality of measured data that is intended for used in real-time applications is of immense importance. Modern technologies to assimilate measured data into forecasting models and processes usually have automatic algorithms that blacklist data that is out of range or in other ways suspicious, because bad data is often worse for the forecast model and processes than no data.

To avoid the potential negative impacts of bad quality data, quality control and clear assessment criteria for the data are important tools for the success of any application using real-time measurements. Section 21.4 details general QC and QA; historic, post real-time data quality assessment is found in section 21.5; real-time data screening is found in section 21.6.1. These measures are all necessary to keep a high quality data standard for the real-time applications and to make sure that instrument failures are found, reported and fixed within a reasonable time.

The following principles are recommended for the quality assurance and control of real-time measurements for forecasting applications in power grid and utility-scale operations:

- High measurement data quality requires continuous maintenance
- Uncertainty in measurements need to be considered (sec. 21.2)
- Quality assurance (QA) and quality control (QC) require a quality assurance project plan (QAPP), i.e. management and documentation of QC and QA procedures including (see sec. 21.4):
  - **(a)** Project description and organization
  - **(b)** QA procedures and monitoring
  - **(c)** Design of QC procedures

Table 22.4 Recommendations for system accuracy and measurement resolution for real-time wind forecasting applications in the power grid and utility-scale operation.

Meteorological Data Requirements for Wind Projects						
Measurement Type	**Units**	**Precision**	**Range**	**Accuracy**	**Height of Instrument**	
					Met Mast	**Alternative**
Wind Speed	Meters /Second (m/s)	0.1 m/s	0 to 50	± 1 m/s	at hub height + lower blade tip height (±10% of rotor diameter)	at 35 m Meters + Nacelle or Lidar
Wind Direction	Degrees from True North	1°	0 to 360	± 5°	at Hub Height + lower blade tip height (±10% of rotor diameter)	At 35 m
Barometric Pressure	Hecto Pascals (HPa)	1 hPa	800 to 1000	± 1.0 hPa at −20 to 50 °C, and ± 1.5 hPa at below −20° C	at or corrected to hub height	
Ambient Temperature	Degree Celsius (°C)	0.1°C	−50 to +50	± 0.2°C	within 10 m of hub height	
Dewpoint	Degrees Celsius (°C)	0.1°C	−50 to +50	± 0.2°C	within 10 m of hub height	at 2 m or 10 m
Relative Humidity	Percentage (%)	1.00%	0 to 100%	± 2%	at hub height	
Ice-up Parameter	Scale 0.0 to1.0	0.1	0 to 1	n/a	within 10 m of hub height	at 35 m
Precipitation	(mm/ min)	0.1	0 to11	2% up to 0.417 mm/min 3% over 0.417 mm/min	at 2 m or 10 m	at 2 m or 10 m

Table 22.5 Recommendations of Accuracy and Resolution requirements for real-time forecasts of solar projects.

Meteorological Data Requirements for Solar Projects

Measurement	Units	Precision	Range	Accuracy	Height of instrument
Wind Speed	Meters /Second (m/s)	0.1 m/s	0 to 50	± 1 m/s	Between 2–10 meters
Wind Direction	Degrees from True North	1 degree	0 to 360	± 5°	Between 2–10 meters
Barometric Pressure	Hecto Pascals (HPa)	1 hPa	800 to 1000	± 1.0 hPa at −20 to 50 °C, and ± 1.5 hPa below −20°C	Between 2-10 meters
Ambient Temperature	Degree Celsius (°C)	0.1°C	−50 to +50	± 0.2°C	Between 2–10 meters
Dewpoint	Degrees Celsius (°C)	0.1° C	−50 to +50	± 0.2°C	Between 2–10 meters
Relative Humidity	Percentage (%)	1.00%	0 to 100 %	± 2%	Between 2–10 meters
Ice-up Parameter	Scale 0.0 to1.0	0.1	0 to 1	n/a	Between 2–10 meters
Precipitation	Millimeters/minute (mm/min)	0.1	0 to11	2% up to 0.417 mm/mon 3% over 0.417 mm/min	Between 2–10 meters
Backpanel Temperature	Degree Celsius (°C)	0.1°C	−50 to +50	± 0.1°C at −27 to +50°C, and ± 0.2°C at below −27°C	Between 2–10 meters
Global Horizontal Irradiance	Watts/Square Metre (W/m2)	0.1	0 to 4000	± 3%	Between 2–10 meters
Diffused Horizontal Irradiance	Watts/Square Metre (W/m2)	0.1	0 to 4000	± 3%	Between 2–10 meters
Direct Normal Irradiance	Watts/Square Metre (W/m2)	0.1	0 to 2000	± 3%	Between 2–10 meters
Sunshine Duration	V	0.1	0 to 1	90.00%	Between 2–10 meters

22.4.3.1 Practical methodology for historic quality control of meteorological measurements

A practical methodology for the validation and quality control of meteorological measurements is a combination of different consistency checks (see details in section 21.5.1.2 and 21.5.1.3):

- Missing values and time stamps
- Forecasted wind speed versus measured wind speed
- Forecasted temperature, wind direction against measured values
- Forecasted power versus active power checked with SCADA MW
- Computed active power from measured wind speed versus actual active power
- Comparison against previous years of the same wind farm
- Comparison to the average error level for wind farms in the same period.

Table 22.6 Practical data screening criteria for data quality control of wind projects.

Variable	Screening Criteria: Flag data if the value
Wind Speed	– is less than zero or greater than 50 m/s – varies less than than 0.1 m/s for 3 consecutive hours – varies less than 0.5 m/s for 12 consecutive hours
Wind Direction	– is less than zero or greater than 360 degrees – varies less than 1 degree for more than 3 consecutive hours – varies less than 10 degrees for 18 consecutive hours
Temperature	– is greater than the local record high – is less than local record low (limit e.g. on monthly basis) – is greater than a 5°C change from the previous hour – varies less than 0.5° for 12 consecutive hours
Temperature Difference	– is greater than 0.1°C/m during the daytime – is less than −0.1°CC/m during the night time – is greater than 5.0°C or less than −3.0°C
Dew Point Temperature	– is greater than ambient temperature for given time period – is greater than a 5°C change from the previous hour – varies less than 0.5°C for 12 consecutive hours – equals the ambient temperature for 12 consecutive hours
Pressure	– is greater than 1060 mb (sea level) – is less than 940 mb (sea level) (values should be adjusted for elevations other than sea level) – changes by more than 6 mb in three hours
Radiation	– is greater than zero at night – is greater than the maximum possible for the date and latitude

22.4.3.2 Data screening in real-time environments

The recommended data screening criteria for wind and solar projects as a practical approach to data quality control and management follow the EPA guideline [107] and are suggested with some limits that are easy to control. Table 22.6 provides some useful and practical limits for the data screening task (more details can be found in section 21.6.3.1).

22.5. Recommendations for real-time measurements for power plant operation and monitoring

The key applications for wind plant operation, where real-time meteorological measurements are required, are:

- **Wind turbine control**
  Due to wake effects on nacelle anemometer, independent site data from a met mast, a LIDAR, or a SODAR can assist the turbine controller to work more safely and efficiently. Information of the turbine's inflow from a nacelle-based LIDAR system can be used to induce blade pitch action, reduce loads and improve turbine power performance.
- **Wind farm control**
  Wake measurements of scanning LIDAR or nacelle-based LIDAR that measure the wake of turbines, can assist to redirect those wakes and thus reduce loads on downstream turbines and increase their power production.
- **Condition Monitoring**
  Knowledge about the wind conditions that affect a wind turbine or wind farm help to estimate the load budget that the turbines have experience during their lifetime. This information can be used for lifetime extension measures thus increasing the energy yield of a wind farm and its profit.

Since measuring wind and other variables at power plant level is not always connected to power forecasting applications, the following recommendations are basic recommendations for high-quality measurements of these variables translated from the available standards. More detailed information can be found in the IEC 61400-12-1 [142], the MEASNET recommendations [98] for wind and the PVPS handbook [91].

It is important to recognize, that the value of measured meteorological data at a wind or solar plant is relevant, not only for the plant operation and the performance monitoring, but also to ensure that the generated electricity can be fed into the power grid in an efficient and environmentally friendly manner.

The principles of ***accuracy*** and ***reliability,*** as described in the key points to this section and the definitions in section 22.1 and section 22.4 for the generation of reliable information about the current weather situation, are all important corner stones for an efficient energy transition. Measurement campaigns are expensive. The benefits of measurements however can only be harvested, if the quality of the measured data is sufficient to be used in modeling, forecasting and verification of performance.

It is for this reason that it is recommended that wind farm control and monitoring design processes be considered together with potential benefits that can assist in the optimal integration of the generated energy into the power grid, by designing instrument deployments that can also be used for grid integration, balancing and/or trading purposes.

Table 22.7 Forecast applications and respective recommended requirements for appropriate instrumentation.

Forecast Application	Requirements for Wind according to IEC 61400 Part 12-1 [142]	Requirements for Solar according to ISO9060: 2018 [148], IEC 61724-1:2021 [144] and WMO Guide No. 8 [106]
Park Control	Class A	Class A
Park/Turbine Monitoring	Class S	Class B or C

22.5.1 Data quality recommendations

22.5.1.1 Requirement recommendations for wind farms

Table 22.7 provides instrument classes for plant operation applications to ensure high-quality measurements. For those applications, where there are two classes provided, the second (lower) class should be understood as minimum requirement and the higher class as a requirement, if high quality is required and the respective budgets justifiable.

The classes for wind projects are in detail defined in the IEC 61400 Part 12-1 [142] and explained in Annex D of the standard. Any further detail on the quality of the instrumentation should be referred to this standard.

A viable alternative option to the classic met masts at hub height, are remote sensing devices (LIDAR, SODAR) and the so-called iSpin technology, where sonic anemometers are mounted at the tip of the turbine. This instrument is described in section 18.1.2. Using new technologies, such as the iSpin technology may or may not lead to better results. It is therefore recommended that pilot projects be carried out (for example, on one turbine) or by analyzing data from turbines that carry such instrumentation. There are open source data and information available for this technology in [130,133].

22.5.1.2 Requirement recommendations for wind farms using remote sensing

The recommended technical requirements for LIDARs and SODARs to ensure high-quality data in long-term real-time operation and as alternatives to met mast measurements are (details supporting the recommendation can be found in sections 18.1.3, 18.1.5, 20.1.3.1, 21.3.1.3 and 22.4.1.2):

- measurements must be raw or technical requirements must include maintenance and software updates
- lightning protection and recovery strategy after lightning measurements should be taken at a height appropriate for the wind farm, either at one of preferable at both hub height and around 30 m
- instruments must be serviced and maintained by skilled staff
- version control must be maintained for signal processing
- LIDAR and SODARs in complex terrain require special consideration.

Table 22.8 Pyranometer classes for different monitoring applications. Note that where there are multiple classes recommended, the classes should always be compared with the requirements and desired outcome (quality of data) at stake. If a sufficient quality can be achieved with a lower instrument class, the "quality of data" criteria should prevail and the lower class chosen.

Forecast Applications	Instrument class	Instrument description
Measurements for high-level monitoring for large commercial scale PV systems	Class B (ISO9060:2018) Class B (IEC 61724-1:2021) Class 2–3 (WMO Guide No. 8)	Good quality
Economic solutions for routine measurements and small PV systems	Class C (ISO9060: 2018) Class C (IEC 61724-1:2021) Class 4–5 (WMO Guide No. 8)	Medium quality Moderate quality

22.5.1.3 Requirement recommendations for solar plants

The recommended technical requirements using pyranometer for solar plant performance monitoring are provided in Table 22.8.

Detailed requirement recommendations and background information can be found in sections 17.2.2 and 20.1.2.

22.5.2 Validation and verification recommendations

In the generally recommended validation of instrumentation as defined in the "ISO Guide to the Expression of Uncertainty in Measurements" [101,102,154] and its two supplements [103,104] from the Joint Committee for Guides in Meteorology (JCGM), two types of measurement uncertainty need to be accounted for in a standardized measurement:

1. **Systematic errors**, which are also known as measurement bias, often associated with offsets of the measured quantity
2. **Random errors**, which are associated with the fact that two measurements of the same quantity are seldom the same

In most cases the validation and verification of instruments and their respective data should be designed for both long-term analysis (e.g. a year) as well as shorter periods such as daily, weekly, monthly or quarterly examination of observational data signals.

Important targets for the validation and quality control:

1. To identify the amount of valid data submitted
2. To produce a comprehensive analysis which will provide the plant owner with a description of the root of the detected error(s) in the signals.
3. To limit the time from when an issue with data signals starts until it is diagnosed and solved
4. To avoid cross correlations between measurements from different sources to fill data gaps

The last item may be canceled from the list above, if there exists a short distance of the generating unit's locations to another generating unit.

Consistency Checks

A practical methodology for the validation and quality control of meteorological measurements is a combination of consistency checks:

- Missing Values and time stamps
- Forecasted wind speed versus measured wind speed
- Forecasted temperature, wind direction against measured values
- Forecasted power versus active power checked with SCADA MW
- Computed active power from measured wind speed versus actual active power

- Comparison against previous years of the same wind farm
- Comparison to average error level for wind farms in the same period

Details and background information on these recommendations can be found in chapter 21 and sections 21.4, 21.5 and 21.6.

22.5.2.1 Statistical test and metric recommendations for the QC process

A practical recommended solution for plant monitoring is to use verification methods to test measurement signal quality similar to the verification of forecast errors, with the exception that a forecast or a forecast range of the respective variable is used as the reference, because it is the measurement that needs validation. The forecast has a known accuracy level, which is used to find changes in quality in the measurement signals. By using ensemble forecasts, for example, the uncertainty of the measurement signals can also be quantified (see e.g. [166,168]).

The validation of different parts of the year, can be used to show whether the error pattern is temporary or exists on a long-term basis.

The use of a set of statistical tests as recommended in part 3 of this recommended practice (see section 15.1) typically provides a data basis that is large enough to reliably interpret the measurement data's accuracy. The following set of statistical metrics (details can be found in section 21.5.1.3, formulas of the metrics are in Appendix F) are recommended:

1. **BIAS:** The BIAS alone does not provide a guarantee or correctness.
2. **MAE:** MAE and BIAS together show, if the data has an offset.
3. **RMSE:** There are few extreme errors, if the ratio RMSE/MAE exceeds 1.3.
4. **CORRELATION:** The correlation allows for easy detection of constant ("locked") measurements as well as sign errors.
5. **Frequency distribution:** The frequency distribution from e.g. a one year data set of 15-min mean values of a wind speed should be a smooth curve with decreasing probability of high wind speeds. A temporary instrument fault will be visible as a skewness of the curve. Comparing the frequency distributions of an ensemble mean forecast against measurements is recommended in this case, as outliers are usually smoothed out in a mean forecast data set.

A graphical analysis of measurement signals with these metrics can then also be used to define acceptance limits for the meteorological variables or to see long-term trends. Examples of such graphical analysis can be found in section 21.5.1.3.

22.5.2.2 Solar specific validation recommendations

Specific validation for solar projects can be found in the PVPS handbook [91] in chapter 9.5 *Solar Resource Data for Plant Operations*. In this section, a variety of approaches for monitoring and measuring the performance of an existing solar power plant are described. Here the handbook says that "..the system is directly linked to the meteorological conditions. For flat-plate thermal collectors and PV, the production is roughly proportional to the incident GTI; for concentrating technologies, the incident DNI is the driving input. In all cases, additional meteorological variables need to be monitored because they play a modulating role."

The handbook concludes that real-time monitoring of the meteorological conditions at the system's location are important for the following applications:

(a) Evaluation of a performance guarantee (acceptance testing)

(b) Assessment of the power plant's performance to improve yield predictions and to gain knowledge toward improvements in future projects

(c) Identification of conditions of poor performance, including evidence of soiling, shading, hardware malfunction, or degradation, which could lead to replacement, etc.

22.5.2.3 Performance control recommendations for hardware and manufacturer production guarantees

Performance control of wind and solar plants and turbine/panels are important in respect to the financial aspects of a project, but also for the predictability of these energy sources, whether this is for system integration, balancing or power trading. In this way, the power performance is directly connected to the efficient usage of the generated power.

And, as described in the previous section, it is a direct recommendation to connect quality control to performance monitoring by designing an instrumentation setup and control mechanism for the performance control to a high standard of data quality. Background information on the definitions and recommendations for power grid applications can be found in section 22.4.

The recommended minimum requirements if the data is only used for performance control are:

1. ***Wind Power Performance Control:***

   Performance control of wind farms and wind turbines is best conducted in the following 3–4 steps:

   a. ***Measuring basic meteorological parameters that can be used to compute power generation output:***
      - wind speed and direction
      - air temperature
      - barometric pressure
      - relative humidity

      It is recommended to measure these parameters in a way that represents the weather conditions at the wind turbine rotor center. At least 2 measurement heights per wind farm with the following measuring recommended heights:

      (a) hub height or within 10 m of hub height

      (b) at approx. 30–35 m above ground (typically first model level of NWP models)

      (c) at 10 m above ground (standard meteorological measuring height)

      If (a) is not possible, a lower height can be measured and corrected for according to ISO 2355 (see chap. 6 [142]).

   b. ***Conversion of the meteorological parameters into a power output:***

      The best and recommended way is the IEC 61400-12-1 standard on power performance measurements, which is based on a physical formula (Equ. 2, chapter 8 [142]).

   c. ***Comparison of power output with measured and forecasted input variables:***

      Additionally, it is recommended to use forecasts from an independent forecasting model that uses power generation output over ideally 1 year, but a minimum of 3 months of various wind conditions and compare these results with the derived measured power output. The improvement from measured parameters should be approximately 3–5% when measured over a minimum of 3 months (see section 21.5.1.3 and e.g. [166–168]).

d. ***Visual Inspection with Ensemble generated Percentiles:***
By using a physical ensemble forecasting system of type b.1 (physical NWP parameterization schemes) or of type "Physical Methods" or "Multi-Scheme Ensemble" (see section 3.10.2 and Fig. 3.2), for example, 10 percentiles can be computed and compared with the computed and measured power output. Changes in performance can be easily seen by visual inspection. This is a straight forward methodology to avoid surprises and prove, with a physical methodology, hardware malfunctioning.

2. ***Solar Power Performance control***[1]
If monitoring of a PV plant's output comprises continuous comparisons to the expected output based on actual meteorological conditions, this leads to 2 main benefits:
   - PV arrays can be cleaned as a function of meteorological conditions
   - Errors and malfunctions of equipment can be detected quicker

   The essential parameters for CST (concentrating solar technologies) plants are [91]:
   a. Real-time DNI
   b. Wind
   c. Temperature

   The best general choice and recommendations for instrumentation are [91]:
   - **Maintenance issues**: a well-maintained reference cell in the POA[2]
   - **Performance assessment**: well-maintained, and regularly cleaned POA pyranometer

   Visual Inspection with Ensemble-generated Percentiles:
   By using a physical ensemble forecasting system of type b.1 (physical NWP parameterization schemes) or of type "Physical Methods" or "Multi-Scheme Ensemble" (see section 3.10.2 and Fig. 3.2), for example, 10 percentiles can be computed and compared with the computed and measured power output. Changes in performance can be easily seen by visual inspection. This is a straight forward methodology to avoid surprises prove, with a physical methodology, hardware malfunctioning.

[1] See details in the PVPS Handbook chapter 9.5.2 [91].
[2] Plane of array, referring to *global tilted irradiance* (GTI) measurements.

22.6. Recommendations for real-time measurements for power trading in electricity markets

Recommendations for real-time measurements for power trading and balancing in electricity markets are very much dependent on the type of trading that is performed. For day-ahead trading, historic measurements are sufficient, and hence also a cleaning strategy to clean out bad data similar to resource assessments, described in the IEC 61400-12-1 standard [142,145] and covered in section 22.4.1.

The following recommendations therefore refer to intra-day trading or trading in rolling markets, where real-time measurements are of immense importance.

To define the need and background for the measurement data quality, the first step is to understand the possibilities trading strategies with the use of real-time measurements provide.

22.6.1 Trading strategies with real-time measurements

In [174] it is reported that "..frequent short-term forecasts based on online data add value not only because they are more accurate than the day-ahead horizon", but also because it enables the trader to trade intelligently within the physical uncertainties of both forecasts and measurements (see also section 21.2).

Nevertheless, trading on intra-day or rolling markets with short-term forecasts that utilize real-time measurements should take place with care, because they also increase the trading volume and thereby the loss compared to the spot market price. This situation can occur, if the short-term forecast errors have opposite sign of the day-ahead error, which statistically occurs with a 50% likelihood, if the error of the day-ahead is small [174].

In most power exchanges, there often is a significant loss on wind and solar power trading on the intra-day or rolling markets. This loss is often associated with the higher expenses when buying short-term power for balancing purposes. Selling surplus wind or solar power generated by a BIAS-free day-ahead forecast is therefore often more beneficial.

However, investigations of this pattern have shown that an efficient trading system should neither deal with imbalances that are traded multiple times, nor that one and the same megawatt (MW) is charged several times with reserve costs [17,18,174]. This can be accomplished by using an approach that uses uncertainty factors, illustrated in Fig. 22.1, and limits the trading of imbalances according to the expected volumes that lie outside a pre-calculated band (that is updated with an uncertainty estimate based on short-term forecasts) around a day-ahead forecast as demonstrated in [17] and explained in more detail in section *3.8.2 The Balancing Challenges on the Intra-day Horizon* [174].

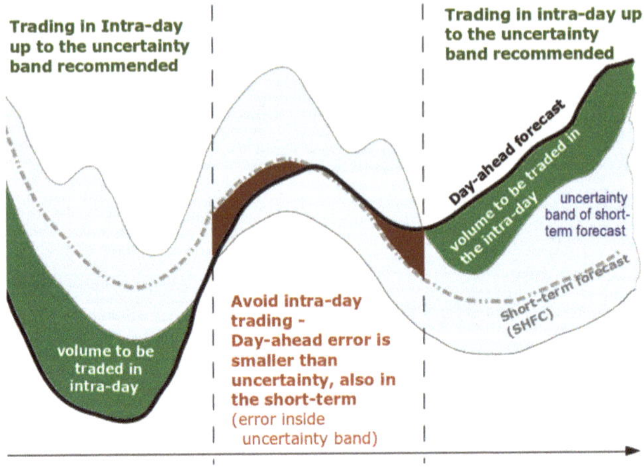

Figure 22.1 Trading principle when the uncertainty band is used for the determination of the volume that is to be traded in an intra-day or rolling market. The dashed grey line is the short-term forecast (SFC), the black line is the day ahead forecast (DFC) and the grey lines are the uncertainty forecast with the upper and lower limit. Image reproduced, modified and translated from Möhrlen et al. [17] with permission from Springer Nature (2012).

22.6.2 Quality recommendations

The quality recommendations follow to a large extent the recommendations for power grid in section 22.4 as the ideal solution, and the instrument classes described in section 20.1 and defined in Table 22.9 for electricity market purposes. Table 22.10 provides the recommended instrument classes for solar projects.

Table 22.9 Forecast applications and respective recommended requirements for appropriate instrumentation.

Forecast Application	Requirements for Wind according to IEC 61400 Part 12-1 [142]	Requirements for Solar according to ISO9060: 2018, EC 61724-1:2021 and WMO Guide No. 8
Electricity Market Trading	Class B	Class B or C (Good to moderate quality)

Table 22.10 Pyranometer class recommendations for different use-cases applied to solar generation forecasting tasks.

Forecast Application	Instrument class	Instrument description
Measurements for high-level monitoring for large commercial scale PV systems	Class B (ISO9060:2018) Class B (IEC 61724-1:2021) Class 2-3 (WMO Guide No. 8)	Good quality
Economic solutions for routine measurements and small PV systems	Class C (ISO9060: 2018) Class C (IEC 61724-1:2021 Class 4–5 (WMO Guide No. 8)	Medium quality Moderate quality

22.6.3 Accuracy and resolution requirement recommendations

It is important to recognize, that the value of measured meteorological data at wind or solar plants is relevant not only for trading the energy from wind and solar plants but also to also ensure that the generated electricity can be efficiently fed into the power grid in a way that minimizes imbalances and the speculation for financial purposes.

The principles of ***accuracy*** and ***reliability,*** as described in the key points to this section and the definitions in section 22.1 and section 22.4 for the generation of reliable information about the current weather situation, are all important corner stones for an efficient energy transition. Measurement campaigns are expensive. And, the benefits of measurements can only be harvested, if the quality of the measured data is sufficient to be used in modeling, forecasting and validation of generation performance.

It is for this reason that it is recommended that the design process for the real-time measurement setup for trading applications not be separate from potential coordination with plant operations, monitoring and grid integration requirements. Only, if measurement strategies are aligned, it is possible that all 4 tiers can benefit from the measurements and share the costs. When making use of these synergies, the integration of the generated energy into the power grid will be more efficient with lower overall costs.

CHAPTER TWENTY-THREE

End note

The fundamental goal of this IEA Wind Recommended Practice guideline is to provide practical guidance for current and prospective renewable energy forecast users for the selection and implementation of an optimal forecast solution for their specific applications. A secondary objective is to provide the energy industry with a scientifically sound basis for the development and adoption of international best business practices in the acquisition and use of renewable energy forecasting information.

This recommended practice guideline has been structured to follow a natural forecast acquisition and implementation cycle and has been divided into four parts that deal with the specifics, aspects and attributes of key stages in this process:

- **Part** 1 (starting at chapter 1): design of a process to select an optimal renewable (wind and solar) energy forecasting solution
- **Part** 2 (starting at chapter 6): maximization of the value of benchmarks or trials to test alternative forecasting solutions
- **Part** 3 (starting at chapter 11): techniques for the meaningful evaluation, verification and validation of forecasts and forecast applications
- **Part** 4 (starting at chapter 16): selection, deployment, maintenance and quality control of meteorological and power data necessary for real-time forecasting solutions

In the **first part**, *Forecast solution selection process*, the design of a customized process to select an optimal forecast solution for a user's specific situation and application is addressed. It provides information on the selection and background information necessary to collect and evaluate when developing or renewing a wind and/or solar forecasting solution for the energy market.

In the **second part**, *Design and execution of benchmarks and trials*, the design, execution and analysis of customized forecasting benchmarks and trials is addressed with the objective of enabling the user to gather information for the selection of the best solution for the user's specific application from a set of alternative solutions.

In the **third part**, *Forecast solution evaluation* methods and guidelines for the meaningful evaluation, verification metrics and framework and validation procedures for wind and solar forecasts or entire forecast solutions, are presented.

IEA Wind Recommended Practice for the Implementation of Renewable Energy Forecasting Solutions
https://doi.org/10.1016/B978-0-44-318681-3.00048-9

In the **fourth part**, *Meteorological and power data requirements for real-time forecasting applications* guidance for the selection, deployment and maintenance of meteorological sensors and the quality control of the data produced by those sensors together with power measurements relevant to real-time forecasting are provided. The objective is to maximize the value of the sensor data and power data for real-time wind and solar power production forecasting.

APPENDIX A

Clarification questions for forecast solutions

In order to define the objectives and possible solutions for a forecasting system, it is recommended to follow an overall structure:

1. Describe your situation
2. Engage vendors, stakeholders and independent consultants
3. Description of the envisioned situation

In this process, it is imperative to describe exactly those processes, where you need forecasting in the future. Here it is essential to get the different departments involved, especially the IT department. The more accurate you can describe the situation you need to solve with forecasting (e.g. which IT restrictions, limitations and methods for data exchange exist, current or future challenges, etc.), the more straight forward it will be to (1) ask questions to the vendors regarding forecasting methodology, but also (2) get clarity of the involved processes enabling forecasting.

Ask questions to the vendors

The questions to the vendors should be of technical character regarding forecast methodology, but also on available data exchange methodologies, required input data for the models and system support.

Typical questions for Part 1

- Processes: Which processes require forecasting
- Data
  - How will the data flow internally be solved: data storage, data exchange, data availability?
  - Which data do we collect that may assist the forecaster to improve accuracy?
- Data Formats:
  - Which formats are required for applications, data exchange and storage?
- Applications

  - Who/which department will use the forecasts, are new applications required to make use of the forecasts?
- Education
  - Is it required to train staff in how to use forecasts?
- Policies
  - Are there policies, political or legal restrictions to be aware of when exchanging data with a forecaster?

Typical questions for Part 2

The following are typical questions to get some overview of what is state-of-the-art in forecasting for renewables and what products are available on the market for a specific purpose.

- Describe the methodology you will use when generating forecast for (wind | solar | . . .).
- How many years of experience do you have in this specific area or related areas?
- Required data fields for the forecasting model for the trial.
- Time scales and IT requirements for the data for the forecasting model.
- Required data for vendor's model, if adopted and used "live".
- Applicable charges for a trial with vendor.
- Vendor's forecast model forecast horizons.

Typical RFI questions prior to or in an RFP

- **Methodology**
  - What unique services can you provide that may address our needs?
  - What input weather data is used?
  - What methodology is used for power generation for the long-term (>1 days ahead) and short-term forecasting (0...24 h)?
  - Can uncertainty forecasts or probability bands be provided? If yes, which methodology is being used.
  - What are the minimum requirements for wind farm site data?
  - Can a Graphical User Interface be provided to visualize forecasts? If yes, please describe it in detail (e.g. platform dependence, user management, in-house installation or web-based).
- **Service Level**
  - What kind of service level does the provider offer (ticket system, personal support, call center, online support, etc.)?
  - What kind of service level is recommended for the specific service?
  - Does the provider have outage recovery guarantee?
- **Contract and Pricing**
  - What are restrictions and preferences on the pricing structure of your service (e.g. price per park, per MW, per parameter, per time increment)?
  - What restrictions/preferences does the provider have in responding to RFPs?
- **Experience**
  - Can the vendor provide minimum of 3 examples of work that are applicable to the end-users needs (e.g. forecast accuracy, references, methodology)?
  - Does the forecast company have significant market shares in the market/area of business? (reason for question: avoidance of correlated errors)
  - Can the forecast company supply products or information that are considered relevant for the end-user when setting out an RFP?

APPENDIX C

Application examples for use of probabilistic uncertainty forecasts

C.1. Example of the graphical visualization of an operational dynamic reserve prediction system at a system operator

Fig. C.1 shows an example of the graphical visualization of an operational dynamic reserve prediction system at a system operator, where operators requested to have various intervals in order to evaluate which of the intervals was economically or from a system security aspect the better choice in a given situation.

The reserve requirement is built with a NWP ensemble approach where the ensemble spread is related and calibrated to the expected forecast error of wind power, demand and an estimated cross-border exchange requirement. The mean of the computed reserve requirement is scaled to zero and the possible positive and negative requirement intervals are plotted in form of 4 percentiles up and down, respectively.

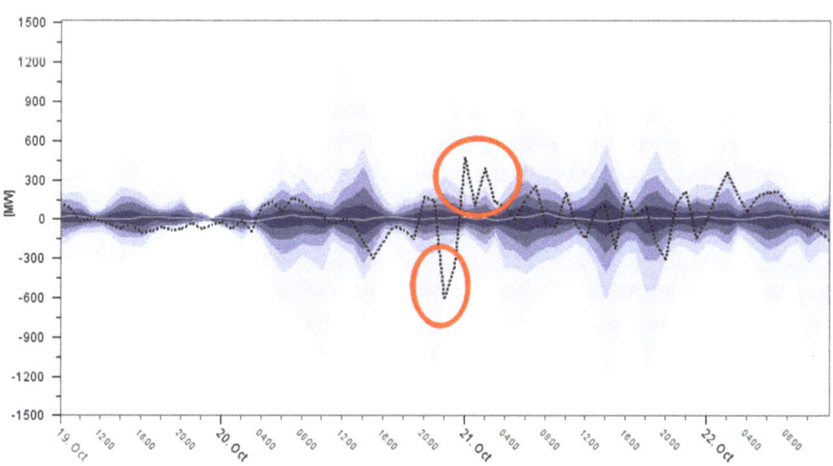

Figure C.1 Example of the graphical visualization an operational dynamic reserve prediction at a system operator.

The red circles indicate areas, where the requirements would have been higher than what e.g. a P20–P80 interval would have covered, if this was the uncertainty range the operators would have requested. It also illustrates why the operators wanted to be "aware" of such outliers, even if they may not pre-allocate reserves according to the outer ranges or boundaries.

C.2. High-speed shut down warning system

In areas where high-speed shutdown is a challenge for the grid security, the development of low pressure systems is typically frequent and the variability of the wind resources is relatively high. Thus, an alert system concerning high-speed shutdown of wind power must be established based on probabilities computed from a probabilistic prediction system that can take the spatial and temporal scales into consideration in order to capture the temporal evolution and spatial scale of such low pressure systems that contain wind speeds leading to large scale shutdown of wind farms.

This can for example be provided by a physical approach based on a NWP ensemble that ideally contains all extreme values inherent in the approach without the requirement of statistical training. Alternative solutions may exist from statistical approaches (see 3.10.2) by employing an extreme event analysis to a statistical ensemble of type 2. This is due to the requirement that such forecasts must be able to provide probabilities of extreme events, where each "forecast member" provides a valid and consistent scenario of the event. The probabilities need to be suitable solutions for a decision process. They can be computed for very critical and less critical events, dependent on the end-users requirements.

Fig. C.2 shows an example of a real-time setup of such a high-speed shutdown warning system. The example exhibits 2 events. The first graph shows the risk index in probability space of a high-speed shutdown event to occur. The second graph shows the wind power forecast with uncertainties inclusive the observations (black dotted line) of what happened. From the upper graph, the operator can directly read out the following:

- Case 1 at 26. January:
  - 10% probability of 50% shutdown
  - 8% probability of 90% shutdown
  - 90% probability of 5% shutdown
- Case 2 on 31. January:
  - 10% probability of 50% shutdown

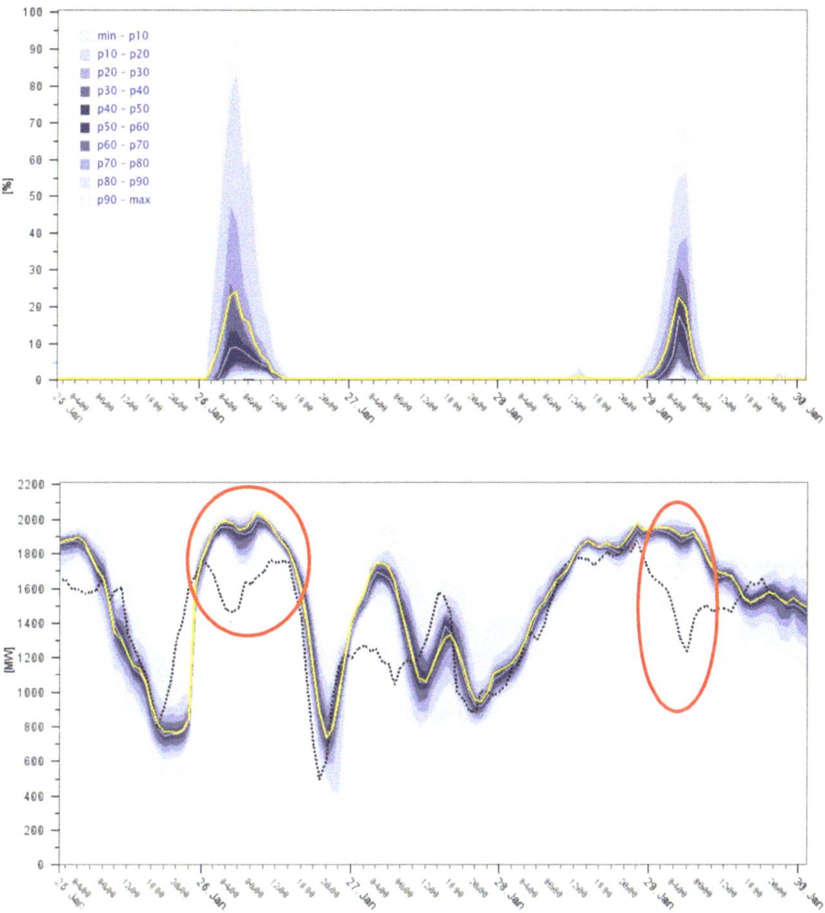

Figure C.2 Example of a high-speed shut-down example, where within 5 days 2 extreme events showed up in the risk index of the system (upper graph), showing the probability of occurrence in terms of probability ranges as percentiles P10...P90 of a high speed-speed shutdown. The second graph shows the 5-day wind power forecast inclusive uncertainty intervals as percentile bands P10...P90 and the observations (black dotted line). The red circles indicate the time frame in which the alarms were relevant.

– 15% probability of 90% shutdown
– 90% probability of 10% shutdown

The reality is shown by the observations in the lower graph of Fig. C.2, where it can be seen that the first case's peak value was 35% high-speed shut-down and the second case exhibited a peak value of 45% of high-speed shut-down.

Practical experience from evaluating high-speed shutdown events and discussing the alert system with the operators, showed that it is absolutely crucial that the operators understand the alerts and are capable of checking and verifying themselves in a graphical way, what they may receive as written alert. Therefore, the impact of a false alarm needs to be evaluated, decided upon and documented in the design phase, so that the operators have a clear reference system to relate an alert to. Technically, the frequency of the alert generation should be adjusted to:

a. lead time of the alert

b. change of severity level since previous alert

c. initial and valid week day and time of the day

d. severity of the event computed from a ramp-rate perspective and actions required

e. the need and possibility to call back and/or revert actions.

The strategy of issuing an alert should include (1) issuing of every alert according to a simple scheme and (2) reduction of the amount of alerts to a level that prevents that critical alerts are not accidentally overlooked.

It was also found that the use of sliding interval from 23–25 m/s was an important introduction into the design to ensure that the warning is issued **before** the event.

APPENDIX D

Metadata checklist

The following checklist (Table D.1), when filled out, will greatly aid Forecast Service Providers (FSPs) in configuring forecasts efficiently. Many of the essential questions relevant to benchmark and trial forecast model configuration are provided here.

Note that the following table is an example and may not contain all necessary information required for the FSP to setup a solution for your purpose. The table is meant to serve as a guideline and can be copied, but should be carefully adopted to the specific exercises before sending out to FSP with questions filled in. If this is done with care, it will expedite forecast configuration and save back and forth communication time.

Table D.1 Wind Power Forecast Trial Checklist.

Metadata	**Input**
Long name of site(s) as it should appear in datafile	
Short name/abbreviation of site(s) as it should appear in datafile	
Latitude and longitude coordinates of sites	
Nameplate capacity of each site	
Graphical web tool required?	
Turbine make/model/rating	
Number of turbines	
Hub height of turbines	
Attachment of suitable plant power curve	
Forecast output information	
Forecast output time intervals (e.g., 15-min, 1-hourly)	
Required length of forecasts	
Timezone of forecast datafile	
Is a local daylight saving time change to be considered?	
Forecast update frequency (e.g., once a day, every hour)	
Value of Forecast	
Which variables will be forecasted and validated?	
Which forecast horizons will be validated?	
Which metrics will be used to validate forecast performance?	
List criteria for determining winning forecast provider	
Will results be shared as a report? Will results be anonymized?	
On what frequency will results be shared with forecast provider?	
Historical Data Checklist	
Is the data in UTC or local time?	
Is the data interval beginning or ending or instantaneous?	
What are the units of the data?	
If met tower histories being provided, indicate height of measurements.	
Real-time Data Checklist (if applicable)	
Email and Telephone number of technical point of contact (POC)	
Email and Telephone of datafeed POC	
Name and email of users that need website access	
Person name and email that filled out this checklist	

Sample forecast file structures

Back and forth communication can sometimes delay the start of a trial or benchmark. One of these delays is getting the forecast file output format just right for the beginning of the trial.

Standardization of the format will make the trial operators life much easier when time comes to validating forecasts. A best practice here is for the trial operator to use a format that is already in use or a format that has already proven to work in operations. See Fig. E.1.

Plant Output	Acme Wind Farm	1.11.2017 4:00	1.11.2017 5:00	1.11.2017 6:00	1.11.2017 7:00
Power	MW	41.43	41.43	41.43	40.89
Windspeed	m/s	11	10	10	10
Time zone: Central European Summer Time (CEST)					
Intervals: hour ending					
Date time format: dd.mm.yyyy hh:mm (e.g., 06.08.1969 08:30)					

Figure E.1 Example forecast file with the first few fields.

E.1. XSD template example for forecasts and SCADA

The following are typical XSDs for forecasts and SCADA data in a b/t, usable also with WebServices

```
<?xml version="1.0" encoding="utf-8"?>
<xs:schema attributeFormDefault="unqualified" elementFormDefault="qualified"
xmlns:xs="http://www.w3.org/2001/XMLSchema">
  <xs:element name="WindForecast">
    <xs:complexType>
      <xs:attribute name="VendorCode" type="xs:string" use="required"/>
      <xs:attribute name="ImportTime" type="xs:dateTime" use="required"/>
      <xs:sequence>
        <xs:element name="CUSTOMER">
          <xs:complexType>
            <xs:attribute name="name" type="xs:string" use="required"/>
```

```
        <xs:sequence>
         <xs:element name="Forecast">
           <xs:complexType>
            <xs:attribute name="MWaggregated" type="xs:double"
            use="required"/>
            <xs:attribute name="time" type="xs:dateTime" use="required"/>
            <xs:sequence>
              <xs:element name="Probability">
                <xs:complexType>
                  <xs:attribute name="P95" type="xs:double" use="required"/>
                  <xs:attribute name="P50" type="xs:double" use="required"/>
                  <xs:attribute name="P05" type="xs:double" use="required"/>
                  <xs:attribute name="max" type="xs:double" use="required"/>
                  <xs:attribute name="min" type="xs:double" use="required"/>
                 </xs:complexType>
               </xs:element>
              <xs:element name="WindFarms">
              <xs:complexType>
            <xs:sequence>
              <xs:element name="WindPark1">
               <xs:complexType>
                   <xs:attribute name="id" type="xs:string" use="required"/>
                    <xs:attribute name="mw" type="xs:double" use="required"/>
                 </xs:complexType>
                 </xs:element>
            </xs:sequence>
                 </xs:complexType>
                 </xs:element>
            </xs:sequence>
             </xs:complexType>
           </xs:element>
         </xs:sequence>
       </xs:complexType>
     </xs:element>
    </xs:sequence>
  </xs:complexType>
 </xs:element>
</xs:schema>
```

E.2. XSD SCADA template for exchange of real-time measurements

```
<?xml version="1.0" encoding="utf-8"?>
<xs:schema attributeFormDefault="unqualified" elementFormDefault="qualified"
xmlns:xs="http://www.w3.org/2001/XMLSchema">
 <xs:element name="WindSCADA">
  <xs:complexType>
    <xs:sequence>
      <xs:element maxOccurs="unbounded" name="WindPark">
        <xs:complexType>
          <xs:attribute name="ID" type="xs:string" use="required"/>
          <xs:attribute name="Time" type="xs:dateTime" use="required"/>
          <xs:attribute name="Mw" type="xs:decimal" use="required"/>
          <xs:attribute name="Availabilty" type="xs:decimal" use="optional"/>
          <xs:attribute name="CurrentActivePower" type="xs:decimal"
          use="optional"/>
          <xs:attribute name="Curtailment" type="xs:string" use="optional"/>
          <xs:attribute name="WindSpeed" type="xs:decimal" use="optional"/>
          <xs:attribute name="WindDirection" type="xs:decimal" use="optional"/>
          <xs:attribute name="AirTemperature" type="xs:decimal" use="optional"/>
```

```
        <xs:attribute name="AirPressure" type="xs:decimal" use="optional"/>
       <xs:attribute name="Outage" type="xs:decimal" use="optional"/>
      </xs:complexType>
     </xs:element>
    </xs:sequence>
   </xs:complexType>
  </xs:element>
</xs:schema>
```

Standard statistical metrics

F.1. BIAS

The BIAS of an estimator is the difference between this estimator's expected value and the true value of the parameter being estimated.

$$BIAS = \frac{1}{N}\sum_{i=1}^{N}(x_1 - y_i) \tag{F.1}$$

The BIAS in itself should be low, but is no guarantee of correctness of the data, because a BIAS can be low for the incorrect reason.

F.2. MAE – mean absolute error

The mean absolute error (MAE) is a quantity used to measure how close forecasts or predictions are to the eventual outcome.

$$MAE = \frac{1}{N}\sum_{i=1}^{N}|x_1 - y_i| \tag{F.2}$$

where N is the number of data points, x are the forecasted values, y are the observations.

In the following test, the MAE and BIAS together show, if the data has an offset.

F.3. RMSE – root mean squared error

The square root of the mean/average of the square of all of the error. RMSE is commonly used as general purpose error metric for numerical predictions. Compared to the similar MAE, RMSE amplifies and severely punishes large errors.

$$RMSE = \sqrt{\frac{1}{N}\sum_{i=1}^{N}(x_1 - y_i)^2} \tag{F.3}$$

where N is the number of data points, x are the forecasted values, y are the observations.

In quality control of measurements, it is considered that there are few extreme errors, if the ratio RMSE/MAE exceeds 1.3.

F.4. Correlation

Correlation is a statistical technique that is used to measure and describe the STRENGTH and DIRECTION of the relationship between two variables.

$$CORRELATION = \frac{COV(x_i, y_i)}{STD_x \cdot STD_y} = \frac{\sum (x - \bar{x}) \cdot (y - \bar{y})}{STD_x \cdot STD_y} \quad \text{(F.4)}$$

where x are the forecasted values, y are the observations, the bars indicate the mean of the time series, COV is the covariance, STD is the standard deviation.

In quality control of measurements, the correlation allows for easy detection of constant measurements as well as sign errors.

F.5. Standard deviation

The standard deviation is a measure of the amount of variation or dispersion of a set of values. A low standard deviation indicates that the values tend to be close to the mean of the set, while a high standard deviation indicates that the values are spread out over a wider range.

$$STDV = \sqrt{\frac{\sum (x_i - \bar{x})^2}{n - 1}} \quad \text{(F.5)}$$

where x are the forecasted values, $\bar{x}$ is the mean of the sample and n the number of forecasts.

F.6. What makes a forecast "good"?

A valuable alternative resource for defining the "goodness" of a forecast has been summarized by the WWRP/WGNE[1] Joint Working Group

[1] World Weather Research Program/Working Group on Numerical Experimentation.

on Forecast Verification Research in the proceedings from their 7th International Verification Methods Workshop in a section called "what makes a forecast good" [59]. The section, dedicated to meteorological verification, coincides with our recommendations on building a framework of verification metrics described in section 15.1 and builds upon the work of Allan Murphy, a pioneer in the field of forecast verification. Murphy's essay from 1993 [175] on what makes a forecast "good" distinguishes three types of "goodness", which we complement here in parentheses with our definitions and the associated links:

- **Consistency** (representative 12.1) – the degree to which the forecast corresponds to the forecaster's best judgment about the situation, based upon his/her knowledge base
- **Quality** (significant 12.2) – the degree to which the forecast corresponds to what actually happened
- **Value** (relevant 12.3) – the degree to which the forecast helps a decision maker to realize some incremental economic and/or other benefit

The nine aspects (called "attributes") Murphy describes in his work that contribute to the quality of a forecast are shown in Table F.1.

Table F.1 Murphy's [175] originally defined nine attributes that contribute to the quality of a forecast and provides explanations [52], including referring links to the associated places in this document.

Attribute/Metric	Description and Meaning	Link
Bias	The correspondence between the mean forecast and mean observation	(F.1, 12.1.2)
Association	The strength of the linear relationship between the forecasts and observations (for example, the correlation coefficient measures this linear relationship)	F.4
Accuracy	The level of agreement between the forecast and the truth (as represented by observations). The difference between the forecast and the observation is the error. The lower the errors, the greater the accuracy.	15.1.2, 14.1.4

continued on next page

Table F.1 (*continued*)

Attribute/Metric	Description and Meaning	Link
Skill	The relative accuracy of the forecast over some reference forecast. The reference forecast is generally an unskilled forecast such as random chance, persistence (defined as the most recent set of observations, "persistence" implies no change in condition), or climatology. Skill refers to the increase in accuracy due purely to the "smarts" of the forecast system. Weather forecasts may be more accurate simply because the weather is easier to forecast – skill takes this into account.	14.11
Reliability	The average agreement between the forecast values and the observed values. If all forecasts are considered together, then the overall reliability is the same as the bias. If the forecasts are stratified into different ranges or categories, then the reliability is the same as the conditional bias, i.e., it has a different value for each category.	14.3.3, 14.3.3.2, 14.5
Resolution	The ability of the forecast to sort or resolve the set of events into subsets with different frequency distributions. This means that the distribution of outcomes when "A" was forecast is different from the distribution of outcomes when "B" is forecast. Even if the forecasts are wrong, the forecast system has resolution if it can successfully separate one type of outcome from another.	22.4.2, 22.6.3, 15.1.4.1, 15.3
Sharpness	the tendency of the forecast to predict extreme probability values (i.e. near 0% or 100%) and is essentially a representation of the estimated forecast uncertainty. To use a counter-example, a forecast of "climatology" has no sharpness. Sharpness is a property of the forecast only, and like resolution, a forecast can have this attribute even if it's wrong (in this case it would have poor reliability).	15.1.4.1, 15.1.3.1
Discrimination	ability of the forecast to discriminate among observations, that is, to have a higher prediction frequency for an outcome whenever that outcome occurs.	14.3.4, 15.1.3.1
Uncertainty	the variability of the observations. The greater the uncertainty, the more difficult the forecast will tend to be.	12, 15.3

APPENDIX G

Validation and verification code examples

G.1. IEA wind task 36 and task 51 specific V&V code examples

The following code examples have been specifically developed under IEA Wind Task 36 "Forecasting for Wind Energy" or Task 51 "Forecasting for a Weather Driven Energy system" projects and build a good basis for the development of a evaluation framework as recommended in chapter 15, section 15.1.

WE-Validate: Python-based code base as a platform to consistently evaluate wind-power forecasts. The tool WE-Validate is meant to gear towards forecast validation using observations and simulations for wind energy ("WE") applications. This infrastructure code enables comparison of time series from arbitrary data sources using user-defined metrics. The tool is designed to be simple, readily usable, open source, publicly available, modularized, and extensible by users. There are detailed instructions for users on its GitHub page, Accessible Online: https://github.com/joejoeyjoseph/WE-Validate.

WE-verify-prob: R-based example code base to verify probabilistic wind energy forecasts. The tool WE-verify-prob is a project initiated within the IEA Wind Task 36 and 51 in order to provide example code to the IEA Wind Recommended Practice for the Implemention of Renewable Energy Forecast Solutions Part 2 *Designing and Executing Forecasting Benchmarks and Trials* and Part 3 *Forecast Solution Evaluation*. Accessible for download at the IEA Wind Task 51 webpage https://iea-wind.org/task51/task51-publications/task51-recommended-practices/.

G.2. Code examples from related projects with relevance to recommendations

The following selection of V&V code examples links from related projects with relevance to the recommendations made in this document.

Weather Forecast Verification Utilities: The R-Package 'verification' [176] has been developed for "verifying discrete, continuous and probabilistic forecasts, and forecasts expressed as parametric distributions" by Eric Gilleland from NCAR Research Applications Laboratory [176]. The Package contains all relevant metrics described in chapter 14 and chapter 22, specifically those described in section 14.3 and those described by [59]. It can be accessed via CRAN https://cloud.r-project.org/web/packages/verification/index.html.

Forecast Verification Routines for Ensemble Forecasts of Weather and Climate: The R-package 'SpecsVerification' [177] is a collection of forecast verification routines developed for the SPECS FP7 project. The emphasis is on comparative verification of ensemble forecasts of weather and climate. The package contains most of the metrics described in chapter 14 and chapter 22, specifically those described in section 14.3 and those described by [59]. It can be accessed via CRAN https://CRAN.R-project.org/package=SpecsVerification.

Ensemble Forecast Verification for Large Data Sets: The R-package 'easyVerification' [178] is a set of tools to simplify application of forecast verification metrics for (comparative) verification of ensemble forecasts to large data sets. The forecast metrics are partially imported from the 'SpecsVerification' R-package, with additional forecast metrics provided within this package. New user-defined forecast scores can be implemented using the example scores provided and applied using the functionality of this package. The package contains all of the metrics described in chapter 14 and chapter 22, specifically those described in section 14.3 and those described by [59]. It can be accessed via CRAN https://CRAN.R-project.org/package=easyVerification.

Ensemble Postprocessing with R: The R-package "ensemblepp" [65] provides postporcessing and verification Data Sets and code examples for the chapter "Ensemble Postprocessing with R" of the book "Statistical Postprocessing of Ensemble Forecasts" by Stephane Vannitsem, Daniel S. Wilks, and Jakob W. Messner (2018), Elsevier, 362 pp. These data sets contain temperature and precipitation ensemble weather forecasts and corresponding observations at Innsbruck/Austria. Additionally, a demo with the full code of the book chapter is provided. Evaluation code is provided as scatter plots, rank histogram, spread skill relationship and histograms. Available Version: 1.0-0 online: https://cran.r-project.org/web/packages/ensemblepp.

APPENDIX H

Examples of system operator met measurement requirements

H.1. Examples of requirements in different jurisdictions

- **AESO**: Alberta Electric System Operator, Calgary, Canada [179]
- **CAISO**: California Independent System Operator, Folsom, USA [180]
- **ERCOT**: Electricity Council of Texas in Austin, USA [181]
- **EIRGRID**: EIRGRID, Irish system operator [182]
- **NYISO**: New York Indep. System Operator, Rensselaer, USA [183]
- **PJM**: Independent System Operator, Audubon, PA, USA [184]
- **HECO**: Hawaiian Electric Company, Maoui, Hawaii [185]

The delivery frequency for meteorological data has a co-dependence to the jurisdicial market structures, especially where wind and solar gernerated electricity is traded in short-term markets, but also, where meteorological information is used in dispatch processes. See Table H.1.

H.2. Met measurement requirement example from California independent system operator in USA

The tables in Figs. H.1 and H.2 are examples from the California Independent System Operator (CAISO) taken from the Appendix Q of their *Eligible Intermittent Resources Protocol* (EIRP) from December 2020 [180].

H.3. Met measurement requirement example from Irish system operator EIRGRID group

Examples from the Met Data Requirement document of the Irish transmission system operator EIRGRID, which is part of the grid code for wind generation units under section WFPS 1.7.1.6 [182]:

Time Delays and Data Quality

Digital signal changes from the Controllable WFPS (Windfarm Power Station) shall be relayed to the TSO Telecommunication Interface Cabinet within 1 second of the associated change of state event. Analogue signal

Table H.1 Summary of technical requirements in other control areas/jurisdictions. Abbreviations for the variables are ws=wind speed, wd=wind direction, T2m=temperature at 2 m, ps=surface pressure, frequency=deliver frequency, threshold=threshold nameplate capacity of the wind farm, where the rules are applicable.

System Operator	threshold [MW]	frequency [sec]	Standing Data: geo-data per farm	Standing Data: geo-data per turbine	Equipment: met mast	Equipment: nacelle	Equipment: other	Met variables to be delivered: ws	wd	T2m	PS	other	location agl.
AESO	5	60	1	0	1	0	0	1	1	1	1	iceup	hub / 2m
CAISO	1/5	4	1	1	1–2	1	2[a]	1	1	1	1	0	hub (+10m) / 2m
ER-COT	1	300	1	0	1	0	0	1	1	1	1	0	hub / 2m
EIR-GRID	10	60	1	0	3[b]	1	1	1	1	1	1	0	35m / 2m
NYISO	1	30	1	0	1	1	0	1	1	1	1	0	hub/2m
PJM	10/100	10/2	1	0	1	0	0	1	1	1	1	0	hub / 2m
HECO	all	900	1	0	1	0	1	1	1	1	1	0	hub + wind-NET

[a] The use of SODAR1 and/or LIDAR2 equipment may be an acceptable substitute for wind direction and velocity only after obtaining prior agreement from the CAISO.

[b] New technologies (e.g. remote sensing LiDARs, SODARs and RADARs) will be allowed to apply as alternative measurement type or in combination with other instruments but will be required to complete and pass a real-time acceptance test of a minimum of three months in a windy period.

Element	Device(s) Needed	Units	Accuracy
Wind Speed (Meter / Second)	Anemometer, wind vane and wind mast	m/s	± 2m/s
Air Temperature (Degrees Celsius)	Temperature probe & shield for ambient temp	°C	± 1°
Barometric Pressure (hecto Pascals)	Barometer	hPA	± 60 hPa

Figure H.1 Wind Eligible Intermittent Resources Telemetry Data Points [180].

Element	Device(s) Needed	Units	Accuracy
Wind Speed (Meter / Second)	Anemometer, wind vane and wind mast	m/s	± 2m/s
Wind Direction (Degrees - Zero North 90CW)	Anemometer, wind vane and wind mast	Degrees	± 5°
Air Temperature (Degrees Celsius)	Temperature probe & shield for ambient temp	°C	± 1°
Barometric Pressure (hecto Pascals)	Barometer	hPA	± 60 hPa
Back Panel Temperature (Degree C)	Temperature probe for back panel temperature	°C	± 1°
Plane of Array Irradiance Watts\Meter Sq.	Pyranometer or Equivalent	W/m²	± 25 W/m²
Global Horizontal Irradiance Watts\Motor Sq.	Pyranometer or Equivalent	W/m²	± 25 W/m²
Direct Irradiance Watts\Meter Sq.	Pyranometer or Equivalent	W/m²	± 25 W/m²

Figure H.2 Solar Eligible Intermittent Resources Telemetry Data Points [180].

changes shall be relayed within 5 seconds and with an error of 0.5% or less, with the exception of the Meteorological Data required as per PPM 1.7.1.2.1, which shall be updated within 5 seconds and with an error of 2.5% or less.

System accuracies and Measurement resolution

The meteorological data signals shall be provided as detailed in the tables shown in Fig. H.3: Meteorological data signal accuracy and resolution and Fig. H.4: Meteorological data variable and their error threshold limit. The Windfarm Power Station (WFPS) shall provide an updated signal every 1 minute.

	Unit	Range	System Accuracy	Measurement Resolution
Wind speed	m/s	0 - 70	≥ 5% improvement	0.1m/s
Wind direction	deg	0 - 360	Statistical and Variance test within acceptable limits as per Table 2	1.0 deg
Air temperature	deg C	-40 - 70		0.1 deg C
Air pressure	mBar	735 - 1060		1 mBar

Figure H.3 Meteorological data signal accuracy and resolution [182].

	Maximum Bias	Maximum MAE	Minimum Correlation	Measurement Unit
Wind speed	3.00	3.00	0.65	m/s
Wind direction	13.00	20.0	0.55	deg
Air temperature	2.00	2.50	0.75	degC
Air pressure	50.00	85.0	0.90	mBar

Figure H.4 Meteorological data variable and their error threshold limit for statistical tests [182].

H.4. Met measurement requirement example from Alberta electric system operator in Canada

Requirements for Wind and Solar Grid Connected Plant Meteorological Data at the Alberta Electric System Operator (AESO) in Canada.

Reference: https://www.aeso.ca/rules-standards-and-tariff/iso-rules/section-304-9-wind-and-solar-aggregated-generating-facility-forecasting/.

Within the ISO Rules Part 300 on System Reliability and 304 on Operations Division for Routine Operations, section 304.9 on *Wind and Solar Aggregated Generating Facility Forecasting* defines the compatibility requirements for wind and solar generating units when operating in the electric grid. See Tables H.2 and H.3.

The rule states on the *Applicability* that "..Section 304.9 applies to: (a) the legal owner of a wind or solar aggregated generating facility connected to the interconnected electric system or an electric system within the service area of the City of Medicine Hat, including a wind or solar aggregated generating facility situated within an industrial complex that is directly connected to the interconnected electric system or to an electric system within the service area of the City of Medicine Hat and that has a gross real power capability equal to or greater than 5 MW; and (b) the ISO."

In section of the rule 304.9 the following requirements apply:

(4) The legal owner of a wind aggregated generating facility must, in response to a request by the ISO under subsection 8(3), provide the following facility data:

1. meteorological tower data collection height in meters (m), with a precision for instantaneous measurements to the nearest 1m;
2. turbin emodel name
3. turbine model capacity in megawatts (MW), with a precision to the nearest 0.1MW
4. turbine wind speed cut-in in meters per second (m/s), with a precision to the nearest 0.1 m/s
5. turbine wind speed cut-out in meters per second (m/s), with a precision to the nearest 0.1 m/s
6. turbine temperature cut-out lower in degrees Celsius (degC), with a precision for instantaneous measurements to the nearest 1 degC and an indicator is required to confirm that the numbers are ambient temperature within the rotor or air temperature
7. turbine temperature cut-out upper in degrees Celsius (°C), with a precision for instantaneous measurements to the nearest 1 deg C and an indicator is required to confirm that the numbers are ambient temperature within the rotor or air temperature
8. site latitude and longitude in degrees; and (i)turbine power curves.

Equivalently, the technical rule states that "..the legal owner of a solaraggregated generating facilitymustin response to a request by the ISO under subsection 8(3), provide the following solar arraydata and records, including:

1. site latitude and longitude in degrees
2. direct current (DC)real power rating
3. alternating current (AC) real power rating
4. inverter manufacturer and model
5. mounting height from ground in meters (m)
6. tilt angle or range of tilt angles to horizontal plane in degrees
7. azimuth angle in degrees; (h) alternating current (AC) real power capacity per solar array in megawatts (MW)
8. mounting type, tracking (fixed, single or dual axis)
9. module type (crystalline, thin-film etc.).

Table H.2 Alberta Electric System Operator's Wind Aggregated Generating Facility Meteorological Data Requirements Technical Rule 304.9.

Wind Aggregated Generating Facility Meteorological Data Requirements

Measurement Type	Units	Precision	Range	Accuracy	Height of instrument	
					Set-1	Set-2
Wind Speed	Meters /Second (m/s)	0.1 m/s	0 to 50	± 1m/s	At Hub Height	At 35m Meters
Wind Direction	Degrees from True North	1 degree	0 to 360	± 5°	At Hub Height	At 35m Meters
Barometric Pressure	Hecto Pascals (HPa)	1 hPa	800 to 1000	± 1.0 hPa at −20 to 50 °C, and ± 1.5 hPa at below −20° C	At Convenient location	At Convenient location
Ambient Temperature	Degree Celsius (°C)	0.1°C	−50 to +50	± 0.2°C	At Hub Height	At 35m Meters
Dewpoint	Degrees Celsius (°C)	0.1°C	−50 to +50	± 0.2°C	At convenient location	At convenient location
Relative Humidity	Percentage (%)	1.00%	0 to 100 %	± 2%	At convenient location	At convenient location
Ice-up Parameter	Scale 0.0 to1.0	0.1	0 to 1	n/a	At convenient location	At convenient location
Precipitation	Millimeters /minute (mm/min)	0.1	0 to11	2% up to 0.417 mm/mon 3% over 0.417 mm/min	At Convenient location	At Convenient location

Table H.3 Alberta Electric System Operator's Solar Aggregated Generating Facility Meteorological Data Requirements Technical Rule 304.9.

Solar Aggregated Generating Facility Meteorological Data Requirements						
Measurement Type	**Units**	**Precision**	**Range**	**Accuracy**	**Height of instrument**	
					Set-1	**Set-1**
Wind Speed	Metres /Second (m/s)	0.1 m/s	0 to 50	± 1m/s	Between 2–10 meters	Between 2–10 meters
Wind Direction	Degrees from True North	1 degree	0 to 360	± 5°	Between 2–10 meters	Between 2–10 meters
Barometric Pressure	Hecto Pascals (HPa)	1 hPa	800 to 1000	± 1.0 hPa at −20 to 50 °C, and ± 1.5 hPa below −20°C	Between 2–10 meters	Between 2–10 meters
Ambient Temperature	Degree Celsius (°C)	0.1°C	−50 to +50	± 0.2°C	Between 2–10 meters	Between 2–10 meters
Dewpoint	Degrees Celsius (°C)	0.1°C	−50 to +50	± 0.2°C	Between 2–10 meters	Between 2–10 meters
Relative Humidity	Percentage (%)	1.00%	0 to 100 %	± 2%	Between 2–10 meters	Between 2–10 meters
Ice-up Parameter	Scale 0.0 to1.0	0.1	0 to 1	n/a	Between 2–10 meters	Between 2–10 meters
Precipitation	Millimeters /minute (mm/min)	0.1	0 to11	2% up to 0.417 mm/mon 3% over 0.417 mm/min	Between 2–10 meters	Between 2–10 meters

continued on next page

Table H.3 *(continued)*

Solar Aggregated Generating Facility Meteorological Data Requirements

Measurement Type	Units	Precision	Range	Accuracy	Height of instrument	
					Set-1	Set-1
Backpanel Temperature	Degree Celsius (°C)	0.1°C	−50 to +50	± 0.1°C at −27 to +50°C, and ± 0.2°C at below −27°C	Between 2–10 meters	Between 2–10 meters
Global Horizontal Irradiance	Watts/Square Metre (W/m2)	0.1	0 to 4000	± 3%	Between 2–10 meters	Between 2–10 meters
Diffused Horizontal Irradiance	Watts/Square Metre (W/m2)	0.1	0 to 4000	± 3%	Between 2–10 meters	Between 2–10 meters
Direct Normal Irradiance	Watts/Square Metre (W/m2)	0.1	0 to 2000	± 3%	Between 2–10 meters	Between 2–10 meters
Sunshine Duration	V	0.1	0 to 1	90.00%	Between 2–10 meters	Between 2–10 meters

Bibliography

[1] R.J. Bessa, Corinna Möhrlen, V. Fundel, M. Siefert, J. Browell, S. Haglund El Gaidi, Bri-Mathias Hodge, U. Cali, G. Kariniotakis, Towards improved understanding of the applicability of uncertainty forecasts in the electric power industry, Energies 10 (9) (Sep. 2017) 1402.

[2] Jan Dobschinski, Ricardo Bessa, Pengwei Du, Kenneth Geisler, Sue Ellen Haupt, Matthias Lange, Corinna Möhrlen, Dora Nakafuji, Miguel de la Torre Rodriguez, Uncertainty forecasting in a nutshell: prediction models designed to prevent significant errors, IEEE Power and Energy Magazine 15 (6) (2017) 40–49.

[3] S.E. Haupt, M. Garcia Casado, M. Davidson, J. Dobschinski, P. Du, M. Lange, T. Miller, C. Mohrlen, A. Motley, R. Pestana, J. Zack, The use of probabilistic forecasts: applying them in theory and practice, IEEE Power and Energy Magazine 17 (6) (2019) 46–57.

[4] Jie Yan, Corinna Möhrlen, Tuhfe Göçmen, Mark Kelly, Arne Wessel, Gregor Giebel, Uncovering wind power forecasting uncertainty sources and their propagation through the whole modelling chain, Renewable and Sustainable Energy Reviews 165 (2022) 112519, https://doi.org/10.1016/j.rser.2022.112519.

[5] Corinna Möhrlen, Gregor Giebel, Ricardo J. Bessa, Nadine Fleischhut, How do humans decide under wind power forecast uncertainty — an IEA wind task 36 probabilistic forecast games and experiments initiative, Journal of Physics. Conference Series 2151 (1) (Jan. 2022) 012014.

[6] Corinna Möhrlen, Ricardo J. Bessa, Nadine Fleischhut, A decision-making experiment under wind power forecast uncertainty, Meteorological Applications 29 (3) (2022) e2077.

[7] Jon Gill, José Rubiera, Claire Martin, Ivan Cacic, Ken Mylne, Chen Dehui, Gu Jiafeng, Tang xu, Munehiko Yamaguchi, Andre Kamnga Foamouhoue, Eugene Poolman, John Guiney, Guidelines on communicating forecast uncertainty, Technical Report WMO/TD No. 4122, World Meteorological Organization, 2008.

[8] Henrik Aa. Nielsen, Torben S. Nielsen, Henrik Madsen, Maria J. San Isidro Pindado, Ignacio Marti, Optimal combination of wind power forecasts, Wind Energy 10 (5) (2007) 471–482.

[9] I. Sańchez, Adaptive combination of forecasts with application to wind energy, International Journal of Forecasting 24 (4) (2008) 679–693.

[10] Aurore N. Porson, Joanne M. Carr, Susanna Hagelin, Rob Darvell, Rachel North, David Walters, Kenneth R. Mylne, Marion P. Mittermaier, Steve Willington, Bruce Macpherson, Recent upgrades to the Met Office convective-scale ensemble: an hourly time-lagged 5-day ensemble, Quarterly Journal of the Royal Meteorological Society 146 (732) (2020) 3245–3265, https://doi.org/10.1002/qj.3844.

[11] IEC 62934:2021 – General requirements for the competence of testing and calibration laboratories, 2021.

[12] Luca Delle Monache, F. Anthony Eckel, Daran L. Rife, Badrinath Nagarajan, Keith Searight, Probabilistic weather prediction with an analog ensemble, Monthly Weather Review 141 (10) (2013) 3498–3516.

[13] George Papaefthymiou, Dorota Kurowicka, Using copulas for modeling stochastic dependence in power system uncertainty analysis, IEEE Transactions on Power Systems 24 (1) (2009) 40–49.

[14] Stefan Möws, Volker Scheffer, Christian Becker, Probabilistic power forecast of renewable distributed generation for provision of control reserve using vine copulas, IET Generation, Transmission & Distribution 14 (25) (2020) 6312–6318.

[15] Pierre Pinson, Henrik Madsen, Ensemble-based probabilistic forecasting at horns rev, Wind Energy 12 (2) (2009) 137–155.
[16] John Bjørnar Bremnes, Probabilistic wind power forecasts using local quantile regression, Wind Energy 7 (1) (2004) 47–54.
[17] Corinna Möhrlen, Markus Pahlow, Jess U. Jørgensen, Untersuchung verschiedener handelsstrategien für wind- und solarenergie unter berücksichtigung der eeg 2012 novellierung, Zeitschrift für Energiewirtschaft 36 (1) (March 2012) 9–25.
[18] Corinna Möhrlen, Markus Pahlow, Jess U. Jørgensen, Author's English translation of (Untersuchung verschiedener Handelsstrategien für Wind- und Solarenergie unter Berücksichtigung der EEG 2012 Novellierung / investigation of various trading strategies for wind and solar power developed for the new eeg 2012 rules.
[19] Pierre Haessig, Bernard Multon, Hamid Ben Ahmed, Stéphane Lascaud, Pascal Bondon, Energy storage sizing for wind power: impact of the autocorrelation of day-ahead forecast errors, Wind Energy 18 (1) (2015) 43–57.
[20] Ricardo J. Bessa, Manuel A. Matos, Ivo C. Costa, Leonardo Bremermann, Ivan Gustavo Franchin, Rui Pestana, Nélio Machado, Hans-Peter Waldl, Christian Wichmann, Reserve setting and steady-state security assessment using wind power uncertainty forecast: a case study, IEEE Transactions on Sustainable Energy 3 (4) (2012) 827–836.
[21] J. Usaola, Probabilistic load flow in systems with wind generation, IET Generation, Transmission & Distribution 3 (December 2009) 1031.
[22] Tiago Soares, Ricardo J. Bessa, Pierre Pinson, Hugo Morais, Active distribution grid management based on robust ac optimal power flow, IEEE Transactions on Smart Grid 9 (6) (2018) 6229–6241.
[23] G. de Jong, O. Franz, P. Hermans, M. Lallemand, Joint tso-dso data management report. Technical report, ENTSO-e, CEDEC, GEODE, EURELECTRIC and EDSO, 2016.
[24] João Silva, Jean Sumaili, Ricardo J. Bessa, Luís Seca, Manuel Matos, Vladimiro Miranda, The challenges of estimating the impact of distributed energy resources flexibility on the tso/dso boundary node operating points, Computers & Operations Research 96 (2018) 294–304.
[25] Matthias A. Bucher, Stefanos Delikaraoglou, Kai Heussen, Pierre Pinson, Göran Andersson, On quantification of flexibility in power systems, in: 2015 IEEE Eindhoven PowerTech, 2015, pp. 1–6.
[26] Clifford W. Hansen, William F. Holmgren, Aidan Tuohy, Justin Sharp, Antonio T. Lorenzo, Leland J. Boeman, Anastasios Golnas, The solar forecast arbiter: an open source evaluation framework for solar forecasting, in: 2019 IEEE 46th Photovoltaic Specialists Conference, PVSC 2019, Conference Record of the IEEE Photovoltaic Specialists Conference, Institute of Electrical and Electronics Engineers Inc., June 2019, pp. 2452–2457, Funding Information: U.S. Department of Energy's National Nuclear Security Administration under contract DE-NA-0003525. Publisher Copyright: © 2019 IEEE.; 46th IEEE Photovoltaic Specialists Conference, PVSC 2019, Conference date: 16-06-2019 Through 21-06-2019.
[27] Mansoor Khan, Muhammad Rashid Naeem, Essam A. Al-Ammar, Wonsuk Ko, Hamsakutty Vettikalladi, Irfan Ahmad, Power forecasting of regional wind farms via variational auto-encoder and deep hybrid transfer learning, Electronics 11 (2) (2022).
[28] Craig Collier, Why do forecast trials often fail to answer the questions for which end-users need answers: a forecaster's point of view, https://iea-wind.org/wp-content/uploads/2021/04/forecast_trials_session_4_uvig2017_ccollier.pdf, 2017.
[29] C. Draxl, L.K. Berg, L. Bianco, T.A. Bonin, A. Choukulkar, A. Clifton, J.W. Cline, I.V. Djalalova, V. Ghate, E.P. Grimit, K. Holub, J.S. Kenyon, K. Lantz, C. Long, J.K. Lundquist, J. McCaa, K. McCaffrey, J.F. Newman, J.B. Olson, Y. Pichugina, J. Sharp,

W.J. Shaw, N.H. Smith, M.D. Toy, The verification and validation strategy within the second wind forecast improvement project (wfip 2), Technical report, National Renewable Energy Laboratory, 2019.
[30] R.J. Bessa, V. Miranda, A. Botterud, J. Wang, 'good' or 'bad' wind power forecasts: a relative concept, Wind Energy 14 (5) (2010) 625–636.
[31] Kenneth R. Mylne, Decision-making from probability forecasts based on forecast value, Meteorological Applications 9 (3) (2002) 307–315.
[32] Glenn W. Brier, Verification of forecasts expressed in terms of probability, Monthly Weather Review 78 (1) (1950) 1–3.
[33] Allan H. Murphy, A new vector partition of the probability score, Journal of Applied Meteorology and Climatology 12 (4) (1973) 595–600.
[34] Ian T. Jolliffe, David B. Stephenson, Proper scores for probability forecasts can never be equitable, Monthly Weather Review 136 (4) (2008) 1505–1510.
[35] Hans Hersbach, Decomposition of the continuous ranked probability score for ensemble prediction systems, Weather and Forecasting 15 (5) (2000) 559–570.
[36] G. Candille, O. Talagrand, Evaluation of probabilistic prediction systems for a scalar variable, Quarterly Journal of the Royal Meteorological Society 131 (609) (2005) 2131–2150.
[37] Tilmann Gneiting, Adrian E. Raftery, Strictly proper scoring rules, prediction, and estimation, Journal of the American Statistical Association 102 (477) (2007) 359–378.
[38] Mathias Blicher Bjerregård, Jan Kloppenborg Møller, Henrik Madsen, An introduction to multivariate probabilistic forecast evaluation, Energy and AI 4 (2021) 100058.
[39] I. Mason, A model for assessment of weather forecasts, Australian Meteorological Magazine 30 (1982) 291–303.
[40] Tom Fawcett, An introduction to roc analysis, Pattern Recognition Letters 27 (8) (2006) 861–874, ROC Analysis in Pattern Recognition.
[41] Receiver operating characteristic, https://en.wikipedia.org/wiki/Receiver_operating_characteristic. (Accessed 11 October 2021).
[42] O. Talagrand, R. Vautard, B. Strauss, Evaluation of probabilistic prediction systems, in: Proc. of the ECMWF Workshop on Predictability, 1999.
[43] Thomas M. Hamill, Interpretation of rank histograms for verifying ensemble forecasts, Monthly Weather Review 129 (3) (2001) 550–560.
[44] Leonard A. Smith, James A. Hansen, Extending the limits of ensemble forecast verification with the minimum spanning tree, Monthly Weather Review 132 (6) (2004) 1522–1528.
[45] H. Madsen, G. Kariniotakis, H.Aa. Nielsen, T.S. Nielsen, P. Pinson, A protocol for standardizing the performance evaluation of short-term wind power prediction models, in: Proc. of AWEA Global WindPower Conference, 2004, pp. 1–16.
[46] Robin Girard, Towards the definition of a standardised evaluation protocol for probabilistic wind power forecasts, Technical report, ARMINES, 2012.
[47] H. Madsen, P. Pinson, G. Kariniotakis, H.A. Nielsen, T.S. Nielsen, Standardizing the performance evaluation of short-term wind power prediction models, Wind Engineering 29 (6) (2005) 475–489.
[48] Tilmann Gneiting, Larissa I. Stanberry, Eric P. Grimit, Leonhard Held, Nicholas Alexander Johnson, Assessing probabilistic forecasts of multivariate quantities with an application to ensemble predictions of surface winds, Test 17 (2008) 211–235.
[49] S.J. Mason, Understanding forecast verification statistics, Meteorological Applications 15 (1) (2008) 31–40.
[50] Wilks, Statistical Methods in the Atmospheric Sciences, third edition, Elsevier B.V, 2011.
[51] T.L. Jensen, T.L. Fowler, B.G. Brown, J.K. Lazo, S.E. Haupt, Metrics for evaluation of solar energy forecasts, Technical report, University Corporation for Atmospheric Research, Boulder, USA, 2016.

[52] WWRP/WGNE Joint Working Group on Forecast Verification Research. Forecast verification methods across time and space scales, 2017.
[53] Jakob W. Messner, Ensemble Postprocessing with R, Elsevier, 2019, pp. 291–329.
[54] Mathias Blicher Bjerregård, Jan Kloppenborg Møller, Henrik Madsen, An introduction to multivariate probabilistic forecast evaluation, Energy and AI 4 (2021) 100058.
[55] Jakob W. Messner, Pierre Pinson, Jethro Browell, Mathias B. Bjerregård, Irene Schicker, Evaluation of wind power forecasts—an up-to-date view, Wind Energy 23 (6) (2020) 1461–1481.
[56] R.S. Mariano, F.X. Diebold, Comparing predictive accuracy, Journal of Business & Economic Statistics 13 (3) (1995) 253–263.
[57] T.M. Hopson, Assessing the ensemble spread–error relationship, Monthly Weather Review 142 (3) (2014) 1125–1142.
[58] E.S. Epstein, A scoring system for probability forecasts of ranked categories, Journal of Applied Meteorology 8 (1969) 985–987.
[59] WWRP/WGNE Joint Working Group on Forecast Verification Research, Forecast verification methods across time and space scales, in: Proc. 7th International Verification Methods Workshop, 2017.
[60] Debbie Hudson, Ensemble verification metrics, Technical report, European Center for Medium Range Forecasting, 2017.
[61] WWRP/WGNE joint working group on forecast verification research, https://www.cawcr.gov.au/projects/verification/#Methods_for_probabilistic_forecasts. (Accessed 11 October 2021).
[62] Creative Commons Corporation. Creative commons attribution non-commercial cc-by-nc v, 4.0 international.
[63] Daniel S. Wilks, Chapter 9 – forecast verification, in: Daniel S. Wilks (Ed.), Statistical Methods in the Atmospheric Sciences, fourth edition, Elsevier, 2019, pp. 369–483.
[64] Stéphane Vannitsem, Daniel Wilks, Jakob Messner (Eds.), Statistical Postprocessing of Ensemble Forecasts, Elsevier, 2019.
[65] Jakob W. Messner, ensemblepp: Ensemble postprocessing data sets, https://cran.r-project.org/web/packages/ensemblepp/, 2019. (Accessed 26 September 2022).
[66] Tilmann Gneiting, Making and evaluating point forecasts, Journal of the American Statistical Association 106 (494) (2011) 746–762.
[67] Irving I. Gringorten, Verification to determine and measure forecasting skill, Journal of Applied Meteorology and Climatology 6 (5) (1967) 742–747.
[68] Allan H. Murphy, Skill scores based on the mean square error and their relationships to the correlation coefficient, Monthly Weather Review 116 (12) (1988) 2417–2424.
[69] Thomas M. Hamill, Josip Juras, Measuring forecast skill: is it real skill or is it the varying climatology?, Quarterly Journal of the Royal Meteorological Society 132 (621C) (2006) 2905–2923.
[70] Joseph Engelberg, Charles F. Manski, Jared Williams, Comparing the point predictions and subjective probability distributions of professional forecasters, Journal of Business & Economic Statistics 27 (1) (2009) 30–41.
[71] D.S. Wilks, A skill score based on economic value for probability forecasts, Meteorological Applications 8 (2001) 209–219.
[72] D.S. Richardson, Skill and relative economic value of the ecmwf ensemble prediction system, Quarterly Journal of the Royal Meteorological Society 126 (2001) 649–667.
[73] Verification of climate forecasts: How is forecast skill or accuracy measured? – What aspects of forecast quality is measured by various scores?, http://indico.ictp.it/event/a09161/session/29/contribution/17/material/0/0.pdf. (Accessed 11 October 2021).
[74] Sabrina Bentzien, Petra Friederichs, Decomposition and graphical portrayal of the quantile score, Quarterly Journal of the Royal Meteorological Society 140 (683) (2014) 1924–1934.

[75] Jooyoung Jeon, James W. Taylor, Using conditional kernel density estimation for wind power density forecasting, Journal of the American Statistical Association 107 (497) (2012) 66–79.

[76] Martyn Clark, Subhrendu Gangopadhyay, Lauren Hay, Balaji Rajagopalan, Robert Wilby, The schaake shuffle: a method for reconstructing space–time variability in forecasted precipitation and temperature fields, Journal of Hydrometeorology 5 (1) (2004) 243–262.

[77] Megan C. Kirchmeier-Young, David J. Lorenz, Daniel J. Vimont, Extreme event verification for probabilistic downscaling, Journal of Applied Meteorology and Climatology 55 (11) (2016) 2411–2430.

[78] Michael Scheuerer, Thomas M. Hamill, Variogram-based proper scoring rules for probabilistic forecasts of multivariate quantities, Monthly Weather Review 143 (4) (apr 2015) 1321–1334.

[79] J.U. Jørgensen, C. Möhrlen, Reserve forecasting for enhanced renewable energy management, in: Proc. 12th International Workshop on Large-Scale Integration of Wind Power into Power Systems, as well as on Transmission Networks for Offshore Wind Power Plant, 2014.

[80] F. Ravazzolo, S. Lerch, T.L. Thorarinsdottir, T. Gneiting, Forecaster's dilemma: extreme events and forecast evaluation, Statistical Science 32 (1) (2017) 106–127.

[81] Didem Sari, Youngrok Lee, Sarah Ryan, David Woodruff, Statistical metrics for assessing the quality of wind power scenarios for stochastic unit commitment, Wind Energy 19 (5) (2016) 873–893.

[82] C. Möhrlen, C. Collier, J. Zack, J. Lerner, Can benchmarks and trials help develop new operational tools for balancing wind power?, in: Proc. of the 16th Workshop on Large-Scale Integration of Wind Power into Power Systems, 2017.

[83] T. Jensen, T. Fowler, B. Brown, J. Lazo, S.E. Haupt, Metrics for evaluation of solar energy forecasts, Technical report, NCAR, 2006.

[84] J. Zhang, A. Florita, B.-M. Hodge, S. Lu, H.F. Hamann, V. Banunarayanan, A.M. Brockway, A suite of metrics for assessing the performance of solar power forecasting, Solar Energy 111 (2015) 157.

[85] S. Vogt, A. Braun, J. Koch, D. Jost, R.J. Dobschinski, Benchmark of spatio-temporal shortest-term wind power forecast models, in: Proc. 17th International Workshop on Large-Scale Integration of Wind Power, 2018.

[86] Allan H. Murphy, Harald Daan, Imparcts of feedback and experience on the quality of subjective probability forecasts: 'Comparison of results from the first and second years of the Zierikzee experiment', Monthly Weather Review 112 (1984), p. 413, International Journal of Forecasting 1 (4) (1985) 313–314.

[87] E. Lannoye, A. Tuohy, W. Hobbs, J. Sharp, Anonymous solar forecasting trial outcomes – lessons learned and trial recommendations, in: Proc. 12th International Workshop on Large-Scale Integration of Solar Power into Power Systems, 2017.

[88] EPRI, Solar power forecasting for grid operations: Evaluation of commercial providers, 2017.

[89] M. Marquis, J. Wilczak, C. Finley, J. Freedman, Wind forecasting improvement project (wfip) final report, Technical report, National Centre of Oceanographic and Atmospheric Administration (NOAA), 2014.

[90] Manajit Sengupta, Aron Habte, Christian Gueymard, Stefan Wilbert, Dave Renné, Thomas Stoffel, Best practices handbook for the collection and use of solar resource data for solar energy applications: Second edition, Technical Report NREL/TP-5D00-68886, National Renewable Energy Laboratory, Golden, Colorado, USA, 2017.

[91] Manajit Sengupta, Aron Habte, Stefan Wilbert, Christian Gueymard, Jan Remund, Best Practices Handbook for the Collection and Use of Solar Resource Data for

Solar Energy Applications: Third Edition, National Renewable Energy Laboratory, Golden, Colorado, USA, IEA PVPS, 2021.

[92] International Electrotechnical Commission (IEC), ISO 17025:2005(E), General requirements for the competence of testing and calibration laboratories, version 2, 2005.

[93] Cup Anemometer Calibration Procedure, Int. network for harmonised and recognized measurements in wind energy (MEASNET), version 2, http://www.measnet.com/wp-content/uploads/2011/06/measnet_anemometer_calibration_v2_oct_2009.pdf, 2009.

[94] J.-Å. Dahlberg, T.F. Pedersen, P. Busche, Accuwind – methods for classification of cup anemometers, Technical report, DTU Wind Energy, May 2006.

[95] T.F. Pedersen, J.-Å. Dahlberg, P. Busche, ACCUWIND – Classification of Five Cup Anemometers According to IEC61400-12-1, version Risø-R-1556(EN), 2006.

[96] P.J. Eecen, F. Mouzakis, A. Cuerva, ACCUWIND Work Package 3 Final Report, version ECN-C-06-047, 2006.

[97] Jeong Wan Lee, Field calibration of wind direction sensor to the true north and its application to the Daegwanryung wind turbine test sites, Sensors 8 (12) (2008) 7783–7791, https://doi.org/10.3390/s8127782.

[98] Measuring Network of Wind Energy Institutes (MEASNET). Evaluation of site-specifc wind conditions v2.0. Procedure, Technical report, Measuring Network of Wind Energy Institutes (MEASNET), April 2016.

[99] IEA Wind Task 32, Task 32. Ground-based vertically-profling remote sensing for wind resource assessment. recommended practice rp 15, Technical report, International Energy Agency TCP Wind https://github.com/IEA-Wind-Task-32/RP15-Ground-Based-Remote-Sensing-for-Wind-Resource-Assessment/releases/tag/1.0, January 2013.

[100] Andrew Clifton, Nicolas Jolin, Alexander Stoekl, Paul Mazoyer, Peter Clive, A Review of Guidance for Using Ground-Based Vertically-Profiling Wind Lidar for Wind Resource Assessment, Technical report, Zenodo, 2020, https://zenodo.org/record/3862384.

[101] Evaluation of measurement data Joint Committee for Guides in Metrology. Evaluation of measurement data – Guide to the expression of uncertainty in measurement, 2008.

[102] Evaluation of measurement data Joint Committee for Guides in Metrology. An introduction to the "Guide to the expression of uncertainty in measurement" and related documents, 2009.

[103] Evaluation of measurement data Joint Committee for Guides in Metrology. Supplement 1 to the "Guide to the expression of uncertainty in measurement" – Propagation of distributions using a Monte Carlo method, 2008.

[104] Joint Committee for Guides in Metrology. The role of measurement uncertainty in conformity assessment, 2011.

[105] M. Sengupta, A. Habte, S. Kurtz, A. Dobos, S. Wilbert, E. Lorenz, T. Stoffel, D. Renné, C. Gueymard, D. Myers, S. Wilcox, P. Blanc, R. Perez, Best practices handbook for the collection and use of solar resource data for solar energy applications: First edition, Technical Report NREL/TP-5D00-63112, National Renewable Energy Laboratory, Golden, Colorado, USA, 2015.

[106] World Meteorological Organisation, WMO guide to meteorological instruments and methods of observation, Technical report, World Meteorological Organisation, 2018.

[107] Meteorological Monitoring Guidance for Regulatory modelling Applications, 2000.

[108] Eweline project: Development of innovative weather and power forecast models for the grid integration of weather dependent energy sources, 2011.

[109] F.T. Ulaby, R.K. Moore, A.K. Fung (Eds.), Microwave Remote Sensing—Active and Passive, Volume I: Microwave Remote Sensing Fundamentals and Radiometry, Addison-Wesley, Reading, Massachusetts, 1981.
[110] C. Matzler, Thermal Microwave Radiation: Applications for Remote Sensing, Chapter 1, The Institution of Engineering and Technology, London, 2006.
[111] V.R. Morris, Ceilometer instrument handbook, doe/sc-arm-tr-020, 2016.
[112] S. Monserrat, A.J. Thorpe, Gravity-wave observations using an array of microbarographs in the alearic islands, Quarterly Journal of the Royal Meteorological Society 118 (1992) 259–282.
[113] Mr. Sean Linehan NOS NGS, the Robinson anemometer, 1899.
[114] S. Basu, F. Porté-Agel, E. Foufoula-Georgiou, J-F. Vinuesa, M. Pahlow, Revisiting the local scaling hypothesis in stably stratified atmospheric boundary-layer turbulence: an integration of field and laboratory measurements with large-Eddy simulations, Boundary-Layer Meteorology 18 (3) (2006) 473–500.
[115] Stéphane Popinet, Murray Smith, Craig Stevens, Experimental and numerical study of the turbulence characteristics of airflow around a research vessel, Journal of Atmospheric and Oceanic Technology 21 (10) (2004) 1575–1589.
[116] L.K. Berg, M. Pekour, D. Nelson, Description of the Columbia basin wind energy study (cbwes), Technical report, Pacific Northwest National Laboratory, 2012.
[117] Julie Lundquist, Eugene Takle, M. Boquet, Branko Kosovic, M.E. Rhodes, Daniel Rajewski, R. Doorenbos, Samantha Irvin, Matthew Aitken, Katja Friedrich, Paul Quelet, Javeria Rana, Clara St. Martin, B. Vanderwende, R. Worsnop, Lidar observations of interacting wind turbine wakes in an onshore wind farm, in: Proc. of the European Wind Energy Association Conference and Exhibition 2014, 2014.
[118] Wikipedia Anemometer, 2022.
[119] Andrew Clifton, Peter Clive, Julia Gottschall, David Schlipf, Eric Simley, Luke Simmons, Detlef Stein, Davide Trabucchi, Nikola Vasiljevic, Ines Würth, Iea wind task 32: Wind lidar identifying and mitigating barriers to the adoption of wind lidar, Remote Sensing 10 (3) (2018).
[120] Ines Würth, Alex Brenner, Maayen Wigger, Po Wen Cheng, How far do we see? analysis of the measurement range of long-range lidar data for wind power forecasting, University of Stuttgart, 2017, https://core.ac.uk/works/50038839, Accepted: 2018-03-15T17:48:48Z.
[121] Axel Albers, K. Franke, Rozenn Wagner, Michael Courtney, M. Boquet, Ground-based remote sensor uncertainty – a case study for a wind lidar, in: Proc. of the European Wind Energy Conference 2013, Copenhagen, 2013.
[122] Stuart Bradley, Yvette Perrott, Paul Behrens, Andy Oldroyd, Corrections for wind-speed errors from sodar and lidar in complex terrain, Boundary-Layer Meteorology 143 (1) (2012) 37–48, https://doi.org/10.1007/s10546-012-9702-0.
[123] Stefan Emeis, Michael Harris, Robert M. Banta, Boundary-layer anemometry by optical remote sensing for wind energy applications, Meteorologische Zeitschrift 16 (4) (2007) 337–347.
[124] Stuart Bradley, Alexander Strehz, Stefan Emeis, Remote sensing winds in complex terrain – a review, Meteorologische Zeitschrift (2015) 547–555.
[125] J. Mann, N. Angelou, J. Arnqvist, D. Callies, E. Cantero, R. Chávez Arroyo, M. Courtney, J. Cuxart, E. Dellwik, J. Gottschall, S. Ivanell, P. Kühn, G. Lea, J.C. Matos, J.M.L.M. Palma, L. Pauscher, A. Peña, J. Sanz Rodrigo, S. Söderberg, N. Vasiljevic, C. Veiga Rodrigues, Complex terrain experiments in the new European wind atlas, Philosophical Transactions of the Royal Society A: Mathematical, Physical and Engineering Sciences 375 (2091) (2017) 20160101.
[126] Martin Hofsäß, Andrew Clifton, Po Wen Cheng, Reducing the uncertainty of lidar measurements in complex terrain using a linear model approach, Remote Sensing 10 (9) (2018).

[127] A. Clifton, M. Boquet, E. Burin Des Roziers, A. Westerhellweg, M. Hofsäss, T. Klaas, K. Vogstad, P. Clive, M. Harris, S. Wilex, E. Osler, B. Banta, A. Choukulkar, J. Lundquist, M. Aitken, Remote sensing of complex flows by Doppler wind lidar: Issues and preliminary recommendations, National Renewable Energy Laboratory, December 2015.
[128] Ines Würth, Laura Valldecabres, Elliot Simon, Corinna Möhrlen Bahri Uzunoğlu, Ciaran Gilbert, Gregor Giebel, David Schlipf, Anton Kaifel, Minute-scale forecasting of wind power—results from the collaborative workshop of iea wind task 32 and 36, Energies 12 (4) (2019) 712, https://doi.org/10.3390/en12040712.
[129] Lars Falbe-Hansen, Review of the spinner anemometer from romo wind ispin, Technical report, DNV GL, 2015.
[130] J.W. Wagenaar, D.a.J. Wouters, P.M.J. Warnaar, Energieonderzoek Centrum Nederland, Evaluation of the romo wind ispin guardian approach, Technical report, Energieonderzoek Centrum Nederland (ECN), 2016.
[131] Troels Friis Pedersen, Giorgio Demurtas, Calibration Procedure for Spinner Anemometer Yaw Error Measurements, Number 0082(EN) in DTU Wind Energy I, This is an internal report and therefore not available in full text DTU Wind Energy, Denmark, 2013.
[132] Troels Friis Pedersen, Paula Gómez Arranz, Spinner anemometer – best practice. Version 2. Number 165 in DTU Wind Energy E, DTU Wind Energy, Denmark, 2018.
[133] Troels F. Pedersen, Paula Gómez Arranz, Spinner anemometry – uncertainty analysis, Technical report, DTU Wind Energy, 2018.
[134] Harald Hohlen, Markus Rühlmann, Achieving performance transparency using spinner anemometry, in: Proc. of Wind Europe Conference, 2017.
[135] Harald Hohlen, Performance monitoring using spinner anemometry, in: Proc. of Duetsche Wind Energie Konferenz DEWEK, 2017.
[136] Romo Wind A/S, Performance transparency project (ptp), Technical report, Romo Wind A/S, 2021.
[137] A. Peña, J. Mann, N. Dimitrov, Turbulence characterization from a forward-looking nacelle lidar, Wind Energy Science 2 (1) (2017) 133–152.
[138] L. Schröder, F. Sehnke, M. Felder, K. Ohnmeiß, A. Kaifel, Pv-kürzestfristvorhersage mit satellitendaten und wolkenkamera, Fachtagung Energiemeteorologie, vol. 5–7, Juni, Goslar, Germany, 2018, 2018.
[139] Sepp Hochreiter, Jürgen Schmidhuber, Lstm can solve hard long time lag problems, in: Advances in Neural Information Processing Systems, 1997, pp. 473–479.
[140] Christelle Rigollier, Mireille Lefèvre, Lucien Wald, The method heliosat-2 for deriving shortwave solar radiation from satellite images, Solar Energy 77 (2) (2004) 159–169.
[141] I.E.A. Wind, Task 36. Iea wind task 36 recommended practice on renewable energy forecast solution selection, Technical report, International Energy Agency Technical Cooperation Programm Wind, 2019.
[142] International Electrotechnical Commission (IEC). Iec standard 61400-12-1:2017 power performance measurements of electricity producing wind turbines, Technical report, International Electrotechnical Commission, 2017.
[143] International Organization for Standardization. Iso 9060:2018 solar energy — specification and classification of instruments for measuring hemispherical solar and direct solar radiation, Technical report, International Organization for Standardization, ISO/TC 180/SC 1, Climate – Measurement and data, 2018.
[144] International Electrotechnical Commission (IEC). Iec standard 61724-1:2021 photovoltaic system performance – part 1: Monitoring, Technical report, International Electrotechnical Commission, 2021.

[145] International Electrotechnical Commission. Iec standard 61400-12-1:2005 power performance measurements of electricity producing wind turbines, Technical report, International Electrotechnical Commission, 2005.
[146] Hukseflux Thermal Sensors B.V., Pv monitoring and meteorological industries prepare for revised pyranometer standard iso 9060:2018, Technical report, Hukseflux Thermal Sensors B.V, 2018.
[147] Ammonit GmbH., Solar measurement knowledge, 2019.
[148] International Organization for Standardization. Iso 9060:1990 solar energy – specification and classification of instruments for measuring hemispherical solar and direct solar radiation, International Organization for Standardization, Technical report, 1990.
[149] N. Kelley, M. Shirazi, D. Jager, S. Wilde, J. Adams, M. Buhl, P. Sullivan, E. Patton, Lamar low-level jet program interim report, Technical report, National Renewable Energy Lab, Golden, CO. (US), 2004.
[150] Alfred K. Blackadar, Boundary layer wind maxima and their significance for the growth of nocturnal inversions, Bulletin of the American Meteorological Society 38 (5) (1957) 283–290.
[151] Shiyuan Zhong, Jerome D. Fast, Xindi Bian, A case study of the Great Plains low-level jet using wind profiler network data and a high-resolution mesoscale model, Monthly Weather Review 124 (5) (1996) 785–806.
[152] World Meteorological Organisation (WMO), Part I – siting and exposure of meteorological instruments, Technical Report 55, Tech. Rep. WMO/TD- No. 589, IOM Report, 2018.
[153] James Wilczak, Cathy Finley, Jeff Freedman, Joel Cline, Laura Bianco, Joseph Olson, Irina Djalalova, Lindsay Sheridan, Mark Ahlstrom, John Manobianco, John Zack, Jacob R. Carley, Stan Benjamin, Richard Coulter, Larry K. Berg, Jeffrey Mirocha, Kirk Clawson, Edward Natenberg, Melinda Marquis, The wind forecast improvement project (WFIP): a public–private partnership addressing wind energy forecast needs, Bulletin of the American Meteorological Society 96 (10) (2015) 1699–1718.
[154] Evaluation of measurement data Joint Committee for Guides in Metrology. The role of measurement uncertainty in conformity assessment, 2012.
[155] Pierre Pinson, Renate Hagedorn, Verification of the ecmwf ensemble forecasts of wind speed against analyses and observations, Meteorological Applications 19 (4) (2012) 484–500.
[156] David Schlipf, Martin Koch, Steffen Raach, Modeling uncertainties of wind field reconstruction using lidar, Journal of Physics. Conference Series 1452 (Jan. 2020) 012088.
[157] Eric Simley, Lucy Pao, Pieter Gebraad, Matthew Churchfield, Investigation of the impact of the upstream induction zone on lidar measurement accuracy for wind turbine control applications using large-eddy simulation, Journal of Physics: Conference Series 524 (2014) 012003.
[158] D. Schlipf, F. Guo, Y. Chen, Comparison of uncertainties in measurements from cup anemometers and lidar systems, in: Proc. Wind Energy Science Conference. Zenodo, May 2021.
[159] A. Borraccino, D. Schlipf, F. Haizmann, R. Wagner, Wind field reconstruction from nacelle-mounted lidar short-range measurements, Wind Energy Science 2 (1) (2017) 269–283.
[160] Susanne Drechsel, Georg J. Mayr, Jakob W. Messner, Reto Stauffer, Wind speeds at heights crucial for wind energy: measurements and verification of forecasts, Journal of Applied Meteorology and Climatology 51 (9) (2012) 1602–1617.
[161] A. Allik, J. Uiga, A. Annuk, Deviations between wind speed data measured with nacelle-mounted anemometers on small wind turbines and anemometers mounted on measuring masts, Agronomy Research 12 (2) (2014) 433–444.

[162] Bo Jing, Zheng Qian, Tianyang Chen, Yan Pei, Dahai Kang, Data-dirven method for wake effect analysis on nacelle anemometer, IOP Conference Series: Earth and Environmental Science 555 (August 2020) 012117.
[163] Dominique Philipp Held, Jakob Mann, Detection of wakes in the inflow of turbines using nacelle lidars, Wind Energy Science 4 (3) (2019) 407–420.
[164] D.A. Smith, M. Harris, A.S. Coffey, T. Mikkelsen, H.E. Jørgensen, J. Mann, R. Danielian, Wind lidar evaluation at the Danish wind test site in høvsøre, Wind Energy 9 (2006) 87–93.
[165] Frederik Zahle, Niels N. Sørensen, Characterization of the unsteady flow in the nacelle region of a modern wind turbine, Wind Energy 14 (2) (2011) 271–283.
[166] Corinna Möhrlen, Ulrik Vestergaard, Eirgrid met mast and alternatives study, Technical report, EIRGRID, 2019.
[167] Corinna Möhrlen, Diarmuid Ó Foghlú, Séamus Power, Gill Nolan, Kenneth Conway, Eric Lambert, John Ging, Eirgrid's met mast and alternatives study, IET Renewable Power Generation (2022) 1941–1954.
[168] C. Möhrlen, D. Ó Foghlú, S. Power, G. Nolan, K. Conway, E. Lambert, J. Ging, Eirgridś met mast and alternatives study, IET Renewable Power Generation 16 (9) (2022) 1941–1954, https://doi.org/10.1049/rpg2.12502.
[169] Michel Journée, Cédric Bertrand, Quality control of solar radiation data within the rmib solar measurements network, Solar Energy 85 (2011) 72–86.
[170] N. Geuder, F. Wolfertstetter, S. Wilbert, D. Schüler, R. Affolter, B. Kraas, E. Lüpfert, B. Espinar, Screening and flagging of solar irradiation and ancillary meteorological data, Energy Procedia 69 (2015) 1989–1998, International Conference on Concentrating Solar Power and Chemical Energy Systems, SolarPACES 2014.
[171] Omaima El Alani, Hicham Ghennioui, Abdellatif Ghennioui, Yves-Marie Saint-Drenan, Philippe Blanc, Natalie Hanrieder, Fatima-Ezzahra Dahr, A visual support of standard procedures for solar radiation quality control, International Journal of Renewable Energy Development 10 (3) (2021) 401–414.
[172] E.E. Lucio-Eceiza, J.F. González-Rouco, J. Navarro, H. Beltrami, Qquality control of surface wind observations in northeastern North America. Part I: data management issues, Journal of Atmospheric and Oceanic Technology 35 (1) (2018).
[173] E.E. Lucio-Eceiza, J.F. González-Rouco, J. Navarro, H. Beltrami, J. Conte, Quality control of surface wind observations in northeastern North America. Part ii: measurement errors, Journal of Atmospheric and Oceanic Technology 35 (1) (2018).
[174] Corinna Möhrlen, J.U. Jørgensen, Integration of Large-Scale Renewable Energy into Bulk Power Systems. from Planning to Operation, Chapter the Role of Ensemble Forecasting in Integrating Renewables into Power Systems: From Theory to Real-Time Applications, Springer Nature, Springer International Publishing AG, Cham, Switzerland, 2008, pp. 79–134.
[175] Allan H. Murphy, What is a good forecast? An essay on the nature of goodness in weather forecasting, Weather and Forecasting 2 (8) (1993) 281–293.
[176] Eric Gilleland, verification: Weather Forecast Verification Utilities, 2015, R package version ≥ 2.10), methods, fields, boot, CircStats, MASS, dtw.
[177] Stefan Siegert, Jonas Bhend, Igor Kroener, Matteo de Felice, SpecsVerification: Forecast Verification Routines for Ensemble Forecasts of Weather and Climate, 2020, License GPL-2 | GPL-3 [expanded from: GPL (≥ 2)].
[178] Jonas Bhend, Jacopo Ripoldi, Claudia Mignani, Rebecca Hiller Irina Mahlstein and, Christoph Spirig, Mark Liniger, Joaqu'in Bedia Jimenez, Andreas Weigel and, Matteo de Felice, Stefan Siegert, Katrin Sedlmeier, easyVerification: Ensemble Forecast Verification for Large Data Sets, 2020, R (≥ 3.0), SpecsVerification (≥ 0.5), stats, utils.
[179] Iso rules part 300 system reliability and operations division 304 routine operations section 304.9 wind and solar aggregated generating facility forecasting, 2019.

[180] Fifth replacement California iso tariff wind technical requirements – appendix q eligible intermittent resources protocol, 2020.
[181] Ercot business practices – ercot and qse operations practices during the operating hour, 2021.
[182] Wfps meteorological equipment requirements, 2022.
[183] Wind plant operator forecast data guide, 2020.
[184] Generator operational requirements manual 14d in rev. 38, 2016.
[185] Information on data requirements, 2016.

Nomenclature

AAP	Available Active Power, a signal indicating the potential power generation, if no contraits are set for the generation unit
AESO	Alberta Electric System Operator
API	Application Interface
BRP	Balance Responsible Party
BS	Brier Score – answers how accurate the probability forecasts are in general
CAISO	California Independent System Operator
CAL	Calibration – part of the Brier Score that answers the question how well does the conditional relative frequency of occurrence of the event match a situation
CFD	Computational Fluid Dynamics
CSV	comma separated values
CRPS	Continuous Ranked Probability Skill
DER	distributed energy resources
ECMWF	European Centre for Medium-Range Weather Forecasts
ENTSO-E	European Network of Transmission System Operators for Electricity
EMS	Energy Management System
EPS	Ensemble Prediction System
ERCOT	Electric Reliability Council of Texas
ES	Energy Score
EU	European Union
FAR	false alarm rate
FTPS	File Transfer Protocol Secure, builds on file transfer protocol (FTP) and adds on a security and encryption layer. See also SFTP
FN	False Negatives
FPR	False Positive Rate
FSP	Forecast Solution Provider
GUM	Guide to the expression of uncertainty in measurement
H	Heaviside function
HR	Hit Rate
HSSD	High-speed Shutdown
IANA	Internet Assigned Numbers Authority
IEA	International Energy Agency
IT	Information Technology
JSON	JavaScript Object Notation
K-Test	The test compares three K values that are ratios of (1) the global irradiance to the extraterrestrial (i.e. top of atmosphere) irradiance, (2) the direct irradiance to the extraterrestrial irradiance and (3) the ratio of diffuse to global irradiance. The test verifies if these values are within specified intervals (see details in chapter 3 "Measuring Solar Radiation" of the PVPS handbook [91] and e.g. [171])
LiDAR	Light detection and Ranging – is a surveying method that measures distance to a target by illuminating the target with pulsed laser light and measuring the reflected pulses with a sensor
LSTM	Long Short Term Memory

MAE	Mean Absolute Error
MEASNET	Measuring Network of Wind Energy Institutes
ML	Machine Learning
MSEPS	Multi-Scheme Ensemble Prediction System
MW	Mega Watt – also used for actual power generation
NOAA	National Oceanic and Atmospheric Administration
NWP	Numerical Weather Prediction
OEM	Original Equipment Manufacturer
PDF	Probability Density Functions
POD	Probability Of Detection
RADAR	RAdio Detection And Ranging – is a detection system that uses radio waves to determine the range, angle, or velocity of objects
RES	Resolution – part of the Brier Score that answers the question how well does the forecast separate events according to whether they occur or dont occur
REST	REpresentational State Transfer; a RESTful API transfers a representation of the state of the resource to the requester or endpoint and can be delivered in several formats via HTTP: JSON (Javascript Object Notation), HTML, XLT, Python, PHP, or plain text. A Web API (or Web Service) conforming to the REST architectural style is a REST API
RMSE	Root Mean Square Error
RPS	Ranked Probability Score
SCADA	Supervisory control and data acquisition is a control system architecture comprising computers, networked data communications and graphical user interfaces for high-level supervision of machines and processes
SFTP	Secure Shell (SSH) File Transfer Protocol that builds on secure shell protocol (SSH) and adds on file transfer capabilities
SODAR	SOnic Detection And Ranging – is a meteorological instrument used as a wind profiler to measure the scattering of sound waves by atmospheric turbulence
StDV	Standard Deviation
t/b	Abbreviation of "trials and benchmarks"
TN	True Negatives
TPR	True Positive Rate
TSO	Transmission System Operator
UNC	Uncertainty – part of the Brier Score that answers the question how difficult/uncertain is the forecast situation
WFIP	Wind Forecasting Improvement Project
WFPS	Windfarm Power Station
WGNE	Working Group on Numerical Experimentation
WWRP	World Weather Research Program
XML	eXtensible Markup Language

Index

F

G

H

I

O

P

Y

FSC
www.fsc.org
MIX
Papier | Fördert
gute Waldnutzung
FSC® C083411

Kolibri 360 GmbH
Ferdinand-Jühlke-Straße 7
99095 Erfurt, Deutschland
produktsicherheit@kolibri360.de